Gym Culture, Identity and Performance-Enhancing Drugs

This book is about gym culture, the pursuit of fit, muscular bodies and the use of drugs as a means to get there.

Building on the international research literature and in-depth interviews with men who have experience of image and performance enhancing drugs (IPEDs), the book explores the fascination with muscles, motivations for using drugs to enhance them, assessments of risks, and experience of side effects. The book examines what the altered body does to the men's identity, self-image and relationships with peers and partners. Taking an evolutionary psychological approach, it also investigates the biological and psychological foundations of the fascination with the muscular body and discusses the notion of precarious manhood. Building on these analyses the book considers the political and regulatory initiatives in place to prevent the use of IPEDs and assesses those strategies' potential to reach their aims.

This is essential reading for anybody with an interest in the issue of drugs in sport, the ethics of sport, sociology of sport, sociology of the body, masculinity or public health.

Ask Vest Christiansen is Associate Professor of Sport Science in the Department of Public Health at Aarhus University in Denmark. He is also Co-Director of the International Network of Doping Research (INDR). Dr Christiansen's research has followed two main branches: doping in elite sport and recreational athletes' use of drugs in gyms, fitness and strength training environments.

Ethics and Sport

Series editors

Mike McNamee, *University of Wales Swansea*
Jim Parry, *Charles University, Prague, Czech Republic*

The *Ethics and Sport* series aims to encourage critical reflection on the practice of sport, and to stimulate professional evaluation and development. Each volume explores new work relating to philosophical ethics and the social and cultural study of ethical issues. Each is different in scope, appeal, focus and treatment but a balance is sought between local and international focus, perennial and contemporary issues, level of audience, teaching and research application, and variety of practical concerns.

Titles in the series:

For more information about this series, please visit: https://www.routledge.com/Ethics-and-Sport/book-series/EANDS

Gym Culture, Identity and Performance-Enhancing Drugs

Tracing a Typology of Steroid Use

Ask Vest Christiansen

Translated by
Heidi Flegal

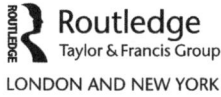

Routledge
Taylor & Francis Group

LONDON AND NEW YORK

First published 2020
by Routledge
2 Park Square, Milton Park, Abingdon, Oxon OX14 4RN

and by Routledge
52 Vanderbilt Avenue, New York, NY 10017

Routledge is an imprint of the Taylor & Francis Group, an informa business

British Library Cataloguing-in-Publication Data
A catalogue record for this book is available from the British Library

Library of Congress Cataloging-in-Publication Data
A catalog record has been requested for this book

ISBN: 978-0-367-86330-2 (hbk)
ISBN: 978-0-367-49764-4 (pbk)
ISBN: 978-1-003-01843-8 (ebk)

Typeset in Goudy
by Taylor & Francis Books

Contents

Illustrations

Figures

Tables

Preface

"Big Benny just bought a whole shipping crate of tuna at Walmart!"

In the early 1990s, I began to notice that some active weightlifters and gym-goers adhered to a very particular lifestyle. I was obviously familiar with the popular film characters Rocky, Rambo and Conan the Barbarian, but as a Danish university student I had never thought of Sylvester Stallone or Arnold Schwarzenegger as anything but distant Hollywood icons. Then a fellow student at the department of sports science at the University of Southern Denmark told me about "Big Benny" and other bodybuilders he hung out with, and I began to wonder: Why would Benny buy canned tuna by the crateload? No matter how good the offer or how long the shelf life of the product, it sounded insane. What kind of physical-training regime could motivate grocery shopping in such bulk? My classmate also lifted weights, and he was extremely fit and had intimate knowledge of the bodybuilding community in our university city, Odense. Being an insider, he knew people who used steroids, but I am sure he was being completely truthful when he told me he had never done so himself. Still, he candidly admitted that he knew the temptations and fully understood what motivated people who did.

Barely a decade later I began doing research on doping in elite sports, although my work focused not on muscle-bound weightlifters but on the greyhounds of professional cycling. While these athletes did not use drugs to gain bulk, they too sought to boost their performance in a sport that demanded strict self-discipline and strong ambitions. The insights I gained into the personal goals and devoted lifestyles underlying the use of performance-enhancing drugs — which rarely coincided with a lack of moral decency — were highly applicable to my later studies of dedicated gym-goers in recreational weightlifting communities. The lifestyle choices of such workout enthusiasts may seem odd to outsiders, but for a researcher (such as myself) studying serious recreational fitness and gym communities, the same basic principles apply as in any academic study of top-level sports: Set aside all prejudice, and let curiosity drive your investigation. In that spirit, my ambition in this book is to shed light on the goals, reasoning and values that motivate people to use image and performance-enhancing drugs (IPEDs), in particular anabolic steroids, to enlarge their muscles. I also hope to offer insights into the psychological mechanisms, social pressures and cultural influences that have made the use of IPEDs among gym-goers far more pervasive than doping in the upper echelons of the sports world — which, truth be told, is a marginal phenomenon. This knowledge also equips us to better understand the challenges law-makers and educators face when addressing these issues.

I began work on this volume in 2009, and the Danish original appeared in 2018. Some of the interviews and discussions have previously appeared in published papers, articles and book chapters. However, along with the Danish original this is the first comprehensive account of my work on the topic.

Along the way I have received valuable and constructive comments to the various chapters of this book from my colleagues at Aarhus University's research unit for Sport and Body Culture at the Department of Public Health. I thank you all. Special thanks are due to Verner Møller and Rasmus Bysted Møller for thoroughly reviewing my manuscript-in-progress and pointing out weak spots in my arguments with uncanny precision. Also, my profound thanks go to Jens Peter Christiansen and Anders Schmidt Vinther, who both read the entire Danish manuscript, corrected errors, brought further relevant literature to my attention and proposed various changes. In addition, Anders Nedergaard offered valuable input to Chapter 3, on effects and side effects, while Anna Lund Christiansen did the same for Chapter 4, on the topic of identity. In the translation, done with Heidi Flegal, we have sought to make my work accessible and relatable to an English-speaking audience, even while embedding it in the original Danish context. That said, any errors and omissions in the finished book are, of course, mine and mine alone.

My greatest debt of gratitude is to the people who were willing to give of their time and share with me their thoughts, experience and personal knowledge about recreational gym and weightlifting communities in Denmark. Without them, neither the underlying research nor the book itself would have existed.

Aarhus, Denmark
April 2020
Ask Vest Christiansen

Chapter 1

Introduction

It really is quite remarkable. Over the past 40 years we have witnessed a veritable media explosion of well-muscled body imagery, accompanied by the invention of new science-based exercise regimens, high-tech workout equipment and sophisticated dietary supplements. Even so, many fitness and weightlifting enthusiasts still regard the Arnold Schwarzenegger of 1975 as the epitome of the perfect body. Since then, advertisements featuring scantily clad soccer players like David Beckham and Cristiano Ronaldo, or fitness icons such as Rich Froning and Jacob Sumana, have brought variation to the image of the ideal male, yet pictures of Schwarzenegger as Mr. Universe still hang on many a gym wall and even appear on fitness-magazine covers. He was also mentioned as an ideal by many of the people I interviewed for this book. A well-proportioned, abundantly muscled body is not merely fascinating to look at. If you can have a body like that yourself, status and other social advantages can be yours.

The fitness industry is acutely aware of this. Today even most small towns have large, well-equipped gyms and health clubs, sometimes with thousands of members. Over the past 20 years the fitness industry has boomed. In Denmark, by way of example, soccer and European handball were the most popular organized physical activities for several generations until fitness and weightlifting leap-frogged to the top of the list some years ago. Statistics show that about one million Danes (of the country's 5.8 million) are members of a health club or gym, and fitness and weightlifting are now the Danes' preferred modes of exercise, outdistancing running and hiking (Asserhøj, 2017; Storm, Toft, & Bang, 2015). Though not all members exercise with equal zeal, the growing number of gyms shows just how popular this type of physical training is. Looking once again at Denmark, in 2006 the country had 306 registered commercial gyms, health clubs and fitness centers. Twelve years later, in 2018, this number had risen to 840 (Bang & van Bedaf, 2018). All age groups are represented, with this flexible exercise option attracting members young and old. Weightlifting is generally quite popular, in commercial gym settings and elsewhere: Over half the 16–29 age group and some 30% of adult Danes aged 30 and older use this type of exercise (IDAN, 2016; Pilgaard & Rask, 2016). In

Europe, "fitness" currently holds a comfortable lead over all other types of sport and exercise, with 56.4 million Europeans holding membership in a gym or fitness-club chain.[1]

Obviously, that does not mean all these people are "bodybuilders" after the style of Schwarzenegger or those who followed his example and joined the black-iron gyms and early clubs of the 1970s. Some gym-goers want to augment their size and strength. Others work out to lose weight, become more attractive, more visibly muscled or healthier, or to increase their physical well-being, gain recognition from their peers, invite attention or be part of a group or community with a shared interest. Although few people really want to end up with a hulking physique, several ideals from the bodybuilding sport have become embedded as values in today's fitness culture, and its methods and techniques have become widespread. Examples are the ideal of the "hard body," sophisticated workout and weight-loss techniques, and the importance of dietary proteins (Klein, 2007; Liokaftos, 2017). Ten to fifteen years ago these values and techniques were mainly used by men, but in recent years women have followed suit. Female workout enthusiasts often post exercise pictures and videos on social media along with catchphrases like "Strong is the new skinny." At Danish championships held by the traditionally male-dominated sports association Danish Bodybuilding and Fitness Federation (DBFF), recent years have seen the category "bikini fitness" swell to the largest discipline by far in terms of participants.

It is a fact that some people in bodybuilding circles use anabolic steroids[2] or other performance-enhancing drugs. This also occurs in the Danish fitness community, where it is less common than among bodybuilders but presumably more common than official numbers tell us. We know this from a number of interview studies, and from the impounding or confiscation of image- and performance-enhancing drugs (IPEDs) by the Danish police and customs authorities. This assumption is further supported by testing conducted in gyms by Anti Doping Danmark, which is Denmark's National Anti Doping Organisation (NADO). Most studies indicate that 3–6% of men who work out in gyms have personal experience with steroid use (Barland & Tangen, 2009; Sagoe, Molde, Andreassen, Torsheim, & Pallesen, 2014; Singhammer & Ibsen, 2010).[3] However, contrary to the 1970s, when bodybuilding arrived in Denmark and the first gyms and clubs opened, today the people involved in competitive bodybuilding, weightlifting and powerlifting make up only a small fraction of IPED users. Rather than seeking to emulate the old-school bodybuilders, most modern-day users of anabolic steroids have a more athletic ideal in mind. They want to be visibly muscular while maintaining a trim, aesthetically pleasing look. Whatever their exact goals, most users want to attain a stronger, more attractive body — and the social advantages that go with it.

In recent years the use of anabolic steroids and other IPEDs in gyms has made politicians, sports organizations, anti-doping authorities and other special-interest groups sound the alarm. In Denmark, high-level concerns about this development led to a 2005 regulation from the Danish parliament that ordered Anti Doping Danmark to carry out random doping controls at Danish gyms and fitness centers, based on the very same rules that apply to professional cyclists and Olympic athletes (Christiansen, 2011; Steele, Bang, Brandt, & Kirkegaard, 2010). At the time, this intervention — testing regular citizens exercising at commercial gyms — was a global first. Since then, other countries, including Belgium, Sweden and Norway, have followed Denmark's example. Concerns about non-athletic IPED use are obviously not limited to Denmark, and several European countries have sought to develop strategies to counteract such practices. Their success has varied considerably, as evidenced in a 2014 study that mapped out existing regulations in the then 28 EU member states. The aim of this study was to make recommendations to the responsible ministers that might conceivably lead to common EU guidelines to handle and combat the use of banned substances outside the world of top-level sports (Backhouse et al., 2014).

Be that as it may, the problem will hardly vanish merely because we implement random testing, laws and regulations. Recognizing the complexity of this issue, in 2012 legislators obliged Anti Doping Danmark to supplement their previous educational and testing agenda with a more proactive, dialogue-based approach that reaches out to involve gyms and fitness facilities. The inability of laws to make much of a difference is evident from the largely uniform prevalence of IPED use across countries that have very diverse legislation on this area (Hibell et al., 1997; Sagoe et al., 2014) and from the tiny variations in the number of users per country over the past 20 years (Pope et al., 2014, and Chapter 2 below). This probably results from a variety of interacting factors, including the fundamental human obsession with strength and muscles, plus four decades of unprecedented growth in the cultural and market-driven focus on our bodies and appearance.

The book's intentions, questions and assumptions

Based on the situation outlined above, my ambition is to offer a framework for understanding what it is that motivates the use of anabolic steroids and other IPEDs among groups of people whose workout activities include serious fitness, bodybuilding and weightlifting.[4] Throughout the chapters of this book I will discuss the factors that motivate some men in weightlifting circles to use such substances. Rather than just seeing the phenomenon from one perspective, my strategy is to include a wide array of psychological, social, cultural and biological explanatory models. Using the Danish model as a starting point, I will also discuss relevant legislation and efforts, to assess how well-suited they are in addressing the situation they aspire to change.

In order to gain an understanding of IPED use (and, in broader terms, of our modern-day body fixation) in the communities described above, I build this book on several assumptions. One is that to understand what is going on behind the scenes, we must include a psychologic and sociological framework that focuses on the type of personal identity formation that is a condition for modern human beings, and which is crucially important during youth and early adulthood, from around 15 to 30 years of age. This age range is precisely where we find the highest incidence of anabolic steroid use, and where the temptation to supplement workouts with muscle-bulking substances seems to be greatest. I explain my use of the identity concept in Chapter 4.

Another assumption is that the increased focus on competition in society — in this case, particularly our traditionally egalitarian Danish society — not only has made its mark on workplaces, educational settings and public institutions, but also affects our relations and interactions with other people. Seen in that light, the body becomes a parameter for our degree of success in life. When people perceive various life contexts as more competitive, they feel an added incentive to improve their appearance by making their bodily manifestation more appealing.

A third assumption in this book is that muscles and masculine identity are intimately linked, and that men often feel a particular need to prove their masculinity — a need that is not as pronounced in women when it comes to their femininity. Expanding on this assumption, I venture to suggest that human biology and the psyche humankind have developed through the processes of evolution play an important role in the topic of this book; more precisely, that they play a far greater role than hitherto appreciated in the quest to achieve an attractive body among the types of serious workout enthusiasts dealt with here. According to this assumption, the link between muscles and masculine identity is no new phenomenon. It is, rather, a link that has always existed, across different ages and different cultures. I therefore also include the perspective of evolutionary psychology to undergird the cultural and sociological framework mentioned above. Note, however, that whereas the first two assumptions focus especially on Western culture, the third is universal.

Geographically, my main focus is on the situation in Denmark and Scandinavia in general, and in Europe and Western culture at large. Certain surveys show widespread use of anabolic steroids among certain fitness and weightlifting communities in non-Western cultures (Sagoe et al., 2014). While I do believe there are some common traits in the ways we can understand IPED use across cultures, it is obvious that any researcher seeking a deeper understanding of, say, steroid use in Afghanistan, Brazil or Kenya must incorporate other culture-specific circumstances and factors than those applying to Denmark. In Western-type cultures, however, the three general assumptions outlined above are indeed linked, since the part of our identity formation that relates to our performance, skills and characteristics has become ever more important, in step with the de-traditionalization of society and increased competitive focus — giving the body a particularly prominent place in the formation of identity.

The book will focus to a much lesser degree on girls and women who use steroids. Even when we look specifically at female members of gyms and health clubs, most studies show that women make only very limited use of anabolic steroids. It is true that although recent years have seen significantly more girls and women involved in bikini-fitness competitions and the like, some of whom may use steroids, few studies have been done on this topic. We do know, however, that girls and women use other substances, including stimulants, to become more well defined and get rid of perceived excess weight. Nevertheless, female users are few and far between when it comes to the most hotly debated substances in bodybuilding and weightlifting circles — namely muscle-bulking anabolic steroids (Kanayama & Pope, 2012; Parkinson & Evans, 2006).

Flaunting the body beautiful on Muscle Beach

Broadly speaking, fixation on bodies and weightlifting only began a good 40 years ago, notably around Muscle Beach in Venice, California. This area was home to the now legendary Gold's Gym, the workout mecca of Arnold Schwarzenegger and a number of other famous bodybuilders from the early 1960s onwards. Attractive bodies had been cultivated along this and other beaches in the Los Angeles and Santa Barbara areas since the late 1940s, but the physical prowess of this new generation of athletes was more extensive and more massive than ever before. Training regimes had been intensified, and a newfound affluence enabled practitioners to increase their intake of dietary protein in the form of meat. The real new difference, however, was that Schwarzenegger and other iconic bodybuilders supplemented their intensive training and strict diets with highly potent pharmaceutical substances called anabolic androgenic steroids to achieve their impressive stature (Liokaftos, 2017). This made the wider world aware of, and interested in, a type of practice which at the time was still a rather peculiar subcultural niche. Interest grew further in 1976, when Schwarzenegger appeared as a live exhibit at the Whitney Museum of American Art, and was then portrayed with charming authenticity in the 1977 documentary *Pumping Iron*. This film quickly became a cult classic, indisputably playing a role in raising bodybuilding out of the shadows of anonymous sports disciplines and eventually making it a part of mainstream culture. Schwarzenegger subsequently took full advantage of his popularity, playing action-hero roles in blockbuster films like *Conan the Barbarian*, *The Terminator* and *Commando*. Here was a modern-day successor to the sword-and-sandal films of yesteryear, offering boys and men around the world a new masculine ideal.

Coinciding with Schwarzenegger's rising popularity, the fitness industry realized the commercial potential in shifting some of the public's awareness away from the world of sports, and towards a perception of physical exercise and fitness as a goal in and of itself. The industry soon began to flourish, with gyms and fitness clubs popping up in virtually every town. Video tapes with Jane Fonda and other exercise gurus sold like hotcakes. Across the Western world, men and women seemed to accept the metaphor that being in control of your body also meant being in control of your life (Klein, 1993; Luciano, 2007). The advertising world used not only slim, bare-skinned women but also strong, bare-chested men to peddle goods of every conceivable kind. The muscular body as a symbol of manliness became popular anew, and the use of muscle-building substances in gym and workout communities spread from competitive bodybuilders and weightlifters to wider groups of active members. This was a new situation, which, in recent years, has also increasingly captured the eye of the media.

Extreme muscle-heads on dope

On the Danish media scene, in November 2012 the respected newspaper *Politiken* launched a whole series of articles focused on recreational and non-athletic doping taking place in the country's gyms and fitness centers. The first was entitled "The Hunt for Mr. Jacob and the Golden Vials," and the two journalists behind the series — Jeppe Laursen Brock and Christian Heide-Jørgensen — later received several awards for their thoroughly researched coverage.[5] One of their angles was to reveal how Danish masterminds in Mumbai were producing drugs in India for the illegal doping market; another showed how new performance-enhancing drugs were flowing into Denmark; and yet another declared that "muscle-fixated exercise fanatics" were ignoring the dangers of using these substances, "even though the side effects of steroid abuse can be fatal." These articles also warned that "steroid abusers are gambling with their lives," explaining that some "muscle-men shoot up bacteria and heavy metals." Not surprisingly, various health complications ensued, with reports from the medical field describing how "muscle-men with bitch tits exploit free medical aid," after observing users who would take calculated risks based on "how they can get the publicly funded [Danish] health system to examine, treat and pay for the damage caused by their doping." The treatment this topic received in *Politiken* elicited reactions from several top-level politicians, including the former World Anti-Doping Agency (WADA) vice-president and conservative minister of justice Brian Mikkelsen, who demanded stricter legislation that would slap "much harder punishments" on those masterminding and facilitating such drug use. The newspaper also focused on the lack of public treatment options for people who "become slaves to doping drugs." The journalists, Brock and Heide-Jørgensen, laid out the harsh realities: "When the dream of the perfect body ends in steroid dependency and psychological collapse, the pumped-up doping addicts must find their own way out of their nightmare."

The *Politiken* articles also covered how the customs authorities frequently impounded doping substances, and how Danish police forces, despite the growing number of reported cases, had to admit they were giving lower priority to "the effort against hardcore doping drugs," despite the fact that "the illegal sale of anabolic steroids helps fund the illegal activities of motorcycle and street gangs." A few months later, the newspaper ran follow-up articles about how steroid use was common among gang members serving time in Danish prisons; about police officers who used and peddled steroids; about steroid theft in pharmaceutical companies; and about the numerous Internet sites involved in IPED sales and brokering. The topic was rounded off by interviews with steroid users who had suffered serious side effects, and with the cardiologists and surgeons at the large specialized public hospital in Copenhagen that provided treatment and heart transplants for the most severely afflicted patients (Brock & Heide-Jørgensen, 2012–2013).

The article series in *Politiken* unquestionably gave the topic in Denmark broad and thorough coverage based on serious research. However, as is apparent above, the journalists also set a certain tone and style in their articles. Steroid users were described as extreme muscle-men or "muscle-heads" who abuse anabolics, ignore side effects, exploit the public-health system, become violent, go to prison and end up as addicts in horrendous abuse scenarios. In short: journalism with an angle and an attitude. Fair enough. But at the same time this sort of journalism communicates an image of weightlifting gym-goers — especially those who use anabolic steroids — as dangerous social deviants. Undoubtedly some steroid users *are* deviants, degenerates, criminals, gang members, weirdos or, on a more serious note, mentally ill. Yet the many other kinds of IPED users receive little media coverage, if any at all, albeit one American study on steroid use found that:

> The typical user [of anabolic steroids] was a Caucasian, highly educated, gainfully employed [male] professional approximately 30 years of age, who was earning an above-average income, was not active in organized sports, and whose use was motivated by increases in skeletal muscle mass, strength, and physical attractiveness.
>
> (Cohen, Collins, Darkes, & Gwartney, 2007)

This group received very little attention in the *Politiken* articles. The same goes for most Danish media coverage of the steroid phenomenon and the majority of scientific studies. When it comes to investigating the use of anabolic steroids outside top-level sports, most research has focused either on adolescent users or competitive bodybuilders. Use among the first group causes outrage, firstly because people so young should not use such potent drugs, and secondly because many stories about this group revolve around "roid rage" and suicide attempts. As for the second group, competitive bodybuilders, many find it easy to distance themselves from such practitioners, regarding their bodies as grotesque. What is more, the large amounts of drugs they use render the probability of their experiencing health problems extremely high. Meanwhile, much evidence suggests that most users fall outside these two groups, as do all of the individuals interviewed in connection with this book.

My research informants and methodology

When touching on the issue of anabolic steroid use in gym and weightlifting circles, many researchers and stakeholders emphasize how difficult it is to obtain factual information. These communities keep to themselves and the very issue is fraught with taboos, meaning that very few users are willing to discuss it openly (Monaghan, 2002; Pope, Phillips, & Olivardia, 2000; Simon et al., 2006). This came as no surprise to me, since it reflected my own earlier experience while researching the use of performance-enhancing drugs among top athletes (Christiansen, 2005; Christiansen & Møller, 2007). The merest suspicion of such practices in these circles can destroy a career, and for that reason alone it is understandable that elite athletes are reluctant to participate in studies that seek frank and truthful information about doping practices.

As it turned out, the situation in Danish gym and weightlifting circles was not like this at all. To my surprise I had little difficulty finding IPED users who were willing to be part of my study as "informants," interviewees prepared to share personal information and experiences with the researcher. Interviewees were recruited partly via a post with an invitation and a link to further information on two websites popular among fitness enthusiasts, and partly via leaflets laid out on the counters of gyms known to have serious weightlifting members. In addition, some informants were recruited by the "snowball" method, where one informant suggested another.

There may be several reasons why the situation was not what I had expected. Perhaps there are simply more users in the non-athletic sports community than in elite sports. Or perhaps the stigmatization of using IPEDs in a non-competitive context is less harsh than in professional sport, or the consequences of being identified are less severe (should the researcher's guarantee of total anonymity miscarry). After all, it is a very different matter for someone to combine IPEDs with lifting weights at a gym than it is for someone to dope themselves to enhance their chances of winning an Olympic medal. All that my informants wanted, beyond guaranteed anonymity, was simply to be sure that by taking part in the study they would not be stereotyped or disparagingly represented as "roid-heads," or expected to show remorse at the life choices they had made.

Bearing the *Politiken* articles in mind, it is easy to understand their concerns. As the British sociologist Lee Monaghan (2001) has rightly pointed out, a person's risk exposure when choosing a lifestyle focused on exercise, strict diets and anabolic steroids not only involves potential side effects from the substances. It also involves a pronounced risk of being stigmatized according to the conventional, stereotypical perception of people who make such choices as violent and intellectually underendowed. A recurring question from the people I contacted for my study was: *"What are you going to use it for?"* After I explained the context, they all expressed their support. One informant even said: *"I've been really keen to do this interview to bring more nuance into the debate, and I think it's really great."* Another explained his willingness to participate as follows:

> You know, I work in the public health system myself, so I know what research is like. You're totally dependent on people agreeing to participate. And that's why I thought to myself: "Okay, I'm not going to hold back. I'm going to give honest answers to the questions you ask." So honesty and openness are absolutely essential. I know that. But then again, I'm confident that this is anonymous.

Most of the people I interviewed made conscious choices about using or avoiding IPEDs. One informant told me how, at one stage, he opted for life in the fast lane, partying and using anabolic steroids, amphetamines and alcohol. At the time of the interview, however, a couple of years after this stage, he was able to reflect on his actions and put them into perspective. Another informant used his well-muscled body to earn some quick money, traveling around to work as a stripper and porn model. A third had for years felt tempted to use anabolic steroids and thoroughly studied the pros and cons, but never dared to take the leap. Not because he was afraid of the physical side effects, but because he was certain he would find the drugs so effective he would be unable to let them go. A fourth and fifth informant became so adamant about their workouts, each in his own way, that they began seriously contemplating competitive activities. Still, neither one mentioned the competitive element as their decisive motivation to use steroids. Like most other users they primarily had workouts and steroids as part of a particular lifestyle. Yet others simply wanted to have a more attractive body, look good on the beach and boost their self-confidence.

The educational and occupational backgrounds of my informants were widely varied. Some were academic students, others were apprentices or craftsmen. One worked in special education, another was a teacher, a third was unemployed. Some had prestigious, well-paid jobs in the IT industry and elsewhere. As my peers have found in Scandinavian and American studies, recreational and non-athletic users of anabolic steroids are difficult to place in any one socio-economic group (Barland & Tangen, 2009; Singhammer & Ibsen, 2010; Skårberg & Engstrom, 2007).[6] But despite their varied backgrounds, naturally my informants are not representative of all IPED users in Denmark. A qualitative study such as mine cannot ensure that sort of statistical representation. People who volunteer for research interviews usually do so after thorough consideration, and because they somehow feel they are getting something in return. Those who see no point in participating never step forward.

As noted, my informant group was mixed. Three features that all interviewees shared, however, was that they were Caucasian and ethnically Danish, and identified as heterosexual. A few maintained they had always been against doping and stayed away from IPEDs for that reason. Others who took a firm stance against doping were once part of the scene and had tried it all. Some took a liberal view and thought people have a right to treat their bodies as they wish, and others had spent years taking doses upwards of 50 times larger than any treatment would ever prescribe. Some had tried every powerful drug on the market but still believed today's young people use steroids without knowing enough about what they are doing. Some of my informants were young men who had never had problems with their self-confidence, whereas others had. Some had little or no luck with the ladies before they started working out, then began to see heads turn as their muscles grew. Others experienced a sort of "steroid kick" that got them hooked, although they could not trace their fascination with muscles and exercise back to any specific circumstance or situation in their childhood, school life, prior athletic pursuits or personality.

For me the aim of this study, and thus my role, was not to tell these people that they were wrong, or that they had gone astray, led unhealthy lives, adhered to the wrong values or ought to change their lifestyle. My task, as I see it, is to understand their perspective to the fullest extent of my abilities. It is not my intention to overlook or neglect potentially harmful health consequences resulting from the use of anabolic steroids, but if we want to understand the people who use these drugs, our basic premise must be built on something other than condemnation. We must instead make an earnest effort to understand what drives them; to understand what they are seeking to achieve; to understand their situation and their ambitions.

As mentioned, I came into contact with my informants partly by placing information folders about the project in a number of gyms and fitness clubs and posting information on two Internet forums, and partly through references from informants with whom I was already in contact. I interviewed a total of 14 people for the study, mainly in the spring of 2009. Although these interviews took place some years ago, in my estimation the informants' experiences with anabolic steroids are just as valid today as they were at the time. Since then, besides following the international literature closely, as a supervisor and examiner on Danish and international master's-degree and PhD theses on the subject I have read a number of interviews with anabolic-steroid users, conducted between 2012 and 2019. None of these have offered any radically new input to user experiences with anabolic steroids. Based on this, I have no reason to assume that the range of views expressed by my informants would have differed in any substantial way, had my interviews been conducted today.

That is not to say I claim to have achieved full data saturation, which would imply that my 14 informants were able to tell me everything there is to say on the matter; a situation that is often presented as a criterion for success in qualitative research studies (Creswell, 2013; Kvale & Brinkmann, 2009).[7] My group of informants was too small and too diverse to ensure this. Even so, I am convinced that by combining my findings with the body of research already done on this topic, I am able to realistically represent the approaches to anabolic steroid use in the recreational workout and weightlifting communities in Denmark.

Naturally, I have done my utmost to avoid convenient cherry-picking when choosing the many quotes that appear throughout this book, although choices did have to be made. I set up selection criteria that would reflect both sides of my own ambition. On the one hand I wanted the quotes to showcase as much variation as possible, and on the other hand I wanted the interview statements to illustrate some sort of general applicability, allowing the analysis to point out patterns, links or trends that transcend the informants' individual experiences.

Doping terminology

A key challenge when discussing IPED use, whether one is looking at top-level competitive sports or non-athletic settings, is that the topic itself is steeped in a witches' brew of moral and ethical questions. This can easily lead to categorical comments and heated debates. As the example from the *Politiken* coverage shows, critical reporting cast in a particular light can set the wider public agenda. The danger in this is, however, that while such an agenda may bring certain disturbing aspects (such as crime, health threats or violence) to the fore in the public debate, the sensational nature of these aspects may make them so prominent that other, less flashy aspects are overlooked.

Linguistic manifestations of this are evident in various terms now widely applied to athletes who use, or have used, performance-enhancing substances: "steroid abusers," "doping sinners" and the like. Such language is practical, since it calls for no further arguments. It nonetheless disregards the fact that the "abuse" (of pills, alcohol, heroin, cocaine, MDMA and so forth) generally weakens the user, whereas "doping" (with performance-enhancing substances) generally fortifies the user. This is a decisive difference, but because the language does not reflect it, the inherent condemnation is unambiguous. Another equally strong mechanism lies in wording that has religious connotations: "sins" or "transgressions," for instance. Some would argue that references to "sinning" imply how diabolically tempting doping is in high-performance environments, but primarily it serves as an effective obstruction to counter-arguments and a springboard for condemnation.

Even without the journalistic angle, the Danish-language equivalent of "abuse" (*misbrug*) has become a common collocation for the word "doping," which has been loaned directly into Danish as a noun and a verb. "Abuse" is used to denote any use of medicine, controlled substances or alcohol that is not in accordance with the intent or prescription (in the case of medicine), or which lies outside socially and culturally acceptable norms (in the case of alcohol, cannabis and other controlled substances). Note that the latter wording implies some flexibility, since what is "acceptable" can and will change, both over time and across various cultural groups. Furthermore, the concept of "abuse" implies a moral judgment that is unfortunate since, objectively speaking, there is a huge difference between, say, an ailing alcoholic on a week-long binge, and a hard-working Tour de France cyclist riding on performance enhancers — both of whom, in these situations, would be termed "substance abusers."

English actually has two terms for what in some languages (including Danish) has only one term. Even so, the English words *misuse* and *abuse* are often used synonymously in the scientific literature and in the media. The World Health Organization (WHO) has attempted to avoid this in its *Lexicon of alcohol and drug terms* by distinguishing between use, misuse and abuse. "Use," in the WHO context, refers to the "self-administration" of a substance with no expression of a normative opinion. "Misuse" applies to substance used "for a purpose not consistent with legal or medical guidelines." Examples of this would be a sprinter using anabolic steroids, or a professional cyclist using the hormone erythropoietin (EPO). The third term, "abuse," refers to

> a maladaptive pattern of use indicated by continued use despite knowledge of having a persistent or recurrent social, occupational, psychological or physical problem that is caused or exacerbated by the use [or by] recurrent use in situations in which it is physically hazardous.
>
> (WHO, 2019)

Abuse also indicates a loss of control, as when a bodybuilder becomes unable to manage the duration of his steroid cycles, or when an alcoholic cannot make it through the day without imbibing strong alcoholic drinks at regular intervals.

Distinguishing in English between "use," "misuse" and "abuse" raises problems of its own. One is that "misuse" also has a normative ring to it, signaling that this too is more than a practice that goes against the original intention. Another problem is that these distinctions do not make it meaningful to talk about "alcohol misuse" among the general population, much less "EPO abuse" among top cyclists. Drinking too much beer is not the same as using beer "for a purpose not consistent with legal or medical guidelines." Nor is it meaningful to talk about EPO used by a famous cyclist as an example of "a maladaptive pattern of use" with associated "social, occupational, psychological or physical" problems. In the latter instance, the consequences would not result from the substance's effects, but from the very revelation that the cyclist was using the substance at all.

A more precise conceptual framework distinguishes between three cate-gories: use, abuse or dependence and off-label use. Here, "use" generally refers to ingesting or injecting a substance, while "abuse" denotes a situation where the use of alcohol, medication or some other substance is out of control, or has negative repercussions as described above and requires treatment. Elsewhere, the third category, "off-label use," is often used synonymously with "sports doping." "Off-label use" refers to the way physical practitioners of various kinds (professional or amateur athletes, and non-athletic or recreational users) functionally employ medication that was originally developed for a purpose other than enhancing performance.[8] Still, in the vast majority of practical situations the distinction between "use" and "abuse" — the two terms I use in this book — is sufficient, given that discussions about a bodybuilder's or a professional cyclist's use of anabolic steroids or EPO will obviously imply "off-label use," or "doping." Hopefully this terminological clarification has also made it obvious that phrases like "doping abuse" or "abusive doping" are not meaningful in most cases that involve top athletes.

The contents of this book

Following this introductory chapter, Chapter 2 looks at the most common explanations for young men's frequent preoccupation with the generously muscled body, and it also deals with workouts, weightlifting, IPED use and media representations of people in gyms and fitness clubs who use illicit substances. I round off with some input on demographics and prevalence: Who uses anabolic steroids, and how common is it? Chapter 3 explains the effects and side effects of using steroids, as I review and discuss physical, psychological and social repercussions based on the scientific literature. Chapter 4 sets out the theoretical foundation of personal identity. Here, I discuss why the issue of identity is pivotal to the theme of this book and how the concept of identity can be applied. I then move on to how steroid use is experienced, understood and justified by users themselves.

In Chapter 5, based on the interviews I conducted, I look at the appeal of muscles and weight training and at what motivates young men and draws them into weightlifting and gym communities. Chapter 6 contains narratives of four people's very different experiences with anabolic steroids. These four accounts show that information levels, attitudes and settings play an impor-tant role in steroid use. They also show how these people have different aims in using steroids and how these aims develop and change as users gain experience or deal with significant life events.

Against this backdrop, Chapter 7 presents an "ideal typology" of anabolic steroid use in gym communities. My work has identified four ideal types: the Expert type, the Well-being type, the YOLO type and the Athlete type. I also argue why the "abuser" is a negative iteration that can occur as a degenerated form under each of the four main types. Chapter 8 revisits the question of side effects, physical and psychological, relating to the use of steroids, this time from the perspective of the steroid users. It also touches upon the way steroids affect users' libido and sex lives. I take a broader view in Chapter 9, examining my informants' strict diets, exercise and self-discipline, and looking at the way partners and parents react to steroid use. This chapter also discusses peer recognition and identity formation. One key driver for serious male gym-goers is the strong tendency to link muscles, manhood and identity. Chapter 10 moves on to include aspects of evolutionary psychology to better explain why humans are basically very attentive to physical attractiveness, and why men and women generally have certain preferences. Along with knowledge about the cultural focus on bodies and appearance, evolutionary psychology allows us to more comprehensively understand the most alluring elements of physical fitness, the modern workout culture and steroids.

In Chapters 11, 12, and 13, I turn my attention to political and regulatory matters, taking my point of departure in Denmark by looking at how Danish organizations and legislators have sought to combat and regulate the use of IPEDs in gym settings. I do this not only because Denmark is my home turf, but also because Denmark was one of the first countries to respond systematically to this issue, and thus is a country with quite a bit of experience. Chapter 11 describes how Anti Doping Danmark has tackled the challenge of fighting steroid use and how this NADO has developed its work. In Chapter 12, my informants voice their views on the anti-doping system and its work, also from personal experience. In Chapter 13, I confront and compare the Danish approach — which evolved out of anti-doping in elite sport — with other strategies, most notably the harm-reduction approach taken in the United Kingdom. Finally, in Chapter 14, I summarize the various discussions and offer general conclusions.

This work draws on an extensive body of literature, so there are numerous bibliographical references throughout. To ease the reader's way, I have decided to limit parenthetical literary references to a maximum of three at a time, placing further information in endnotes after each chapter.

Notes

1 The European Health and Market Report, by Deloitte. See (EuropeActive, 2019).
2 The most accurate term is "anabolic-androgenic steroids." This denotes a group of synthetically manufactured hormones that simulate the effects of the male sex hormone testosterone. Chapter 3 presents in detail the effects and side effects of such substances. To make for smoother reading, in this book I generally refer to both testosterone and synthetic androgens as "anabolic steroids" or simply "steroids."
3 See also (Simon, Striegel, Aust, Dietz, & Ulrich, 2006; Singhammer, 2013; Striegel et al., 2006).

4 Bodybuilders and serious weightlifters and gym-goers are averse to being identified as part of the "fitness" segment. They prefer not to be included in "the fitness community," which they associate with spinning and exercise classes, whereas their activity is not about fitness but about building bulk or lifting weights. I have done my best to use the terms "serious gym-goers," "weightlifters," "the weightlifting community" and the like, reserving "bodybuilding" and related terms for those with a competitive profile. Further, because Anti Doping Danmark often uses the words "fitness center," "fitness culture" and "fitness communities," I occasionally use these terms as well when speaking of wider groups in Denmark and abroad. As a result, the terminology in this book varies to reflect what is most appropriate to the context.
5 In 2018, the UK National Crime Agency (NCA) was able to announce that "Mr. Jacob" was, in fact, the Danish citizen Jacob Sporon-Fiedler, and the case that began in *Politiken* turned out to be possibly the largest ever on smuggling anabolic steroids, with seizures that totaled in excess of GBP 40m. The two Danish journalists were witnesses in the case, during which it was estimated that Sporon-Fiedler and his associates had smuggled some 42 tons of illicit anabolic steroids into the UK; drugs which were then sold on the black market in the UK and the European mainland. As Rob Burgess, NCA regional head of investigations, said: "We believe this organised criminal group to be the most prolific of its kind ever uncovered, probably the biggest global players in the illicit anabolic steroid market" (Forrest, 2019).
6 See also (Cohen et al., 2007).
7 Had I aspired to achieve such data saturation, I would have been obliged to narrow down my group of informants considerably, and to apply criteria such as "males aged 19–21, with 1–2 years of anabolic steroid use" or alternatively "males over 30, with long-term, varied use of IPEDs." I considered narrowing the group but found this incompatible with the very concept of the project. Instead, in cases where I deemed my own material to be insufficient as documentation, I looked for support elsewhere in the research literature, Danish and international.
8 Danish substance-abuse consultants continue to work on categorizing a Danish vocabulary along the same lines as the prevailing English terminology, which distinguishes among various levels of use, recreational or casual use and actual abuse, measured by frequency. Even so, no consistent terminology has yet found its way into Danish usage.

References

Asserhøj, T. L. (2017). *Danskernes fitnessvaner og brug af kommercielle idrætstilbud* Retrieved from København: www.idan.dk/vidensbank/downloads/danskernes-fitnessvaner-og-brug-af-kommercielle-idraetstilbud/b499a51a-dce1-439a-8ee8-a6ff00bcb9bc.
Backhouse, S., Collins, C., Defoort, Y., McNamee, M., Parkinson, A., & Sauer, M. (2014). *Study on doping prevention. A map of legal, regulatory and prevention practice provisions in EU 28.* Retrieved from Luxembourg: http://ec.europa.eu/assets/eac/sport/news/2014/docs/doping-prevention-report_en.pdf.
Bang, S., & van Bedaf, A. (2018). Stadig vækst blandt de kommercielle fitnesscentre. Retrieved from: www.idan.dk/nyhedsoversigt/nyheder/2018/b153_stadig-vaekst-blandt-de-kommercielle-fitnesscentre.
Barland, B., & Tangen, J. O. (2009). Kroppspresentasjon og andre prestasjoner – en omfangsundersøkelse om bruk av Doping. Retrieved from Oslo: https://antidoping.no/sitefiles/1/dokumenter/pdf/omfangsundersokelsen.pdf.

Brock, J. L., & Heide-Jørgensen, C. (2012–2013). Politiken undersøger doping i Danmark, Artikelserie. *Politiken.*

Christiansen, A. V. (2005). The Legacy of Festina: Patterns of drug use in European cycling since 1998. *Sport in History,* 25(3), 497–514.

Christiansen, A. V. (2011). Bodily Violations: Testing citizens training recreationally in gyms. In M. McNamee & V. Møller (Eds.), *Doping and anti-doping. Ethical, legal and social perspectives* (pp. 126–141). London: Routledge.

Christiansen, A. V., & Møller, V. (2007). *Mål, medicin og moral: Om eliteatleters opfattelse af sport, doping og fairplay* (Ambitions, drugs and morality: On athletes' perceptions of sport, doping and fair play). Odense, Denmark: Syddansk Universitetsforlag.

Cohen, J., Collins, R., Darkes, J., & Gwartney, D. (2007). A league of their own: Demographics, motivations and patterns of use of 1,955 male adult non-medical anabolic steroid users in the United States. *J.Int.Soc.Sports Nutr.,* 4(12). doi: doi:10.1186/1550-2783-4-12.

Creswell, J. W. (2013). *Qualitative inquiry and research design: Choosing among five approaches* (3 ed.). London: Sage publications.

EuropeActive. (2019). *Who we are.* Retrieved from: www.europeactive.eu/who-we-are.

Forrest, A. (2019, 6 June). London man convicted over role in £40m international steroid smuggling gang. *The Independent.* Retrieved from: www.independent.co.uk/news/uk/crime/steroid-smuggling-gang-gurjaipal-dhillon-london-guilty-a8946356.html.

Hibell, B., Andersson, B., Bjarnason, T., Kokkevi, A., Morgan, M., & Narusk, A. (1997). The 1995 ESPAD report. Alcohol and other drug use among students in 26 European countries. Retrieved from Stockholm: www.espad.org/sites/espad.org/files/The_1995_ESPAD_report.pdf.

IDAN. (2016). Styrketræning hitter blandt børn og voksne. Retrieved from: www.idan.dk/nyhedsoversigt/nyheder/2016/a828_styrketraening-hitter-blandt-boern-og-voksne.

Kanayama, G., & Pope, H. G. (2012). Illicit use of androgens and other hormones: Recent advances. *Current Opinion in Endocrinology, Diabetes and Obesity,* 19(3), 1–9. doi: doi:10.1097/MED.0b013e3283524008.

Klein, A. M. (1993). *Little big men: Bodybuilding subculture and gender construction.* Albany, NY: State University of New York Press.

Klein, A. M. (2007). Size matters: Connecting subculture to culture in bodybuilding. In J. K. Thompson & G. Cafri (Eds.), *The muscular ideal: Psychological, social, and medical perspectives* (1 ed., pp. 67–83). Washington, DC: American Psychological Association.

Kvale, S., & Brinkmann, S. (2009). *Interviews: Learning the craft of qualitative research interviewing.* Thousand Oaks, CA: Sage Publications.

Liokaftos, D. (2017). *A Genealogy of male bodybuilding: From classical to freaky.* New York & Oxon: Routledge.

Luciano, L. (2007). Muscularity and masculinity in the United States: A historical overview. In J. K. Thompson & G. Cafri (Eds.), *The muscular ideal: psychological, social, and medical perspectives* (1 ed., pp. 41–65). Washington, DC: American Psychological Association.

Monaghan, L. F. (2001). *Bodybuilding, drugs, and risk.* London: Routledge.

Monaghan, L. F. (2002). Vocabularies of motive for illicit steroid use among bodybuilders. *Soc.Sci.Med.,* 55(5), 695–708.

Parkinson, A. B., & Evans, N. A. (2006). Anabolic androgenic steroids: A survey of 500 users. *Medicine & Science in Sports & Exercise*, 38(4), 644–651. doi: doi:10.1249/01.mss.0000210194.56834.5d.

Pilgaard, M., & Rask, S. (2016). Danskernes motions- og sportsvaner 2016. Retrieved from København: www.idan.dk/vidensbank/udgivelser/danskernes-motions-og-sportsvaner-2016/03e7c32f-151c-44d2-a678-a69400850057.

Pope, H. G., Phillips, K. A., & Olivardia, R. (2000). *The Adonis complex: How to identify, treat, and prevent body obsession in men and boys*. New York: Free Press.

Pope, H. G., Wood, R. I., Rogol, A., Nyberg, F., Bowers, L., & Bhasin, S. (2014). Adverse health consequences of performance-enhancing drugs: An Endocrine Society scientific statement. *Endocr Rev*, 35(3), 341–375. doi: doi:10.1210/er.2013-1058.

Sagoe, D., Molde, H., Andreassen, C. S., Torsheim, T., & Pallesen, S. (2014). The global epidemiology of anabolic-androgenic steroid use: A meta-analysis and meta-regression analysis. *Annals of Epidemiology*, 24(1873–2585 (Electronic)), 383–398.

Simon, P., Striegel, H., Aust, F., Dietz, K., & Ulrich, R. (2006). Doping in fitness sports: Estimated number of unreported cases and individual probability of doping. *Addiction*, 101(11), 1640–1644. doi: doi:10.1111/j.1360-0443.2006.01568.x.

Singhammer, J. (2013). Attitudes toward anabolic-androgenic steroids among non-competing athletes in various types of sports: A cross-sectional study. *Sport Science Review*, 22(1–2), 109–128. doi: doi:10.2478/ssr-2013-0006.

Singhammer, J., & Ibsen, B. (2010). Motionsdoping i Danmark: En kvantitativ undersøgelse om brug af og holdning til muskelopbyggende stoffer. Retrieved from Denmark: www.antidoping.dk/media/1243/motionsdoping_i-danmark_sdu_2010.pdf

Skårberg, K., & Engstrom, I. (2007). Troubled social background of male anabolic-androgenic steroid abusers in treatment. *Subst Abuse Treat Prev Policy*, 2, 20. doi: doi:10.1186/1747-597X-2-20.

Steele, R., Bang, S., Brandt, H. H., & Kirkegaard, K. L. (2010). Indsatsen mod motionsdoping i kommercielle motions- og fitnesscentre – en evaluering af mærkningsordningen (The fight against doping in commercial fitness centres: An evaluation of the labelling scheme). Retrieved from København: www.idan.dk/vidensbank/forskningoganalyser/stamkort.aspx?publikationID=bbd99a70-1a98-4232-a6e9-9e3000e57a68&/Vidensbank/Forskningoganalyser.aspx?currentstart=0&ResultPrPage=5&Kortvisning=False&emneID=873805be-6673-4d78-b326-25899e74736f.

Storm, R. K., Toft, D., & Bang, S. (2015). Motionsdoping i Danmark. Evaluering af indsatsen mod motionsdoping i kommercielle motions- og fitnesscentre (Use of IPEDs in Denmark: An evaluation of the intervention in commercial gyms in Denmark). Retrieved from København: www.idan.dk/vidensbank/downloads/motionsdoping-i-danmark/382b209b-fd84-4c04-9a6a-a50f0113101b.

Striegel, H., Simon, P., Frisch, S., Roecker, K., Dietz, K., Dickhuth, H. H., & Ulrich, R. (2006). Anabolic ergogenic substance users in fitness-sports: A distinct group supported by the health care system. *Drug Alcohol Depend*, 81(1), 11–19. doi: doi:10.1016/j.drugalcdep.2005.05.013.

WHO. (2019). Lexicon of alcohol and drug terms published by the World Health Organization. Retrieved from: www.who.int/substance_abuse/terminology/who_lexicon/en/.

Chapter 2

IPEDs as a cultural phenomenon

In sports, the use of performance-enhancing drugs can usually be explained by the ambitious athlete's desire for a competitive advantage. However, in gym communities this explanation is of little value, given that few gym-goers take part in competitions. Most studies indicate that the use of anabolic steroids and similar IPEDs in non-competitive environments is motivated by a wish to achieve or move closer to an ideal physique — be it more muscular, larger, stronger or slimmer (Backhouse, McKenna, Robinson, & Atkin, 2007; McVeigh, Bates, & Chandler, 2015; Monaghan, 2001).[1] This absence of the usual competitive motivation may be a common denominator for users of anabolic steroids in gyms, but beyond this there are few shared traits. What is more, steroid users today have a wider variety of driving factors than 30 years ago. Recurring themes in the various studies of what motivates IPED use are the desire to increase muscle mass, lose fat, become stronger and get into better shape. Meanwhile, some users embark on a systematic workout and doping regimen to replace or overcome problems with other addictive substances (Barland, Tangen, & Johannesen, 2010), and another group of respondents state, among their motives, a wish to improve their sex drive (Bates & McVeigh, 2016; Begley et al., 2017).

Such a drive or ambition to change one's bodily appearance hardly comes out of the blue, so there must be historical, cultural and social reasons that can explain why people work to achieve their body ideals, more today than ever before. Creating a backdrop for the book's further discussions, in this chapter we will look at the most broadly supported explanations of this trend, and at what we know about steroid users and the prevalence of IPED use.[2]

Historical background

As I already mentioned, the exposure Arnold Schwarzenegger was able to achieve helped make it legitimate for men to strive for a muscular body. In parallel with this, in the early 1970s the mainstream media also began to take an interest in the strong male body. This was a new development. Although strong-man competitions and public spectacles featuring strong men had enjoyed some attention from the 1890s onwards, throughout the first half of the twentieth century they were associated with the proletarian background from which they first arose. Eugen Sandow (1867–1925) is arguably the most famous figure among the early titans of physical fitness. This German-born icon deliberately strove to refine his mode of expression, and his performances focused not only on strength but on bodily aesthetics as well. That is why he is frequently referred to as the father of modern bodybuilding (Liokaftos, 2017). Still, in his day he was regarded as something of an anomaly, and he was not an ideal for the men of the middle class — a group that generally did not find their identity in sports or physical work but primarily in non-physical activities, mainly as bread-winners for their families. This is evidenced in the male role models from the silver screen in the 1940s and 1950s, who rarely had a muscular frame. Even so, the figure of the strong man was not absent in popular culture in the mid-twentieth century. For instance, the famous advertisements for Charles Atlas and his self-improvement program held a particular appeal for insecure teenage boys.

One of these ads, which appeared in several versions, features a cartoon strip of a young man being harassed on the beach by a sand-kicking bully while his girlfriend looks on passively. Back in his room he angrily kicks a chair, "gambles a stamp" and orders physical-fitness material from Charles Atlas. "Later" he returns to the beach with his new, impressive physique. It's pay-back time: He punches the bully in full public view, and his girlfriend and the other beach-goers celebrate him as the "Hero of the beach!" (see for instance Alcott, 2014; Wikipedia, 2019). This ad ran in magazines and similar publications for decades. Its success was undoubtedly due to the narrative motif of physical and mental transformation, a message with a universal appeal that continued to resonate with readers and audiences. Although today no company would dream of using physical violence and potential revenge as an incentive to make customers buy an exercise program, we basically see the same figure used by the companies promoting health-club chains, training concepts and dietary supplements as they advertise their product offerings with archetypal "before and after" pictures and testimonials.

Although "the strong man" had a presence, generally the adult population in the 1950s preferred tall, slim men with a physique that was not too pronounced. The 1960s hippie movement and its renunciation of traditional gender roles underscored the rejection of aggressive muscular masculinity. Instead, the hippie generation explored models for alternative living, music genres and psychedelic drugs, also demonstrating against the Vietnam War and the soldiers fighting abroad by dressing in loose-fitting, gender-neutral clothing and wearing flowers in their free-flowing hair (Luciano, 2007).

Then, from the 1970s, things gradually began to change. Chronicling these developments in detail lies outside the scope of this book. Still, briefly told, several factors — the oil crisis in the early 1970s, growing unemployment and a new wave of exercise zeal and health awareness — combined to form what would crystallize into "the me generation" around the early 1980s. These factors and others brought about a new situation and also led to an interest in cultivating the more masculine, muscular body (Lasch, 1980; Luciano, 2007). It was against this cultural backdrop that Arnold Schwarzenegger, Jane Fonda and a slew of other health and exercise gurus captivated a new audience as the interest in weightlifting, bodybuilding and physical fitness spread throughout most of the Western world.

In the context of the Olympic Games, the use of sports doping in the form of various more or less effective performance-enhancing drugs has been discussed since the 1930s (Gleaves & Llewellyn, 2013). However, it was only later, at the 1960 Olympic Games in Rome, that more effective drugs like anabolic steroids began to play a role (Dimeo, 2007). Weightlifters were among the first athletes to understand the potentially revolutionizing impact of steroids on muscle strength. Obviously, the use of such drugs caused alarm, at least to the extent that it became known (Woodland, 1980). Meanwhile, few people were interested in what was going on in the small, subcultural bodybuilding community in Southern California, so it was not until the late 1970s that the general public gradually become aware of ana-bolic-steroid use among athletes outside the world of elite sports (Brohm, 1978; Goldman, Bush, & Klatz, 1984; Taylor, 1985). Sport organizations and researchers were primarily concerned with doping among top athletes, so the use of such drugs in non-competitive and recreational environments was treated in cursory form, chiefly in incidental comments about this regretta-ble spin-off effect of elite-sports doping. Only in the 1980s did attention turn towards non-sports doping, as a more general cultural shift of interest in the male body became observable.

One of the first researchers to draw attention to the spread of steroid use to gyms and health clubs was the American sport historian Terry Todd. His article, evocatively entitled Anabolic Steroids: The Gremlins of Sport,[3] included quotes from an interview with a dealer who described how easy it was to procure steroids in the early 1980s: "Most people don't understand how easy it is to buy steroids. All you have to do is to go into almost any gym in the US and inside of a day you can score." As the dealer explained,

> The largest group of users would be bodybuilders, of course, and I don't mean competitive bodybuilders. I mean average guys who just wanted to be bigger and stronger as fast as they can. The last three or four years, the use of the stuff has just exploded.
>
> (Todd, 1987, p. 104)

Gone were the days when anabolic-steroid use was confined to a small group of top-level professional athletes — which brought a whole new reason for concern.

The Adonis Complex

In the early 1990s, a group of American researchers led by the Harvard professor Harrison Pope began to take an interest in what they described as millions of young men who, due to growing dissatisfaction with their bodies, spent many hours lifting weights at gyms. While most researchers in this field had, thus far, primarily studied girls and women's body dissatisfaction (which typically focused on fat aversion, body size and perceived excess weight), some now redirected their attention to boys and men and their preoccupation with muscle. Pope and his group claimed that, combined with the generally increasing exposure of the male body, the reason for the widespread use of steroids in gym communities had to be understood in light of the enormous contemporary focus on body and appearance, along with greater steroid accessibility. Investigating American culture, Pope and his colleagues pointed to the exposure of buff bodies on television, films, ads and other sites of popular culture as a key factor in understanding the apparently widespread use of anabolic steroids in gyms. To support their claims they showed, among other things, how the presence of male models in popular magazines, ads and elsewhere had grown over a period of 25 years. But perhaps more importantly, they further documented that the male models also showed more skin than before and were more muscular and well-defined. Having studied male models featured as centerfolds in *Playgirl* magazine, the researchers traced the gradual development towards a more muscular physique from the early 1970s up to the late 1990s (Pope et al., 2000).

Yet this development is not global. A Taiwanese study, which counted the number of semi-nude men portrayed in women's magazines, found a much higher incidence of nudity and far more muscular men in Western European and American magazines than in corresponding Taiwanese publications (Yang, Gray, & Pope, 2005). In the Western world, however, the trend was clear. In keeping with this, Pope's group also noted how, over a period of 30 years, boys' action-figure toys like Superman, Batman and G.I. Joe had undergone a transformation from resembling well-proportioned but easily recognizable men to exhibiting muscular frames unrivaled by even the most steroid-enhanced bodybuilders. Just as Barbie dolls had been criticized in the 1980s for giving girls an unrealistic image of the female body, the researchers found that these action figures could give the boys who played with them an unrealistic image of the ideal male body (Baghurst, Hollander, Nardella, & Haff, 2006; Pope, Olivardia, Gruber, & Borowiecki, 1999).

Based on their observations, Pope and his colleagues therefore began discussing what they called "the Adonis Complex," a phrase they coined to denote a culturally rooted, excessive preoccupation with one's body and appearance. "Unlike healthy men and boys," they concluded, those suffering from the Adonis Complex "have an unrealistic view of how they should look — and so they may abuse drugs, exercise excessively and spend millions on products that are often worthless" (Pope et al., 2000, p. xiii). They found that such an unhealthy fixation with the body and its appearance adversely affected the social lives of people with this complex, fearing that the worst cases of men suffering from the Adonis Complex would cause them to develop mental illness. Envisioning a scenario inversely mirroring the critics' claim that Barbie dolls could give young girls anorexia, there was now talk of action figures causing a distorted body image in boys and leading to the opposite phenomenon in men. Stories began to surface of steroid-using weightlifters who felt they were too small, even though everyone else could plainly see they were huge.

According to the researchers, the experience of not being muscular enough would sometimes become so dominant in these men that they would develop the opposite of anorexia, initially termed *bigorexia*. Psychologists have since agreed on the less colorful term *muscle dysmorphia* — literally, fear of not being muscular enough (Pope, Gruber, Choi, Olivardia, & Phillips, 1997; Pope et al., 1999; Pope et al., 2000). At any rate, a large-scale study that summed up findings from several independent studies (a metastudy) showed that although muscle dysmorphia occurs more frequently in bodybuilders than among average gym-goers, the correlation between muscle dysmorphia and anabolic steroid use is quite weak. Looking at the links between these two phenomena it is impossible to determine whether steroids cause muscle dysmorphia, or whether steroids are simply used by certain people who have that condition already. Likewise, it is impossible to determine whether bodybuilding leads to muscle dysmorphia, or whether people who are predisposed for the condition are attracted to bodybuilding as an activity (Hildebrandt, Alfano, & Langenbucher, 2010; Mitchell et al., 2017). Hence, using the diagnosis "muscle dysmorphia" as a general explanation for steroid use in gym communities is not very helpful. Rather than finding, or inventing, a diagnosis that can explain steroid use, there is good reason to investigate what other cultural, social and historical changes may have exerted an influence on the altered body perception among men, and among women.

Cultural shifts

Consumer culture

Looking at advertisements, one can easily get the impression that it is actually possible to buy an identity. As we shall see in Chapter 4, however, this does not work in practice. Even so, several sociologists have pointed out that consumer culture has led people to believe they can create themselves, and their identity, through consumption, and in this connection shaping the body is a key component. It is not enough to own an expensive wardrobe, a cool car or a designer kitchen. You have to have a gorgeous body too

(Bauman, 2001; Featherstone, Hepworth, & Turner, 1993). The body as a symbol of the successful life can be purchased at gyms and health clubs, and as a multitude of performance-enhancing products. The covers of health and fitness magazines often display beautiful, physically fit men and women, while the contents of these magazines include a veritable flood of advertisements for pills, powders, drinks, gels and energy bars conducive to physical change (Hoff, 2016). Although it is true that these ads do not peddle drugs, the message at their core is unmistakable: Besides exercise and training, it takes performance-enhancing products to achieve a beautiful body, and if you use them you will more easily reach your goal.

Television and social media

In recent years the number of television channels and services has exploded, and today, with the right subscription package, viewers can watch continuous sports programming, uninterrupted, day and night. In April 2016 the Danish newspaper *Politiken* did a viewership survey that showed how the average live-sports TV offering for Danes had risen from 14 hours in 1996, across an average 116 hours in 2006, to an overwhelming 267 hours per week in 2016 (Sinnbeck, 2016). Many of these broadcast hours display sportspeople who train far more than the average Olympic athlete did just 40 years ago. In other words, televised exposure of the athletic body, which many hold as their ideal, has significantly increased. But that is not all. Over the past four decades the athletic bodies we see have undergone a qualitative shift, towards ever greater perfection and trimness. Obviously, athlete's bodies are very diverse. First, different sports select for different body types. Second, countless hours of training alter athletes' bodies to suit the sport they perform. No surprise, then, that a marathon runner and a weightlifter look hugely different. Having said that, what people often refer to as "an athletic build" is the body type seen in team ballplayers, swimmers, cross-country skiers, sprinters and decathletes (Barland & Tangen, 2009; Dixson, Halliwell, East, Wignarajah, & Anderson, 2003; Etcoff, 1999). Swimmers, for example, are often regarded as an athletic group that represents the classic, well-trained, athletic body with narrow hips and broad shoulders. If we then compare pictures of the best male swimmers from the 1972 Olympic Games in Munich with those from the 2016 games in Rio de Janeiro, the difference is striking. The world's best, most superbly trained athletes have become even more physically fit and muscular than before, and so the body ideal they represent has become harder to achieve today than it was 40 years ago. On top of this, some of the most successful reality-TV shows, which have hundreds of thousands of young viewers, use the beautiful body as a central marketing tool. Shows like *Love Island* and *Paradise Hotel*, are built around a simple concept: young, tanned, well-trained, attractive contestants are accommodated in luxury hotels, where they drink, have sex and argue — most often dressed in little more than swimwear. However, this apparently innocuous concept has an impact on young viewers, who may feel less perfect than their on-screen peers. According to a YouGov survey of 4,505 UK adults, almost one in four (24%) of those aged 19 to 24 say "reality TV makes them worry about their body image." The survey thus suggests that *Love Island* and similar programs could leave thousands of young adults feeling worried about their own bodies. In line with this, 34% of respondents in the same survey said images used in advertising and promotions on social media made them worry about their body image (Mental Health Foundation, 2019).

In recent years, technological developments have given us new ways to share information about exercise, training, diets and steroids. This has almost certainly contributed to the greater diversity in people's motives to use steroids and other IPEDs. Social media conduits like Instagram and Facebook are teaming with more or less manipulated images showing the effects of the contributors' training and dietary regimes. The online super-stars of personal training and physical fitness have hundreds of thousands of Instagram followers, who find inspiration in the results posted by their idols. Eminent examples are the crossfit athletes Sara Sigmundsdóttir from Iceland and Rich Froning Jr from the United States, who both have online commu-nities of over 1.3 million followers (as of September 2019).

Health

During the same period, health has become an ideal in almost every phase and walk of life. Among many others, the British sociologist Ivan Wad-dington (2000) and the Australian sociologist Deborah Lupton (Lupton, 1995) have both pointed out that being healthy, in itself, has become an imperative for modern human beings. We associate a wide variety of posi-tive values with health, ranging from lifestyle to work issues to moral and ethical qualities. We not only talk about the value of a healthy body or healthy food, but also about the value of healthy homes, relationships, friendships, workplaces, cities, economies, and so on and so forth. This makes it attractive to be, and not least to be *perceived* as being, healthy. A salient point here is that our assessment of a person's state of health is rarely based on biomedical facts about what actually *is* healthy, but more often relies on what *looks* healthy; in other words, on the visual expression of health (Etcoff, 1999). This means that although bodybuilding and intensive strength training are practiced in a way that does not always follow official health recommendations, these activities have been astutely marketed with images of beautiful, physically toned men and women who *signal* healthiness. In this way the fitness industry has used, or exploited, our intuitive percep-tion of healthiness. Herein lies one key to explaining the success of the fit-ness industry: The activities they market have been represented as elements that are imperative for a healthy lifestyle (Klein, 2007).

Masculinity in crisis

In addition to these issues there are wider social and societal trends that tie in with the women's liberation movement from the 1960s onwards. With the liberation of women in the Western world, men no longer enjoy the same privileges or status in society as in earlier times. Consequently, some men have felt threatened in terms of their manhood, experiencing what is sometimes called a "crisis of masculinity." When it comes to steroid use and the upsurge of fitness culture, the hypothesis is that some men, in order to at least partially win back their lost masculine appeal, have sought recourse in hypermasculinity as expressed in muscularity. The point is that although women can certainly become police chiefs, pilots, professors and presidents, they can never attain the same muscle bulk as men can — no matter how liberated they are (or how doped on steroids). That is why, to a man, working with his muscles is one of the most original, primal expressions of his personal status of manhood (Cafri et al., 2005; Gray & Ginsberg, 2007; Klein, 1993).

As is true of the other cultural theories mentioned here, the masculinity-crisis hypothesis cannot stand alone as an explanation for the interest in muscular bodies or the rise in steroid use. This becomes evident when we consider the interest in bodybuilding and steroids found in countries where women's liberation has not moved into the mainstream, like it has in Scandinavia, Western Europe and North America. This is the case, for instance, in Afghanistan, Iran and also in several Middle Eastern countries where bodybuilding has become immensely popular, with steroid use following suit (Dalsgaard & Winding, 2006; Sagoe, Molde, Andreassen, Torsheim, & Pallesen, 2014; Tahtamouni et al., 2008).

Surgical and pharmaceutical aid

Beyond the strictly cultural developments, various other options are available so people can buy their way to profoundly altering their appearance. These actions are not just symbolic, like paying a gym membership or consuming protein powder and energy bars. They are extremely concrete. Four decades ago, prominent ears, a small bosom or a crooked nose was something you simply had to grin and bear for life. Basically, you were stuck with your looks. This changed with the advent of elective plastic surgery (building on reconstructive techniques pioneered after World War I) and hormone treatments. The body could be altered, laying the foundation for a billion-dollar industry in beauty products, cosmetic surgery and legal hormone therapies (Gray & Ginsberg, 2007; Hoberman, 2005). In this context it is interesting to note that while men and women accept that such alterations are purchasable commodities, women prefer to have them done surgically — as breast implants, liposuction procedures and the like — whereas men more often find it reasonable to strive for their goals by pharmaceutical means — not least, taking anabolic steroids (Breivik, Hanstad, & Loland, 2009).

While the use of anabolic steroids in gyms and among athletes is stigmatized and widely condemned, cultural acceptance of steroid use in other contexts is broadly found acceptable. An example of this is testosterone as used in "anti-aging therapy." The American sports and cultural historian John Hoberman has illustrated this by referring to the 500% increase, between 1993 and 2003, in prescription-based testosterone sales in the US. He underscores that this increase was not due to a higher incidence of reduced testicular function (hypogonadism) in men who therefore needed the drug to remedy their disorder. But even that increase did not level off. According to the *New York Times*, the number of testosterone prescriptions in 2002 had risen a further 260% by 2010, swelling in that period from 1.75 million to 4.5 million (Kettmann, 2011). One probable explanation lies in the aggressive marketing campaigns launched by pharmaceutical companies in the US, targeting men who ostensibly suffer from testosterone insufficiency, which the advertising industry euphemistically calls "low T."

One firm, AbbVie, spent some 80 million US dollars in 2012 alone on marketing their testosterone cream AndroGel (Rosenthal, 2013). As Hoberman wrote about developments in the US in 2005, "testosterone had already become a predominantly off-label drug" (Hoberman, 2005, p. 285). This development frames a cultural paradox: On the one hand, the use of performance-enhancing drugs in sports and gyms is condemned and leads to stigmatization. On the other hand, societies and Western culture at large show widespread acceptance — and in some instances even encouragement — of the use of various performance enhancers to improve quality of life and the ability to perform, at school, at work, in the army or in bed.

Market forces

If a culture is to grasp and accept this duality, it takes a supportive premise or two. In one domain, we accept that competition has become a fundamental norm for virtually all activities in society. And given that a multitude of pharmacological substances can contribute to improving or maintaining peoples' ability to perform and compete well into old age, it is acceptable to employ these drugs (Møldrup & Hansen, 2006). In the other domain, to justify and uphold stigmatization we maintain that sport — by definition an activity based on competition in its purest form — is nevertheless a sacrosanct field that lies beyond the logic of pharmacology. Sport, like a nature preserve, must be kept pure and untainted.

Besides the legal medical market, a gray market and a black market serve as important supply channels for users in gym environments. In 2007 in a report commissioned by the World Anti-Doping Agency (WADA), the Italian doping investigator Alessandro Donati documented the huge amounts of anabolic steroids entering the world market. Donati concluded that among the 790 million Europeans he had looked at in his survey, the number of anabolic steroid users was a staggering 15.5 million. This clearly illustrates that steroid use goes far beyond the tiny circles of top-level sports. According to Donati, users included "athletes of various levels, bodybuilders and other gym-goers, people in the military and various types of police officers, bodyguards and various types of private surveillance agents, people involved in show business, and victims of the improper administration of drugs" (Donati, 2007, p. 103). Using Italy as a case study, Donati and one of his colleagues, the Italian criminologist Letizia Paoli, also investigated the market to determine who was supplying and distributing doping drugs. The general preconception is that the sale of doping substances is associated with organized crime. Meanwhile, the Italian investigators found that the suppliers were by no means hard-boiled criminals from the Italian Mafia. On the contrary, they were typical male Italian citizens with regular administrative jobs or similar employment, no criminal record and little prior history of violence. Paoli and Donati also pointed out how the accessibility of various doping drugs, notably anabolic steroids, had dramatically increased over the past 20 years. Importantly, the Internet has brought radical change, "so much so that users can nowadays bypass the whole domestic distribution chain and comfortably order doping products on the internet and have them delivered by mail at home" (Paoli & Donati, 2013, p. 19).

Anabolic steroid users

A global market that enables people to discreetly order products online understandably makes it very hard to gauge just how many people use anabolic steroids, and who they are. Beyond the general picture that they are most often men aged 18 to 35 who work out in gyms and health clubs, it is difficult to profile a typical steroid user. As mentioned earlier, the vast majority of studies show that just a small proportion of steroid users in gym settings participate in competitions. There was, however, one large study that found a deviation from this pattern. The study cohort consisted of 8,238 people from nine European countries who filled in an electronic questionnaire about drug use in gym communities. Of these respondents, 2.5% (n=208) had personal experience with illegal performance-enhancing substances, and 42% of this subgroup stated they were active in another sport besides fitness. But as in other studies, the numbers here are small, and because the variations among countries were large the margin of uncertainty was considerable (EHFA, 2012). In the 1980s and 1990s the group of users was more homogeneous, consisting mainly of bodybuilders, whereas today both users and their motives are more numerous and more diverse (McVeigh et al., 2015).

Studies on the topic show a variety of socio-economic profiles for users, depending on the study design. In the Scandinavian countries, even across various studies we, in general, identify none of the conventional socio-economic variables such as (parental) education, (parental) residential setting or (parental) financial situation, which otherwise are clear explanatory indicators for steroid use.

In the UK, on the other hand, English studies indicate differences between various geographical areas. The Northwest, which is characterized by higher unemployment rates and lower levels of education, has a higher prevalence (the percentage of users in a given population) of steroid users than, say, the eastern regions (Shaw, Hurst, McVeigh, & Bellis, 2012).

One study did, however, find a significant difference in user profiles. Instead of being population-based, it contrasted 545 men who in the years 2006–2017 had tested positive (predominantly for anabolic steroids) in the Danish doping control program for gyms and fitness centers, with a control group of 5,450 individuals who matched on all relevant parameters. The mean age for both groups was 26. The Danish health and administrative system contains numerous comprehensive data registers, which enabled researchers to trace a significant difference in education. They found that just 3% of the steroid users had 15 years or more of schooling, as opposed to 13% in the control group. Even so, when the study was published, media attention focused not on this but on the difference in the groups' criminal records: Just 5% (n=267) in the control group had a prison sentence, whereas the figure for steroid users was 30% (n=161) (Christoffersen, Andersen, Dalhoff, & Horwitz, 2019). The result is quite significant, but it is also worth noting that the steroid users included in the study were those caught by control measures in Danish gyms. They likely stood out from the crowd, attracting the attention of doping-control officers and gym staff (for reasons described in connection with more on the Danish anti-doping program in Chapter 11). Consequently, the people caught by control measures are not necessarily representative of Danish steroid users at large.

Even so, the result does contrast with what has been reported elsewhere. Such variations in researchers' conclusions can be illustrated by comparing results from an American study and a Norwegian study. Based on information from nearly 2,000 American steroid users recruited through Internet portals and exercise and steroid sites, Jason Cohen and his colleagues concluded that the average anabolic steroid user was a 31-year-old, well-educated Caucasian man with an income above the American average, who worked out 4 to 5 times a week and described himself as competitive but did not participate in organized sports. His primary motives for taking steroids were increasing muscle volume and strength, and improving his appearance (Cohen et al., 2007). By comparison, a Norwegian study of almost 4,500 young Norwegian males aged 19 showed that those who had personal experience with doping substances (2.9%, or 129 of the Norwegian cohort) were also more likely to have experience with pills, heroin, ecstasy, marijuana, alcohol and tobacco than the youths with no doping experience. The 2.9% were also more frequently involved in fights and other disorderly conduct, and they more rarely had a clean criminal record than those without doping experience (Barland & Tangen, 2009). Undoubtedly, the differences in the two studies' participant ages and recruiting methods play a major part in explaining the differences in their findings, for whereas those respondents who had steroid experience in the Norwegian study had already acquired it at the age of 19 or younger, the average age of initial steroid experience in the American study was just shy of 26 years. In other words, it is highly probable that if a person begins using anabolic steroids as a teenager, that behavior will be part of their experimenting, risk-prone youth, whereas if a person has their steroid debut in their mid-twenties, it will be more of a conscious, calculated, goal-oriented choice. A survey done in Denmark has shown that while less than 1% of male adolescents in academic high schools had experience with "anabolic steroids or similar substances," the corresponding number for male adolescents at Denmark's vocational schools was 3.4% (Bendtsen, Mikkelsen, & Tolstrup, 2015). Given the clear socio-economic differences between academic and vocational students in Denmark, this survey indicates corresponding socio-economic differences among teenage steroid users.

Against this background we can conclude that the answers given about socio-economic profiles for anabolic steroid users are highly dependent on whom you ask. And as for the question of the negative effects of steroids on other aspects of one's life, it seems to make a vital difference whether a person began using in their teens or in their twenties. International studies show that less than 1 in 100 users have their steroid debut before they turn 16, and that about 1 in 5 begin using before they turn 20, while the majority begin using after they turn 20 (typically at 22–24 years of age). We see, then, that young people's first steroid experience occurs much later than in the typical pattern for using other drugs like marijuana and cocaine (Pope, Kanayama, et al., 2014; Pope, Wood, et al., 2014). In keeping with these findings, an extensive European study showed that recreational drug use was lower among people who were members of a gym or health club than among the rest of the population (EHFA, 2012).

Be that as it may, if one takes a broader look at anabolic steroid users, the single factor that most distinctly cuts across a wide range of studies is that they also use other substances (such as cannabis, alcohol and cocaine) more often than people who do not use steroids (McVeigh et al., 2015; Pope, Kanayama, & Hudson, 2012; Simon, Striegel, Aust, Dietz, & Ulrich, 2006).[4] As we saw above, however, this correlation is particularly clear among the youngest group of users, which also agrees with the finding that, more often than non-users, young steroid users have experimented with other drugs before embarking on steroids (Sagoe et al., 2015).

Apart from these findings, it is difficult to identify common traits. The widespread view that steroid users are either criminals or uneducated individuals whose socio-economic circumstances lie below the general population average has some backing in Danish data (Christoffersen et al., 2019), but they cannot be unequivocally confirmed (Barland & Tangen, 2009; Cohen et al., 2007; Skårberg, Nyberg, & Engstrom, 2010).[5] Bear in mind that Cohen and his group found steroid users to be relatively better educated than the American average; typically well-paid, competitive, Caucasian men who exercised and took steroids to attain a stronger, more attractive physique (Cohen et al., 2007). Meanwhile, a Swedish study of steroid users receiving medical treatment for steroid dependence (or abuse) found that more respondents in this group had a problematic social background, and some even reported poor-quality relations with their parents (Skårberg & Engstrom, 2007). What is more, international surveys show that each of the factors, being a man, having a short education and doing multiple workouts per week, independently increases the probability of a person having doping experience (DuRant, Escobedo, & Heath, 1995; Pedersen, 2010; Zelli, Lucidi, & Mallia, 2010).

Still, no one begins taking steroids without somehow having been led down that road. As demonstrated for other types of youth-culture drugs, when it comes to anabolic steroids, researchers can see that willingness to try out steroids comes gradually, in the sense that using a less potent substance increases the probability that a person will later try using a more potent one. This is known as the "gateway hypothesis." An American study that Bryan Karazsia and his colleagues conducted among 448 college students showed that people who had used protein powder were six times more likely, later, to use creatine than people who had not used protein powder. Further to this, creatine users were eight times more likely than people who had not used creatine to also try out drugs that had a more potent anabolic effect (Karazsia, Crowther, & Galioto, 2012). Due to the nature of these findings, we cannot deduce any clear cause-and-effect from them. The same applies to creatine use as to the use of alcohol or marijuana, namely that a person's use of such a substances is not, in and of itself, a reliable indicator of whether or not they will later use a more potent substance. It goes without saying that many people who use protein powder will never use anabolic steroids. All these findings suggest is that some sort of higher-level link exists, showing that users of anabolic steroids have tried other drugs more frequently than non-users have. Similar types of general links or probabilities can be set out for a range of social and cultural variables. Thus, Karazsia and his group also found that people who had espoused an athletic body ideal were more likely to use protein powder, that people dissatisfied with the muscularity of their body were more likely to use creatine, and that people who often compared their body with others were more likely to use substances with a more potent anabolic effect (Karazsia et al., 2012). Naturally, these are not cause-and-effect correlations either, merely patterns and higher probabilities.

While such patterns can certainly help us identify various general trends, broad correlations and probabilities that indicate why some young people choose to try steroids, they cannot tell us much about how such factors manifest in an individual's life. To find out more about these, we must seek more specific explanations, as I will do from Chapter 5 onwards.

Quantifying steroid use

When discussing the number of anabolic steroid users, it is difficult to state precise figures. This is because no standardized, reliable, validated indicators exist that can tell us how many people in a given population illicitly use IPEDs — in athletic circles and among non-competitive and recreational users. In recent years, however, new query techniques applied by research groups in Germany and elsewhere have shown promising results. The topic of IPED use is generally investigated using traditional questionnaire surveys. However, like any survey that asks about socially stigmatizing behavior or touches on taboos, IPED surveys often run into well-known problems with under-reporting, high respondent drop-out and low response rates. All this makes it difficult to reach any conclusions that can indicate, with reasonable certainty, what percentage of the population uses such drugs. What is more, in questionnaire surveys it is impossible to make sure that all respondents understand the questions in the same way as the researcher asking them. Imagine asking a population whether they have used "doping substances" or "muscle-building drugs." How can the researcher be sure that respondents understand these concepts in precisely the same way as the person who phrased the question? One option is to list examples of potentially relevant names, but the market is huge, and product names vary from one brand manufacturer to another. The above-mentioned Norwegian study ran into this very problem. It found that 2.9% of the male respondents had experience with "doping substances," but although the researchers had listed a variety of drugs so as to prompt respondents to answer more specifically about which type of substances they had used (including testosterone, anabolic steroids, growth hormone, insulin and clenbuterol), 50% of those who stated they had experience with "doping substances" still ticked off the category "other" when asked to specify the nature of their experience (Barland & Tangen, 2009). With this in mind, one cannot help but ask whether the percentage of young Norwegians who use doping drugs may actually be smaller than the 2.9% found in the study.

In Denmark, the most recent and largest-ever study on this topic found that 1.5% of respondents aged 15–60 had first-hand experience with "muscle-building drugs." Extrapolated to the entire population, this would mean that "44,000 people at some point have used, or are currently using, muscle-building drugs." Firstly, however, 15–25-year-olds were over-represented in the study. Secondly, of the total 5,010 potential respondents contacted, only 1,703 answered the survey questionnaire. Out of this group, 25 individuals had experience with "muscle-building drugs," whereas just four were currently using such drugs (Singhammer, 2013; Singhammer & Ibsen, 2010). This material is much too small for us to make any conclusions that can quantify IPED users in Denmark as a whole.

One promising way to investigate the problem of underreporting is a method introduced to doping research by a few German research groups (Pitsch & Emrich, 2012; Simon et al., 2006; Ulrich et al., 2018). Known as the Randomized Response Technique (RRT), the methodology is well known from the social sciences as a way to ask respondents about sensitive issues like tax evasion or infidelity.[6] After conducting an RRT-based study of 500 people from 49 German gyms and health clubs, researchers found that 12.5% had used "doping substances" at some point in their life (Simon et al., 2006). By comparison, a Danish study from 1999 using conventional query methods looked at 1,036 members of gyms and fitness centers and found that 5% had used doping drugs (Danish Ministry of Culture, 1999; Pedersen, 2010). The difference of 7.5 percentage points can hardly express a factual difference in the German and Danish gym members' views on IPEDS, so it is far more likely to show the sizeable margins for measurement uncertainty in studies of this type. Confirmation that such uncertainty does exist seems to be given in a study from the Netherlands that compared results from a traditional questionnaire survey with the RRT methodology. While the traditional method found a prevalence rate of about 0.4%, the RRT methodology showed prevalence levels of 4–8%, depending on whether stimulants were included or not (Stubbe, Chorus, Frank, de Hon, & van der Heijden, 2014).

The problems relating to measurement methods, and the discrepancies that can occur between different population groups, are evident in the fluctuating prevalence numbers for anabolic steroid use found in international studies in this field.

As Table 2.1 shows, there are even considerable differences in the numbers found for relatively homogeneous cultures like the three Scandinavian countries. Table 2.2 shows a largely corresponding pattern for examples outside Scandinavia. A few studies have attempted to track developments over several years to find out whether use is rising, falling or remaining stable. A commentary by the Danish doping researcher Anders Schmidt Vinther containing an aggregated analysis of prevalence studies from Scandinavia, USA, Australia and the UK shows only minor fluctuations in prevalence from the early 1990s up to 2015, with no indication that steroid use is generally on the rise (Vinther, 2016). Here, too, it is important to remember that the respondent groups are often small, meaning that the modest changes observable are not easy to interpret. In other words, they do not necessarily express a rise or fall in use, and, random fluctuations aside, they can also be caused by the way the questions are posed (McVeigh et al., 2015). Based on these

Table 2.1 Lifetime prevalence of anabolic steroid use among Scandinavian men[7]

First author	Year	Country	Population	Lifetime prevalence among men
Nilsson	2001	Sweden	Teenagers (n=5,827)	2.9%
Kindlundh	2001	Sweden	High-school students (n=2,742)	2.1%
Leifman	2008	Sweden	Population, 18–50 years (n=3,144)	0.6%
Leifman	2011	Sweden	Health-club members (n=1,752)	3.8%
Pallesen	2006	Norway	High-school students (n=1,351)	3.6%
Barland	2009	Norway	19-year-olds at military pre-service (n=5,332)	2.9%
Danish Ministry of Culture	1999	Denmark	Fitness-center members (n=1, 035)	5%
Singhammer	2010	Denmark	Population, 15–60 years (n=1,703)	1.5%

Table 2.2 Lifetime prevalence of anabolic steroid use among men outside Scandinavia[8]

First author	Year	Country	Population	Lifetime prevalence among men
Hoare	2010	UK	Population, 16–24 years (n=26,500)	0.9%[9]
Hibell	1997	26 European countries	School pupils, 15–16 years (n=approx.2,400 per country)	~2%[10]
Dunn	2011	Australia	High-school students (n=21,361)	2.4%
Johnston	2009	USA	Population, 19–30 years (n=2,300)	4.1%
van Rooij	2009	Netherlands	Population (n=5,769)	1.6%[11]
Tahtamouni	2008	Jordan	College students (n=503)	4.2%
Sagoe	2014	Global	Literature study, many diverse populations (n=187 studies)	6.4%[12]
Pope et al.	2014	USA	College students	2.9–4.0%

considerations, a cautious guess would be that, for men, lifetime prevalence (how many respondents have used anabolic steroids at some point in their life) is 1–4%, wherever one investigates this phenomenon in the Western world. Point prevalence (how many respondents are actively using at the given point in time) is significantly lower than lifetime prevalence — probably by a factor of 8 to 10 (Pope, Kanayama, et al., 2014).

It is worth noting that despite the methodological difficulties and the observable fluctuations in results, for studies conducted both in Scandinavia and elsewhere in the Western world, the prevalence rates in a given area drop by some 1–4% depending on the group surveyed.[13] Although cultural values in Western countries largely resemble each other, the policies and regulatory measures that have been put into practice differ immensely. Although I have investigated potential correlations, I remain unable to identify any systematic links between the prevalence rates found and national antidoping policies. This would seem to suggest there is a lower limit to what policies and regulation can do to bring prevalence down (see Chapter 13), meaning culture and politics are not the only factors affecting the use of muscle-building drugs. Rather, as I will discuss in Chapter 10, it seems that traits general to Western culture — and to human nature itself — are also part of this complex equation.

Notes

1 See also (Barland & Tangen, 2009; Begley, McVeigh, & Hope, 2017; Bojsen-Møller & Christiansen, 2010; Cohen, Collins, Darkes, & Gwartney, 2007; Gray & Ginsberg, 2007; Parkinson & Evans, 2006; Pope, Phillips, & Olivardia, 2000; Thompson & Cafri, 2007).
2 As will become clear in this and the following chapters, steroid use exists within complex physical and social systems, and therefore user motivations cannot be pinpointed to a few individual factors. A widely recognized idea, which led Geoff Bates and his colleagues at Liverpool John Moores University to develop a sociological framework that includes the interaction of a range of factors at the individual, social-network, institutional, community and societal levels (Bates, Tod, Leavey, & McVeigh, 2019). While my book does not explicitly apply the model in its analyses, it certainly does so implicitly, which is recognizable in the book's overall ambition (see Chapter 1) and in this and subsequent chapters.
3 The word "gremlins" alludes to the eponymous 1984 American horror-comedy film about a young man who receives an odd pet — a mogwai — as a gift. This adorable, good-natured little creature has one serious drawback: If it accidentally comes into contact with water, it propagates into a number of destructive little monsters called "gremlins," which are extremely hard to eliminate.
4 See also (Barland & Tangen, 2009; Dodge & Hoagland, 2011; Dunn & White, 2011; Hakansson, Mickelsson, Wallin, & Berglund, 2012; Ip, Barnett, Tenerowicz, & Perry, 2011; Kanayama, Cohane, Weiss, & Pope, 2003; Mattila, Parkkari, Laakso, Pihlajamaki, & Rimpela, 2010; Molero, Bakshi, & Gripenberg, 2017; Nilsson, Baigi, Marklund, & Fridlund, 2001; Pallesen, Josendal, Johnsen, Larsen, & Molde, 2006).

5 See also (Paoli & Donati, 2013; Singhammer & Ibsen, 2010; Skårberg & Engstrom, 2007).
6 The RRT method is by no means infallible. For some, the questioning technique is difficult to get a firm grip on, which can lead to underreporting and reporting errors. RRT does, however, have the advantage that people who confirm a stigmatizing behavior do not feel divergent, and at the same time the method is a good way to anonymize respondents. The RRT query mechanism works like this: The questionnaire begins by instructing the respondent how to answer before the question is posed. The questionnaire could read like this, with the instruction first: "If your mother was born in either January February March or April, please answer 'Yes' to the next question, no matter what you are asked. If she was born in one of the other eight months of the year, please answer honestly." Then comes the question: "Have you used doping substances within the past 12 months?" The whole point of the RRT method is that when respondents can see that at least every third person who is asked the question will answer "Yes" (provided the group's maternal birthdays show normal distribution over the 12 months of the year), respondents are more likely to answer honestly when asked to do so. On the face of it, the method seems simple, yet it involves quite sophisticated statistical mathematics that seek, among other things, to reflect the probability that not all respondents will follow the instructions.
7 Sources for Table 2.1: (Barland & Tangen, 2009; Danish Ministry of Culture, 1999; Kindlundh, Hagekull, Isacson, & Nyberg, 2001; Leifman & Rehnman, 2008; Leifman, Rehnman, Sjoblom, & Holgersson, 2011; Nilsson, Baigi, Marklund, & Fridlund, 2001; Pallesen, Josendal, Johnsen, Larsen, & Molde, 2006; Singhammer & Ibsen, 2010).
8 Sources for Table 2.2: (Dunn & White, 2011; Hibell et al., 1997; Hoare & Moon, 2010; Johnston, O'Malley, Miech, Bachman, & Schulenberg, 2016; Pope et al., 2014; Tahtamouni et al., 2008; van Rooij, Schoenmakers, & Mheen, 2011).
9 This number is for men and women jointly, as the study had no gender-specific data. However, findings from other studies show that men use anabolic steroids much more often than women do.
10 Most countries reported prevalence rates of 1–3%. Certain countries reported rates above 3% (Croatia 6%; Italy, Malta and the UK 4%)
11 The Dutch term used in phrasing the question corresponds to "performance-enhancing drugs."
12 This study, which at the time of writing is the only meta-analysis, includes interview-based surveys and qualitative studies, studies with respondents selected randomly by drawing lots and studies with strategically selected respondents. There are great differences in the prevalence rates found in these various types of studies. The questionnaire surveys taken alone, for instance, make for a prevalence rate of 3.0%. However, the strength of this review study lies not in its aggregating the numbers (given the problems that arise from attempts to add or collate numbers across different study designs and methodologies) but in its grouping of many studies from widely varying periods and geographical regions.
13 Prevalence is significantly lower in countries such as Japan, China and South Korea.

References

Alcott, R. (2014). The man who knew Charles Atlas. Retrieved from: www.youtube.com/watch?v=w3r1c4I2j00&t=.
Backhouse, S., McKenna, J., Robinson, S., & Atkin, M. (2007). International literature review: Attitudes, behaviours, knowledge and education – drugs in sport:

Past, present and future. Retrieved from: www.wada-ama.org/rtecontent/docum
ent/Backhouse_et_al_Full_Report.pdf.
Baghurst, T., Hollander, D. B., Nardella, B., & Haff, G. G. (2006). Change in sociocultural ideal male physique: An examination of past and present action figures.
Body Image, 3(1), 87–91. doi: doi:10.1016/j.bodyim.2005.11.001.
Barland, B., & Tangen, J. O. (2009). Kroppspresentasjon og andre prestasjoner – en
omfangsundersøkelse om bruk av Doping. Retrieved from Oslo: https://antidop
ing.no/sitefiles/1/dokumenter/pdf/omfangsundersokelsen.pdf.
Barland, B., Tangen, J. O., & Johannesen, C. A. (2010). Doping, muskler, mestring og
mening. En kvalitativ studie av unge menns bruk av muskelbyggende medikamenter. Retrieved from Oslo: https://brage.bibsys.no/xmlui/handle/11250/175072.
Bates, G., & McVeigh, J. (2016). Image and performance enhancing drugs – 2015
survey results. Retrieved from Liverpool: www.ipedinfo.co.uk/resources/downloa
ds/2015%20National%20IPED%20Info%20Survey%20report.pdf.
Bates, G., Tod, D., Leavey, C., & McVeigh, J. (2019). An evidence-based socioecological framework to understand men's use of anabolic androgenic steroids and
inform interventions in this area. *Drugs: Education, Prevention and Policy, 26*(6), 484–
492. doi: doi:10.1080/09687637.2018.1488947.
Bauman, Z. (2001). *The individualized society.* Cambridge: Polity Press.
Begley, E., McVeigh, J., & Hope, V. (2017). Image and performance enhancing
drugs – 2016 national survey results. Retrieved from Liverpool: www.wales.nhs.uk/
sitesplus/documents/888/IPED%20report%202017.%20FINAL.pdf.
Bendtsen, P., Mikkelsen, S. S., & Tolstrup, J. S. (2015). Ungdomsprofilen 2014. Sund-
hedsadfærd, helbred og trivsel blandt elever på ungdomsuddannelser. Retrieved from
København: www.sdu.dk/da/sif/publikationer/2015/ungdomsprofilen_2014.
Bojsen-Møller, J., & Christiansen, A. V. (2010). Use of performance- and image-
enhancing substances among recreational athletes: a quantitative analysis of inquiries submitted to the Danish anti-doping authorities. *Scandinavian Journal of Medicine & Science in Sports, 20*(6), 861–867.
Breivik, G., Hanstad, D. V., & Loland, S. (2009). Attitudes towards use of performance-enhancing substances and body modification techniques. A comparison
between elite athletes and the general population. *Sport in Society, 12*(6), 737–754.
doi: doi:10.1080/17430430902944183.
Brohm, J.-M. (1978). *Sport, a prison of measured time: Essays.* London: Ink Links.
Cafri, G., Thompson, J. K., Ricciardelli, L., McCabe, M., Smolak, L., & Yesalis, C.
(2005). Pursuit of the muscular ideal: Physical and psychological consequences and
putative risk factors. *Clinical Psychology Review, 25*(2), 215–239. doi: doi:10.1016/j.
cpr.2004.09.003.
Christoffersen, T., Andersen, J. T., Dalhoff, K. P., & Horwitz, H. (2019). Anabolic-
androgenic steroids and the risk of imprisonment. *Drug Alcohol Depend, 203,* 92–
97. doi: doi:10.1016/j.drugalcdep.2019.04.041.
Cohen, J., Collins, R., Darkes, J., & Gwartney, D. (2007). A league of their own:
demographics, motivations and patterns of use of 1,955 male adult non-medical
anabolic steroid users in the United States. *J.Int.Soc.Sports Nutr., 4,* 12. doi:
doi:1550-2783-4-12.
Dalsgaard, A., & Winding, O. (Writers). (2006). *Afghan Muscle.* Cinema Guild (USA).
Danish Ministry of Culture. (1999). Doping i Danmark: En hvidbog. Retrieved
from København: https://kum.dk/publikationer/1999/doping-i-danmark-en-hvid

bog. English summary: https://kum.dk/uploads/tx_templavoila/Doping_in_denma rk_a_white_book.pdf.

Dimeo, P. (2007). *A history of drug use in sport 1876–1976: Beyond good and evil.* London: Routledge.

Dixson, A. F., Halliwell, G., East, R., Wignarajah, P., & Anderson, M. J. (2003). Masculine somatotype and hirsuteness as determinants of sexual attractiveness to women. *Archives of Sexual Behavior*, 32(1), 29–39. doi: doi:10.1023/A:1021889228469.

Dodge, T., & Hoagland, M. F. (2011). The use of anabolic androgenic steroids and polypharmacy: A review of the literature. *Drug Alcohol Depend*, 114(2–3), 100–109. doi: doi:10.1016/j.drugalcdep.2010.11.011.

Donati, A. (2007). World traffic in doping substances. Retrieved from Montreal: http s://wada-main-https://www.wada-ama.org/sites/default/files/resources/files/WADA_ Donati_Report_On_Trafficking_2007.pdf.

Dunn, M., & White, V. (2011). The epidemiology of anabolic-androgenic steroid use among Australian secondary school students. *J.Sci.Med.Sport*, 14(1), 10–14. doi: doi:10.1016/j.jsams.2010.05.004.

DuRant, R. H., Escobedo, L. G., & Heath, G. W. (1995). Anabolic-steroid use, strength training, and multiple drug use among adolescents in the United States. *Pediatrics*, 96(1), 23–28.

EHFA. (2012). Fitness against doping: Executive summary of the FINAL REPORT for the Copenhagen Fitness Anti-Doping Conference. Retrieved from Bruxelles, Belgium: www.ehfa.eu.

Etcoff, N. (1999). *Survival of the prettiest: The science of beauty*. London: Little, Brown.

Featherstone, M., Hepworth, M., & Turner, B. S. (1993). *The body: Social process and cultural theory* (2 ed.). London: Sage Publications.

Gleaves, J., & Llewellyn, M. (2013). Sport, drugs and amateurism: Tracing the real cultural origins of anti-doping rules in international sport. *The International Journal of the History of Sport*, 31(8), 839–853. doi: doi:10.1080/09523367.2013.831838.

Goldman, B., Bush, P. J., & Klatz, R. (1984). *Death in the locker room: Steroids & sports.* London: Century Publishing.

Gray, J., & Ginsberg, R. (2007). Muscle dissatisfaction: An overview of psychological and cultural research and theory. In K. J. Thompson & G. Cafri (Eds.), *The muscular ideal: Psychological, social, and medical perspectives* (1 ed., pp. 15–39). Washington, DC: American Psychological Association.

Hakansson, A., Mickelsson, K., Wallin, C., & Berglund, M. (2012). Anabolic androgenic steroids in the general population: User characteristics and associations with substance use. *European Addiction Research*, 18(2), 83–90.

Hibell, B., Andersson, B., Bjarnason, T., Kokkevi, A., Morgan, M., & Narusk, A. (1997). The 1995 ESPAD report. Alcohol and other drug use among students in 26 European countries. Retrieved from Stockholm: www.espad.org/sites/espad.org/ files/The_1995_ESPAD_report.pdf.

Hildebrandt, T., Alfano, L., & Langenbucher, J. W. (2010). Body image disturbance in 1000 male appearance and performance enhancing drug users. *Journal of Psychiatric Research*, 44(13), 841–846. doi: doi:10.1016/j.jpsychires.2010.01.001.

Hoare, J., & Moon, D. (2010). Drug Misuse Declared: Findings from the 2009/10 British Crime Survey, England and Wales (13/10). Retrieved from London: http:// webarchive.nationalarchives.gov.uk/20110220142329/http://rds.homeoffice.gov.uk/ rds/pdfs10/hosb1310.pdf.

Hoberman, J. M. (2005). *Testosterone dreams: Rejuvenation, aphrodisia, doping*. Berkeley, CA: University of California Press.

Hoff, D. (2016). Reflections on "doping in sport" and "doping in society". In N. Ahmadi, A. Ljungqvist, & G. Svedsäter (Eds.), *Doping and public health* (pp. 49–63). Oxon & New York: Routledge.

Ip, E. J., Barnett, M. J., Tenerowicz, M. J., & Perry, P. J. (2011). The Anabolic 500 survey: Characteristics of male users versus nonusers of anabolic-androgenic steroids for strength training. *Pharmacotherapy*, 31(8), 757–766. doi: doi:10.1592/phco.31.8.757.

Johnston, L. D., O'Malley, P. M., Miech, R. A., Bachman, J. G., & Schulenberg, J. E. (2016). Monitoring the future: National survey results on drug use, 1975–2015. Overview. Key findings on adolescent drug use. Retrieved from U.S. Department of Health and Human Services: http://monitoringthefuture.org/pubs/monographs/vol2_2009.pdf.

Kanayama, G., Cohane, G. H., Weiss, R. D., & Pope, H. G. (2003). Past anabolic-androgenic steroid use among men admitted for substance abuse treatment: an underrecognized problem? *J Clin Psychiatry*, 64. doi: doi:10.4088/JCP.v64n0208.

Karazsia, B. T., Crowther, J. H., & Galioto, R. (2012). Undergraduate men's use of performance-and appearance-enhancing substances: An examination of the gateway hypothesis. *Psychology of Men & Masculinity*, 14(2), 129.

Kettmann, S. (2011, December 17). Are we not man enough? *New York Times*. Retrieved from: www.nytimes.com/2011/12/18/opinion/sunday/are-we-not-man-enough.html.

Kindlundh, A. M., Hagekull, B., Isacson, D. G., & Nyberg, F. (2001). Adolescent use of anabolic-androgenic steroids and relations to self-reports of social, personality and health aspects. *Eur J Public Health*, 11(3), 322–328.

Klein, A. M. (1993). *Little big men: Bodybuilding subculture and gender construction*. Albany, NY: State University of New York Press.

Klein, A. M. (2007). Size matters: Connecting subculture to culture in bodybuilding. In J. K. Thompson & G. Cafri (Eds.), *The muscular ideal: Psychological, social, and medical perspectives* (1 ed., pp. 67–83). Washington, DC: American Psychological Association.

Lasch, C. (1980). *The culture of narcissism: American life in an age of diminishing expectations*. London: Abacus/Sphere Books.

Leifman, H., & Rehnman, C. (2008). Studie om svenska folkets användning av dopningspreparat (34). Retrieved from Stockholm: https://dokodoc.com/studie-om-svenska-folkets-anvndning-av-dopningspreparat.html.

Leifman, H., Rehnman, C., Sjoblom, E., & Holgersson, S. (2011). Anabolic androgenic steroids. Use and correlates among gym users: An assessment study using questionnaires and observations at gyms in the Stockholm region. *International Journal of Environmental Research and Public Health*, 8(7), 2656–2674. doi: doi:10.3390/ijerph8072656.

Liokaftos, D. (2017). *A Genealogy of male bodybuilding: From classical to freaky*. New York & Oxon: Routledge.

Luciano, L. (2007). Muscularity and masculinity in the United States: A historical overview. In J. K. Thompson & G. Cafri (Eds.), *The muscular ideal: Psychological, social, and medical perspectives* (1 ed., pp. 41–65). Washington, DC: American Psychological Association.

Lupton, D. (1995). *The imperative of health: Public health and the regulated body.* London: Taylor & Francis.

Mattila, V. M., Parkkari, J., Laakso, L., Pihlajamaki, H., & Rimpela, A. (2010). Use of dietary supplements and anabolic-androgenic steroids among Finnish adolescents in 1991–2005. *Eur.J.Public Health*, 20(3), 306–311. doi: \t "_blank" 10.1093/eurpub/ckp124.

McVeigh, J., Bates, G., & Chandler, M. (2015). Steroids and Image Enhancing Drugs: 2014 Survey Results. Retrieved from Liverpool: www.ipedinfo.co.uk/resources/downloads/SIEDs%20Survey%20report%202014%20FINAL.pdf.

Mental Health Foundation. (2019, 3 June). Mental Health Foundation criticises new series of Love Island as it releases new statistics about body image and reality TV. Retrieved from: www.mentalhealth.org.uk/news/mental-health-foundation-critici ses-new-series-love-island-it-releases-new-statistics-about.

Mitchell, L., Murray, S. B., Cobley, S., Hackett, D., Gifford, J., Capling, L., & O'Connor, H. (2017). Muscle dysmorphia symptomatology and associated psychological features in bodybuilders and non-bodybuilder resistance trainers: A systematic review and meta-analysis. *Sports Med*, 47(2), 233–259. doi: doi:10.1007/s40279-016-0564-3.

Molero, Y., Bakshi, A. S., & Gripenberg, J. (2017). Illicit drug use among gym-goers: A cross-sectional study of gym-goers in Sweden. *Sports Med Open*, 3(1), 31. doi: doi:10.1186/s40798-017-0098-8.

Monaghan, L. F. (2001). *Bodybuilding, drugs, and risk.* London: Routledge.

Møldrup, C., & Hansen, R. R. (2006). Public acceptance of drug use for non-disease conditions. *Current Medical Research and Opinion*, 22(4), 775–780. doi: doi:10.1185/030079906X100258.

Nilsson, S., Baigi, A., Marklund, B., & Fridlund, B. (2001). The prevalence of the use of androgenic anabolic steroids by adolescents in a county of Sweden. *Eur J Public Health*, 11(2), 195–197.

Pallesen, S., Josendal, O., Johnsen, B. H., Larsen, S., & Molde, H. (2006). Anabolic steroid use in high school students. *Subst Use Misuse*, 41(13), 1705–1717. doi: doi:10.1080/10826080601006367.

Paoli, L., & Donati, A. (2013). The supply of doping products and the potential of criminal law enforcement in anti-doping: An examination of Italy's experience. Executive summary. Retrieved from Montreal: www.wada-ama.org/en/resources/world-anti-doping-program/paoli-and-donati-report.

Parkinson, A. B., & Evans, N. A. (2006). Anabolic androgenic steroids: A survey of 500 users. *Medicine & Science in Sports & Exercise*, 38(4), 644–651. doi:doi:10.1249/01.mss.0000210194.56834.5d.

Pedersen, I. K. (2010). Doping and the perfect body expert: Social and cultural indicators of performance-enhancing drug use in Danish gyms. *Sport in society*, 13(3), 503–516.

Pitsch, W., & Emrich, E. (2012). The frequency of doping in elite sport: Results of a replication study. *International Review for the Sociology of Sport*, 47(5), 559–580.

Pope, H. G., Gruber, A. J., Choi, P., Olivardia, R., & Phillips, K. A. (1997). Muscle dysmorphia: An underrecognized form of body dysmorphic disorder. *Psychosomatics*, 38(6), 548–557. doi: doi:10.1080/1532502 4.2018.1428484.

Pope, H. G., Kanayama, G., Athey, A., Ryan, E., Hudson, J. I., & Baggish, A. (2014). The lifetime prevalence of anabolic-androgenic steroid use and dependence in

Americans: Current best estimates. *Am J Addict*, 23(4), 371–377. doi: doi:10.1111/j.1521-0391.2013.12118.x.

Pope, H. G., Kanayama, G., & Hudson, J. I. (2012). Risk factors for illicit anabolic-androgenic steroid use in male weightlifters: A cross-sectional cohort study. *Biological Psychiatry*, 71(3), 254–261. doi: doi:10.1016/j.biopsych.2011.06.024.

Pope, H. G., Olivardia, R., Gruber, A., & Borowiecki, J. (1999). Evolving ideals of male body image as seen through action toys. *International Journal of Eating Disorders*, 26(1), 65–72.

Pope, H. G., Phillips, K. A., & Olivardia, R. (2000). *The Adonis complex: How to identify, treat, and prevent body obsession in men and boys*. New York: Free Press.

Pope, H. G., Wood, R. I., Rogol, A., Nyberg, F., Bowers, L., & Bhasin, S. (2014). Adverse health consequences of performance-enhancing drugs: An Endocrine Society scientific statement. *Endocr Rev*, 35(3), 341–375. doi: doi:10.1210/er.2013-1058.

Rosenthal, E. (2013, October 15). A push to sell testosterone gels troubles doctors. *New York Times*. Retrieved from: www.nytimes.com/2013/10/16/us/a-push-to-sell-testosterone-gels-troubles-doctors.html?ref=elisabethrosenthal&_r=0.

Sagoe, D., McVeigh, J., Bjørnebekk, A., Essilfie, M.-S., Andreassen, C. S., & Pallesen, S. (2015). Polypharmacy among anabolic-androgenic steroid users: A descriptive metasynthesis. *Substance Abuse Treatment, Prevention, and Policy*, 10(1), 1–19. doi: doi:10.1186/s13011-015-0006-5.

Sagoe, D., Molde, H., Andreassen, C. S., Torsheim, T., & Pallesen, S. (2014). The global epidemiology of anabolic-androgenic steroid use: A meta-analysis and meta-regression analysis. *Annals of Epidemiology*, 24(1873–2585 (Electronic)), 383–398.

Shaw, C., Hurst, A., McVeigh, J., & Bellis, M. A. (2012). Indications of public health in the English regions. 10: Drug use. Retrieved from Centre for Public Health: www.cph.org.uk/publication/indications-of-public-hea lth-in-the-english-regions-10-drug-use-3.

Simon, P., Striegel, H., Aust, F., Dietz, K., & Ulrich, R. (2006). Doping in fitness sports: Estimated number of unreported cases and individual probability of doping. *Addiction*, 101(11), 1640–1644. doi: doi:10.1111/j.1360-0443.2006.01568.x.

Singhammer, J. (2013). Attitudes toward anabolic-androgenic steroids among non-competing athletes in various types of sports: A cross-sectional study. *Sport Science Review*, 22(1–2), 109–128. doi: doi:10.2478/ssr-2013-0006.

Singhammer, J., & Ibsen, B. (2010). Motionsdoping i Danmark: En kvantitativ undersøgelse om brug af og holdning til muskelopbyggende stoffer. Retrieved from Denmark: file:///C:/Users/au220550/Downloads/Motionsdoping_i%20Danmark_inkl_s.pdf

Sinnbeck, P. (2016, 27 April 2016). Der er uendelige mængder sport i tv – men er der overhovedet nogen, der ser det? *Politiken*. Retrieved from: http://politiken.dk/maga sinet/premium/ECE3177701/der-er-uendelige-maengder-sport-i-tv—m en-er-der-overhovedet–nogen-der-ser-det.

Skårberg, K., & Engstrom, I. (2007). Troubled social background of male anabolic-androgenic steroid abusers in treatment. *Subst Abuse Treat Prev Policy*, 2, 20. doi: doi:10.1186/1747-597X-2-20.

Skårberg, K., Nyberg, F., & Engstrom, I. (2010). Is there an association between the use of anabolic-androgenic steroids and criminality? *European Addiction Research*, 16(4), 213–219. doi: doi:10.1159/000320286.

Stubbe, J. H., Chorus, A. M. J., Frank, L. E., de Hon, O., & van der Heijden, P. G. M. (2014). Prevalence of use of performance enhancing drugs by fitness centre members. *Drug Testing and Analysis*, 6(5), 434–438. doi: doi:10.1002/dta.1525.

Tahtamouni, L. H., Mustafa, N. H., Alfaouri, A. A., Hassan, I. M., Abdalla, M. Y., & Yasin, S. R. (2008). Prevalence and risk factors for anabolic-androgenic steroid abuse among Jordanian collegiate students and athletes. *Eur.J.Public Health*, 18(6), 661–665. doi: doi:10.1093/eurpub/ckn062.

Taylor, W. (1985). *Hormonal manipulation: A new era of monstrous athletes*. London: McFarland.

Thompson, J. K., & Cafri, G. (Eds.). (2007). *The muscular ideal: Psychological, social, and medical perspectives* (1 ed.). Washington, DC: American Psychological Association.

Todd, T. (1987). Anabolic steroids: The gremlins of sport. *J.Sport Hist*, 14(1), 87–107.

Ulrich, R., Pope, H. G., Jr., Cleret, L., Petroczi, A., Nepusz, T., Schaffer, J., ... Simon, P. (2018). Doping in two elite athletics competitions assessed by randomized-response surveys. *Sports Med*, 48(1), 211–219. doi: doi:10.1007/s40279-017-0765-4.

van Rooij, A., Schoenmakers, T., & Mheen, D. (2011). Nationaal Prevalentie Onderzoek Middelengebruik 2009: De kerncijfers [National Prevalence Study on Substance Use 2009: Core Statistics].

Vinther, A. S. (2016). The steroid "epidemic" myth. *INDR Newsletter, Commentary*. Retrieved from: http://ph.au.dk/en/research/research-units/sport-and-body-culture/research-unit-for-sport-and-body-culture/international-network-of-doping-research/newsletters/december-2016/indr-commentary-anders-schmidt-vinther.

Waddington, I. (2000). *Sport, health and drugs: A critical sociological perspective*. London: E & FN Spon.

Wikipedia. (2019). Charles Atlas. *Wikipedia*. Retrieved from: http://en.wikipedia.org/wiki/Charles_Atlas.

Woodland, L. (1980). *Dope: The use of drugs in sport*. Newton Abbot, UK: David and Charles.

Yang, C. F., Gray, P., & Pope, H. G., Jr. (2005). Male body image in Taiwan versus the West: Yanggang Zhiqi meets the Adonis complex. *Am J Psychiatry*, 162(2), 263–269. doi: doi:10.1176/appi.ajp.162.2.263.

Zelli, A., Lucidi, F., & Mallia, L. (2010). The relationships among adolescents' drive for muscularity, drive for thinness, doping attitudes, and doping intentions. *Journal of Clinical Sport Psychology*, 4(1), 39–52.

Chapter 3

Effects and side effects of anabolic steroids

Anabolic androgenic steroids are synthetically manufactured hormones that simulate the effects of the male sex hormone testosterone.[1] Testosterone is present everywhere in the animal kingdom, occurring in every animal species, from crustaceans to birds and mammals. Basically, it has just a single function: to promote sex and help male individuals reproduce. But the really interesting thing about testosterone is the numerous spin-off effects of this single function. The fact is that semen production and lust, by themselves, cannot ensure reproduction. As Joe Herbert, a professor emeritus at Cambridge University, eloquently explains in his book *Testosterone: Sex, Power, and the Will to Win*, males must be attractive to females in order to gain access to them. In other words, they must be willing to run risks, and they must be physically strong and have a propensity for competition in every shape and form.

In an adult male specimen of the human race and the great apes (and other large mammals), testosterone essentially does three things: (1) It brings about sexual maturity. (2) It stimulates certain physical characteristics — body hair, facial hair and muscles — which increase his sexual attractiveness while also preparing him for a more competitive and risk-oriented adult life. (3) It affects his brain, making him not merely interested in sex and prone to seek it out, but also endowing him with the psychological and emotional qualities that improve his chances of success in such endeavors (Herbert, 2015). Testosterone basically works the same way in humans and great apes, stimulating risk-willingness, muscle growth and a competitive mindset. However, while these factors unfold in relatively uniform conditions in nature, among human beings they are very specifically expressed in terms of culture. Humans are subject to the same stimuli from testosterone, but they have many more layers of sophisticated behavior in which to respond.

Testosterone is a steroid hormone. In men it is primarily produced in the testicles, along with negligible amounts produced in the adrenal cortex. Women also produce testosterone, in their ovaries and adrenal cortex, but in much smaller amounts than men (about 10% as much). This hormone plays a crucial role in the development of the primary sexual characteristics in males, namely the testicles and prostate gland, and it is also responsible for the physical features that typify the male body. As mentioned, anabolic androgenic steroids mimic the effects of testosterone. These substances build tissue because, as the medical term "anabolic" denotes, they increase protein synthesis. This is the effect coveted by most non-competitive users and athletes who take anabolic androgenic steroids. Then there is the term "androgenic," which means that such substances promote the secondary sexual characteristics for males outlined above, including the growth of facial and body hair, a deeper voice, skeletal musculature, bone size and density, and body-fat distribution. Distinguishing between the anabolic and the androgenic effects of such substances may be conceptually useful, but it is also imprecise, given that testosterone — and hence also anabolic androgenic steroids — effect virtually all tissues in the body and therefore play a key role in a wide array of physiological, psychological and behavioral processes that fall outside the scope of the classic "anabolic–androgenic" distinction (Guyton & Hall, 2006; Herbert, 2015). Examples would be the way testosterone affects the intensity and development of sexual experiences in men and women, and the way it affects the production of red blood cells. Also, testosterone is essential to the health and general well-being of men, and its influence on personality is not insignificant (Pinker, 2002).

Generally the interest in anabolic steroids lies in their capacity to mimic the effects of testosterone. However, in a medical context they are also, and most often, deemed interesting because of their tissue-building anabolic qualities (except when used therapeutically to remedy a condition called "hypogonadism," meaning inadequate testosterone production). That is why early modern medicine quickly began research to invent synthetic hormones with the desired qualities. The first of these substances was ready for use in the 1930s, and by the 1950s various drugs had already become available in injectable and oral form (Evans-Brown & McVeigh, 2009; Hoberman, 2005). It soon became clear that anabolic steroids increase growth and performance, which is why athletes soon became interested in them, and from the 1950s onwards steroid use quickly spread to a variety of sports (Dimeo, 2007; Hoberman, 1992; Voy, 1991). One direct consequence of the Cold War between East and West was that competition between the US and the USSR intensified after World War II. According to popular legend, at the weightlifting world championships in Vienna in 1954 the American team's physician, John B. Ziegler, observed how Soviet athletes had to use catheters to urinate. He knew that an enlarged prostate gland and the attendant difficulty urinating was one side effect of using testosterone. What followed from this, according to Ziegler, was that because he also knew of testosterone's muscle-building effects, he pieced together the puzzle of what he had seen and returned from the championship intent on producing a synthetic version of testosterone that could level the playing field between the Eastern and Western athletes, and at the same time avoid the undesirable effects of prostate-gland enlargement. His efforts resulted in a drug known as Diana-bol, which Ziegler manufactured in collaboration with the pharmaceutical company CIBA.[2] The effects of this drug were less androgenic and more anabolic than earlier synthetic versions of testosterone, and it gradually won popularity among athletes (Voy, 1991). CIBA no longer produces Dianabol, but the substance is still available as a variety of generic drugs known in gym and bodybuilding circles under names like "D-bol," "Thai Anabol tablets" (referring to their manufacturing origin in Thailand) and "Arnold's break-fast," because reputedly they were a standard component in Arnold Schwarzenegger's hormone cycles.[3]

Obviously, athletes have known for decades that steroids enhance perfor-mance. Nevertheless, it was not until the first study on this topic, published in 1996 by the Indian-American medical researcher Shalender Bhasin and his colleagues, in which test subjects had received testosterone doses far above natural levels, that science began to take the performance-enhancing effects of steroids seriously. Their work has been followed by several other studies, and today there is a broad consensus that anabolic steroids increase not only muscle strength but also the body's fat-free volumes, muscle size, protein metabolism, bone metabolism and collagen synthesis — even *without* physi-cal training (Bhasin et al., 1996; Bhasin, Woodhouse, & Storer, 2001; Hart-gens & Kuipers, 2004).

For athletes and non-professional users, anabolic steroids are most often taken orally or through the skin, or injected directly into muscle tissue. Over the past 20 years this third option has become the most popular. When ingested the drug has a short half-life, meaning oral tablets must normally be taken daily. Injectable steroids, on the other hand, can be administered weekly or every two weeks. More recently a number of tes-tosterone preparations have become available for absorption through the skin as patches, gels or creams. Large doses of testosterone are difficult to administer by this route, but some users supplement pills and injections with transcutaneous gels to receive a constant low dose of testosterone (Pope et al., 2014).

Physical side effects

Educational campaigns intended to make young men, in particular, averse to steroid use have traditionally emphasized the physical side effects. Like many other National Anti Doping Authorities (NADOs), the Danish body Anti Doping Danmark has descriptions of steroid side effects on their website (www.antidoping.dk), outlining risks for male and female users. They read as follows: "The issues are development of pimples (acne), liver damage and rapid weight increase." In addition, among men researchers have found "decreased insulin sensitivity and increased cholesterol, which can result in diabetes, increased vascular stiffness and increased blood pressure, as well as decreased cardiac output even several years after the use of AAS [anabolic androgenic steroids]." Furthermore, the administration of steroids have been associated with: "the risk of shrinking testicles, impaired sperm quality and consequently decreased reproductive capacity, as well as enlarged prostate gland" (Anti Doping Danmark, 2019).

These are all alarming side effects, which ought to make most people think twice about starting to use such drugs. Nonetheless, the problem from an educational perspective is that although these effects are upsetting, people who take even large doses of anabolic steroids do not necessarily experience their own side effects as serious, or as threats to their health. One of the most extensive questionnaire studies ever conducted among seasoned heavy users of anabolic steroids clearly illustrates this point.

Working through Internet sites where steroids were discussed, researchers recruited 500 anabolic-steroid users who, using an online link, filled in a comprehensive questionnaire. The results were both frightening and surprising. Frightening because 60% of respondents stated using doses in excess of 1,000 mg per week, with 13% of respondents exceeding 2,000 mg. Now bear in mind that the highest dose given in the Bhasin group's 1996 study was 600 mg per week, which is six to ten times higher than the therapeutic doses given to hypogonadic men whose own testosterone production had ceased (Bhasin et al., 1996). What is more, 95% of respondents combined several types of steroids to achieve these megadoses in a practice often referred to as "stacking," and 96% used other drugs besides steroids. These were mainly stimulants, fat-burners, sedatives and remedial drugs meant to reduce the side effects of anabolic steroids, but in some cases users took growth hormone and insulin as well. The element of surprise was that although 99% reported experiencing side effect symptoms, with 70% reporting three or more side effects which (they assessed) were caused by their steroid use, they did not regard these side effects as serious. Although 61% were, admittedly, concerned that their use of anabolic steroids could have serious repercussions, they did not experience any. Furthermore, with the exception of gynecomastia (benign enlargement of the male breast), the side effects respondents did experience were actually reversible, gradually disappearing after steroid use stopped. The most common side effects were shrinking testicles (64%), acne (63%), fluid retention (52%), insomnia (51%), pain at the injection site (49%), stretch marks (44%), mood swings (43%), sexual dysfunction (25%) and gynecomastia (23%). The fact that respondents "only" experienced less serious side effects was not due to their being neophytes, and therefore as yet being unaffected by the more detrimental effects of the drugs: 43% had used steroids for at least four years, and 12% had been going through steroid cycles for more than ten years (Parkinson & Evans, 2006).

A cautious approach to self-reported data reminds us not to take all the reported side effects at face value. In keeping with this, obviously the researchers were unable to confirm that their respondents had experienced the side effects they reported, and also unable to investigate whether respondents had experienced other, potentially more serious side effects that they had refrained from reporting or simply not reported because they were unaware of them. Likewise, such studies based on self-reporting are unable to tell us whether the reported doses are correct, and whether the products reportedly used actually contained the amounts of active drug the users thought they did. The reason for this is that steroids are often imported illegally, so the type and amount of active ingredient is often mislabeled (Evans-Brown, Kimergård, & McVeigh, 2009; Graham et al., 2009). Then again, insofar as respondents had side effects they were aware of, there does not seem to be any particular reason for them *not* to report them, not least because respondents neither veiled nor hid the use of illegal substances, risky injection techniques, illegal procurement methods (89%) or other side effects. The remarkable thing about the results is that these veteran heavy steroid users did not experience worse side effects than they did, which was especially surprising because they used not only anabolic steroids but also a number of other drugs, including ancillary anabolic drugs such as insulin (25%) and insulin-like growth factor-1 (IGF-1; 10%). In addition to potentially causing hypoglycemia (an acute drop in blood-sugar levels) and coma, using these drugs can lead to type 2 diabetes (Kanayama & Pope, 2012).

Quite apart from this, the fact that virtually all respondents (96%) took a number of other substances besides steroids makes it even more difficult to interpret the reported side effects, for although the side effects correspond to those presented, for instance, on Anti Doping Danmark's website, we do not know enough about the cocktail effects when users take different types of anabolic steroids, or between anabolic steroids and all the other drugs users take. Consequently we are unable to reconstruct the causal links for the individual side effects with any certainty. Not that this makes the side effects any less relevant, or less alarming, but it does obscure the picture of how dangerous anabolic steroids are, in and of themselves.

The findings presented in the Parkinson and Evans study are not unique. Cohen and his colleagues conducted a study of 1,955 anabolic steroid users and got comparable results, and a study from a Dutch clinic treating steroid users likewise showed all the same acute but transient side effects, while no serious side effects emerged (Cohen, Collins, Darkes, & Gwartney, 2007; Smit & de Ronde, 2018). Also, a popular-science book entitled *The Adonis Complex*, written by a group of long-time researchers in the field (Pope, Phillips, & Olivardia, 2000, treated elsewhere), refers to an interview with one user who describes going through anabolic-steroid cycles for at least 36 months, all told, but who has never experienced a single side effect. "This is typical," the authors wrote. "Of the hundreds of steroid users we've interviewed, most have never been conscious of a serious medical problem, nor do they know of any friends who have." Some get pimples that take a long time to go away, and others develop gynecomastia ("bitch-tits"), but "for most men the increase in breast tissue isn't visible to the naked eye" (Pope et al., 2000, p. 110). While some young people might be scared away from steroids by the threat of pimply skin or the risk of developing breasts, many are willing to take the risk, as long as the steroids and training deliver the goods, boosting their muscles, strength and self-confidence (Bates, 2019).

As in the Parkinson and Evans study, many of the users referenced in *The Adonis Complex* had reported shrinking testicles, which is to be anticipated when the body is given artificial testosterone, as this inhibits the signal to the testicles to produce their own testosterone. Pope and his colleagues wrote, back in 2000,

> But when one stops taking steroids, the body's own system comes back "on line," and the testicles grow back to their original size after a while. We've never heard of a case in which permanent impairment of testicular functioning occurred as a result of steroid use.
>
> (Pope et al., 2000, p. 111)

That may well be, but 20 years later there is evidence showing that users' testicles may not always return to their original size, and newer research suggests that functioning may be permanently impaired (Rasmussen et al., 2016). Still, there are doubts about just how much young people are deterred from steroid use by information campaigns with an overly dramatic message; indeed, some studies have even found that scare tactics have the opposite effect (Bates et al., 2017). The fact of the matter is, users themselves rarely worry about the temporary side effects that occur.

Beyond the ambition of giving educational campaigns the desired clout, such dramatization of side effects is undoubtedly caused by the way reporting and registration take place: Most reports of severe side effects stem from observational studies and individual case reports by physicians confronted with serious and sometimes life-threatening situations (Evans-Brown & McVeigh, 2009; Hartgens & Kuipers, 2004; Thiblin & Petersson, 2005). Even so, it is logical that physicians do not see the many steroid users who do not experience problems that would motivate them to consult their doctor. Therefore, a potential overestimation of the harmfulness of these drugs may well be caused by a skewed selection of cases emphasized by influential medical doctors and researchers (Hoffman & Ratamess, 2006). Indeed, there are numerous indications that such cases have been over-represented in anti-doping and educational campaigns about steroids. As pointed out by the sports historian John Hoberman, such campaigns with their moral outset have emphasized the dangers of using anabolic steroids far more than the corresponding medical literature has. Yet another problem in assessing the risk of using anabolic steroids is that we know little about the long-term effects. The side effects mentioned above, for instance in the

Parkinson and Evans study, are all acute and, in most cases, reversible. In one of the few studies that has attempted to illustrate the long-term effects of anabolic steroids, researchers compared mortality among powerlifters with the general population. They assessed that these powerlifters had, most probably, used anabolic steroids, given that they were active between 1977 and 1982 and doping control was not implemented in their sport until 1984. The scientific comparison showed that after 12 years the mortality rate among these power-lifters was 12.9%, compared to 3.1% among the general population. In other words, the risk of dying during that period in the powerlifter group was 4.6 times higher than in the control group. Powerlifting in itself is not dangerous, so the findings show that using anabolic steroids may have serious long-term effects (Pärssinen, Kujala, Vartiainen, Sarna, & Seppälä, 2000; Pärssinen & Seppälä, 2002). A Danish study compared 545 Danish men who, between 2006 and 2018, tested positive (predominantly for anabolic steroids) in the anti-doping program in Danish gyms with 5,450 matched control individuals (another study on the same population is mentioned in Chapter 2). Researchers found an increased mortality rate of 3.0 among the steroid users, as well as a median number of annual hospital contacts of 0.81 in the steroid group versus 0.36 in the control group (Horwitz, Andersen, & Dalhoff, 2019).

A large study of the literature, likewise done by experienced researchers in the field, has investigated illness histories and mortality rates of steroid users who debuted in the 1980s and therefore had reached middle age in the 2000s. Based on their study design, the researchers expected not only to collect information about acute side effects, but also to capture potential long-term effects of the drugs. They concluded that "long-term use of supraphysiologic doses of AAS [anabolic androgenic steroids] may have adverse effects on a number of organ systems, leading to both medical and psychiatric pathology," and that this damage could persist long after steroid use had ceased. They also concluded, however, that knowledge was still lacking about the influence of steroids on increased mortality rates, due to the relatively young age of the earliest large groups of users (Kanayama, Hudson, & Pope, 2008, p. 8). More recently, studies have shown that long-term use involves a greater-than-normal risk of dying of cardiovascular diseases (Baggish et al., 2017; Pope et al., 2014; Rasmussen et al., 2016; Thiblin et al., 2015).[4]

Mental side effects

In recent years campaigns, education and information about steroids have increasingly emphasized the mental side effects. So too with the Danish campaign launched in 2009 by Anti Doping Danmark and entitled "Steroids are stronger than you," illustrating a man in three phases of increasing mental distress as his body gradually grows larger (see Figure 11.1). Steroids may well cause pimples, bitch tits and small testicles, but as discussed above, if users feel they can live with the side effects as long as they achieve the desired increase in muscle mass and strength, such campaigns will hardly be effective against steroid use. If one can point to mental side effects of the drugs, however, and adverse consequences not just for the user but for those around him, that is a different matter. This could illustrate that the steroid user is not making a purely personal choice with personal consequences, but a choice that has social consequences as well.

The main issue for researchers and authorities is whether steroids lead to violence and aggression, and it has also been pointed out that some steroid users develop depression and psychosis. In 2017 Anti Doping Danmark wrote about the mental side effects:

> The more testosterone you take, the greater the mental changes. As a user of anabolic steroids you will find it hard to control your temper. Mood swings, violent reactions, uncontrollable behavior, psychotic tendencies and changes in sex drive are among the most frequent side effects. Some users become so severely depressed that they commit suicide.
> (quoted from Christiansen, 2018, p. 47, my translation).[5]

Here, too, most of the information underlying the description stems from formally reported side effects in specific patients seen by medical doctors, meaning the information suffers from the same lack of scientific rigor that besets the information about physical side effects. Not that this rules out a link between steroids and aggression, but there is no demonstration of direct causality in humans. As noted earlier, most studies asking respondents to state their side effects get numerous reports of shrinking testicles, pain at injection sites and high blood pressure (Begley, McVeigh, & Hope, 2017; Cohen et al., 2007). As for mental side effects, many users report mood swings, but the findings vary greatly, and only a small group experience serious symptoms with episodes of rage and aggression (Bates & McVeigh, 2016; Pope et al., 2014; Rowe, Berger, & Copeland, 2016).

Researchers and police can nevertheless cite countless cases where people with no previous record of criminal conduct or violent behavior suddenly became violent while taking a course of steroids. Many of these cases had to do with sudden, uncontrollable rage in traffic, violence against women or violence in prison. A few cases involved homicide (Eisenegger, Naef, Snozzi, Heinrichs, & Fehr, 2010; Pope et al., 2000). Hence, this phenomenon has become known as "roid rage," but the question is whether there really is a cause-and-effect relationship between steroids and violent behavior. One Swedish group tested the hypothesis that anabolic-steroid use among people held in police custody coincided with a higher probability that they had committed violent crime, compared with other types of crime. Their study did find that police detainees reporting anabolic-steroid use showed a higher likelihood of violent crime than those not reporting steroid use. However, a surprising finding was that this was true whether users reported steroid use within the last month, the last year, the last 1–5 years or more than 5 years prior, or even just at some point in their life. All of these groups had a 34–38% probability of having committed violent crime, compared to a 26% probability among those who reported never using steroids. The greatest surprise was the lack of evidence of any chronological link between when detainees had taken steroids and when they had committed the violent criminal act — making it impossible to unequivocally document a cause-and-effect correlation between steroids and violence (Lundholm, Kall, Wallin, & Thiblin, 2010).

What is more, as with all other side effects, not everyone reacts mentally to steroids. Far from it. In a randomized clinical study conducted on healthy American men by the National Institute of Mental Health, 20 subjects received a placebo, and 20 subjects received 240 mg of methyltestosteron daily (1,680 mg weekly), which is at the very high end of what most body-builders take. Two of the 20 in the latter group had "bad reactions," one losing control so severely he asked to be voluntarily sequestered in his room (Pope et al., 2000, p. 115). In real life, outside university laboratories, people do not undergo a selection process, and the situations in which they find themselves are not controlled as they are in a lab. Also, the researcher rarely knows which substances these people have taken, and in what doses. Even so, one of the most astonishing things about steroid studies is that only a small minority of men develop severe depressive conditions after using. Referring again to the work of Pope and his colleagues, they are convinced that "Even though only a minority of men have this predisposition, and even fewer men reach the point of having dangerous reactions, we are still looking at a significant public health problem" (Pope et al., 2000, p. 117). In the wake of this, others have claimed that rather than *causing* negative character traits, steroids *reinforce* traits that already exist. In the words of Carlon Colker, an American physician and consultant for the food-supplement industry: "If you're a jerk, and you take steroids, then you're a super-jerk" (Bell, Buono, & Rawady, 2009).

Laboratory studies

Although we do not know precisely what it is about steroids that triggers aggression, there are few indications that steroids lead to aggressive behavior or violence — all other things being equal, and in unprovoked situations. Some studies suggest that steroids initiate or intensify a feeling seated deep in the male brain of the need to protect one's sexual territory. Other studies indicate that social context and the perception of being provoked are of significance, or that the chemical structure of the specific anabolic steroid is decisive.

The most scientifically solid findings in this field come from randomized, controlled studies, like the one described above. "Randomization" is typi-cally ensured by having two groups: one that gets the active substance, and another that gets an inactive "placebo" substance. During the study, no one knows who is getting what; neither the researchers administering the drugs nor the test subjects.

A Zurich-based research group has questioned the basic premise of what they call "the folk hypothesis," which says that testosterone leads to anti-social, egoistic, aggressive or violent behavior. So, the scientists asked, what if testosterone is primarily involved in status-related behavior? This alternative hypothesis — "the social status hypothesis" — would still enable them to explain the many individual reported cases concerning violence and steroids, and it would also explain why higher testosterone levels have been found among people committing rape, murder or armed robbery than among control groups. The proposed explanation is this: The social status hypothesis says that the hormone testosterone plays a role when an individual challenges social interactions. However, in seeking to understand testosterone in the context of status-related behavior, an experiment had to be designed that could confirm (or refute) the social status hypothesis. This design had to keep the two hypotheses separate and also ensure that higher testosterone levels would be observable as more prosocial behavior, rather than as the aggressive or negative behavior assumed in the folk hypothesis. That is precisely what the Zurich researchers did. They had individuals who had received either placebo or testosterone play out a scenario from game theory called "the ultimatum game." This involves two people, A and B, who must agree on how to divide 10 dollars.[6] Person A can choose to offer B either 5, 3, 2 or 0 dollars, the fairest bid of which, obviously, would be 5 dollars. Person B cannot negotiate this amount; only accept or refuse it. If B accepts A's offer, the money is split according to the bid. If B refuses A's proposition, neither of the parties gets anything and all the money is lost — therein lies the "ultimatum."

Now, based on the folk hypothesis, one would expect that the subjects who were given testosterone would make a lower offer, in order to maximize their own gain (egoistic behavior). Based on the social status hypothesis, however, one would expect the subjects on testosterone to make the highest offer, in order to increase their status. But the results were surprising, because they confirmed the status hypothesis while at the same time clearly showing that the test subjects were under the influence of the folk hypothesis. When the experiment was over, the subjects were asked whether they believed they had received placebo or testosterone. Lo and behold, the results showed that their behavior was strongly affected by what the subjects *thought* they had been getting. Subjects who believed they had been getting testosterone bid far less than those who thought they had received placebo. But the test also showed that subjects who had received testosterone bid an average of 3.9 dollars, whereas the placebo group bid an average of 3.4 dollars, regardless of whether they believed they had been getting testosterone or placebo. The subjects who most frequently offered their opponent 5 dollars (the fairest bid) were those who had received testosterone but *thought* they had received placebo. Conversely, the subjects who most frequently offered their opponent 0 or 2 dollars (the unfairest bids) were those who had received placebo but *thought* they had received testosterone. In other words, although the folk hypothesis seems to cause an anticipatory effect, based on the findings of this randomized study it is fair to call the folk hypothesis into question, given that the people who actually received testosterone — regardless of what they *thought* they were getting — offered the fairest bids in the ultimatum game (Eisenegger et al., 2010).[7]

Researchers have attempted to clarify the correlation between anabolic steroids and the factors that bring on aggression by studying various situations in animal-model experiments. Using mainly rats as test animals, scientists have sought to isolate the importance of various factors in triggering normal aggressive behavior. Such experiments are based on the assumption that results from studies involving rats (animals whose brains correspond, in size, to a mere smidgen of a human brain and have no prefrontal cortex — the area often described as the seat of reason, which deals with our more sophisticated cognitive processes) can be transferred to humans. Employing this assumption also implies that one believes aggression is a very fundamental phenomenon shared by humans and animals. There is a consensus among ethologists (scientists who study animal behavior) that aggressive behavior is a result of evolutionary development that aids survival and regulates social behavior in humans and animals, particularly when it comes to territorial defense, ranking and dominance (Herbert, 2015; Mazur, 2005). In that sense, studies based on rats may actually help us to gain some basic understanding of how anabolic steroids affect aggression.

The many studies of this kind notably include a review study done by two prominent researchers in the field, the American pharmacologists Augustus Lumia and Marilyn McGinnis, who investigated the behavior of male rats under the influence of anabolic steroids (Lumia & McGinnis, 2010). One key finding was that the animals' behavior depended on the surroundings in which they were placed. The rats given testosterone reacted differently depending on whether they were tested in their home cage, in an opponent's cage or in a neutral cage. The individual rats were most aggressive when a rival turned up in their home cage, whereas their aggression level was elevated yet lower when they were in an opponent's cage or a neutral cage. In a different study design, the scientists showed that male rats that had received testosterone were able to distinguish between castrated and non-castrated rivals, showing no aggression towards castrated competitors. This finding supports the idea that while testosterone probably lowers the threshold for triggering aggression, the aggression itself is context-dependent and influenced by the social signals triggered when competitors meet.

Lumia and McGinnis also found that rats given testosterone had a higher aggression level when provoked, which leads researchers to suggest that testosterone lowers the reaction threshold for individuals facing an external threat. The test animals' prior experience also played an important role. One study demonstrated that male rats given the anabolic steroid nandrolone exhibited more aggression, whereas nandrolone did not lead to aggression in a number of subsequent studies. To explain this discrepancy, Lumia and McGinnis proposed that the rats in the first study had received two weeks of "fight training" before they were given nandrolone. In the subsequent studies, however, the rats did not have this experience, and nandrolone did not lead to increased aggression. Based on these studies, Lumia and McGinnis maintain that the behavioral consequences of anabolic steroids are not exclusively determined by the presence of very high levels of the drug. Rather, they say that the aggressive response is affected by a wide range of factors, including environment, social signals, physical provocation and prior experience, and they conclude that "Anabolic androgenic steroids do not induce indiscriminate and unprovoked aggression or violence" (Lumia & McGinnis, 2010, p. 201).

The most unanticipated finding may be that the rats' aggression levels depended on the type of anabolic steroid administered. We know that as a performance enhancer, testosterone is coveted among some gym-goers, thanks to its dual capacity as an androgenic (masculinizing) drug *and* a potent anabolic (muscle-building) drug. Another favorite of users in gyms is stanozolol, a drug with strong anabolic but less pronounced androgenic effects. Incidentally, this was the substance for which the Canadian sprinter Ben Johnson tested positive at the Seoul Olympic Games in 1988. A third frequently used steroid is nandrolone, which, like other steroids, has anabolic and androgenic properties. All three of these drugs have been used in animal studies. The ability of testosterone to produce aggression and other masculine behavior in animals, including mating and territory-marking, is thoroughly documented. By contrast, stanozolol actually inhibits aggression and other androgenic, sensitive behavior. Treatment with nandrolone, on the other hand, seems to cause little behavioral change in rats. Males treated with this drug generally exhibited the same behavior in terms of sexual acts and aggression as the animal control group (Lumia & McGinnis, 2010).

One study has looked at the effects of these three substances when they are "stacked," or used in combination, as often seen in gym and weightlifting circles. Intriguingly, the researchers found that the aggression-inhibiting properties of stanozolol were canceled out when it was used along with testosterone, whereas this was not the case when it was combined with nandrolone. Based on this, Lumia and McGinnis concluded that "the chemical composition of individual AAS [anabolic androgenic steroids] is an important factor in determining AAS's effects on behavior" (Lumia & McGinnis, 2010, p. 202).

Animals and humans

There are enormous differences between animals and humans. If rats are given free access to steroids, they will self-administer doses until they die, due to the positive reinforcement this gives the brain's reward system. Few steroid users, no matter how obsessive they are, would go that far. What is more, even though humans and animals are under the influence of testosterone, human beings have become ever more peaceful as civilization has progressed, whereas the use of violence in the animal kingdom is the same today as it was millennia ago. The way humans approach aggression and status, and handle related problems, are far more complex than what we see in animals (Herbert, 2015; Pinker, 2011).

We cannot generalize or extrapolate results from animal studies to humans without huge reservations. Nevertheless, such studies can serve as a window to some of the processes also at work in humans. One example is the observations that testosterone, in particular, can lead to aggressiveness in rats, which tie in with anecdotal accounts from steroid-using athletes. As early as 1987 the American sports historian Terry Todd, a pioneering researcher of anabolic steroids in sports, reported behavioral changes experience by people who replaced Dianabol, one of the earliest anabolic steroids, with testosterone. One description came from the wife of an American football player who related changes she observed in her husband: "He's so impatient when he's on steroids, so easily annoyed. He becomes vocal and hostile real fast and he was never that way before." As the athlete himself said: "It definitely makes a person mean and aggressive. And I was always so easygoing. On the field I've tried to hurt people in ways I never did before" (Todd, 1987, p. 98).

Testosterone is probably one of the commonly used steroids with the highest tendency to produce self-assertive and aggressive behavior. However, as we saw in the study mentioned above, where test subjects were given 240 mg of methyltestosterone a day, only 10% of the subjects developed "bad reactions." Seemingly, the conclusion is that the people who can *not* be talked out of using anabolic steroids should at least be advised against using testosterone or substances (such as trenbolone) with a corresponding structure and affect, and be encouraged to choose less potent drugs like stanozolol instead.

At any rate, anabolic steroids do, indisputably, exert an effect. People experience benefits, including increased muscle growth, greater strength, more fat-free volume, quicker restitution and heightened libido. However, these effects act at a level that is stronger and more pervasive than we can explain using dry, objective references to the pharmacological and physiological effects on the body. The fact is, steroids also affect the way a person relates to their surroundings, which is why steroids hold the potential to alter self-image and identity.

Notes

1 I am extremely grateful to the Danish muscle physiologist Anders Nedergaard for his comments and constructive suggestions to improve this chapter.
2 Many sources have retold this story, but my choice of the word "legend" is a very conscious one. The account as represented here follows a well-known template with "the Russians" cast as the bad guys who devised a method of cheating; a tactic to which the Americans were obliged to respond in kind to reestablish the status quo, meaning fair competition. In this way the Americans have successfully related the story of inventing Dianabol as a defense measure necessary to contain the Soviet Union's foul play. It is implicit from the contours of this template that if the Soviets had not upped the ante, the Americans would never have followed suit, and sports doping might not have developed into the problem it has since become. But actually the Americans were already well on their way to developing Dianabol before the weightlifting world championship in 1954. Some sources even say that Ziegler was giving testosterone preparations to American athletes as early as 1953. The reason the story as rendered here has gained such a strong foothold is that Ziegler's version fits hand in glove with the subsequent historiography of the roles of the USSR and the US in the sports race of the Cold War. See (Gleaves & Llewellyn, 2018).
3 The Internet has a number of websites showing the anabolic-steroid cycles used by various high-profile bodybuilders, including Arnold Schwarzenegger. See, for instance, "The Arnold Schwarzenegger cycle" at: www.isteroids.com/steroids/a rnold-schwarzenegger-cycle.html (accessed on 27 October 2019).
4 See also (Herman, Conlon, Rubenfire, Burghardt, & McGregor, 2014; Horwitz et al., 2019).
5 As is the nature of such websites, Anti Doping Danmark recently changed the text, so that in October 2019 it reads: "Abuse of AAS also involves a risk of a number of psychological side effects including depressive symptoms and mood swings." (Anti Doping Danmark, 2019).
6 Participants in this experiment played the game using Swiss francs, but these had been abstracted into ten Money Units (MUs) per game. The test subjects were allowed to offer 5, 3, 2 or 0 MUs — which, to be practical, I have rendered here as "dollars."
7 Later studies have replicated the design of this study while also including an opportunity for B to reward or punish A, depending on whether B was satisfied with the bid or not. Researchers found that low bids combined with high testosterone levels made for harsher punishments. Conversely, rewards were also larger when the bid was satisfactory and testosterone levels high. See (Dreher et al., 2016).

References

Anti Doping Danmark. (2019). Anabole androgene steroider. Retrieved from: www.antidoping.dk/undervisning/dopingstoffer-og-metoder/anabole-androgene-steroider.
Baggish, A. L., Weiner, R. B., Kanayama, G., Hudson, J. I., Lu, M. T., Hoffmann, U., & Pope, H. G., Jr. (2017). Cardiovascular toxicity of illicit anabolic-androgenic steroid use. *Circulation*, 135(21), 1991–2002. doi: doi:10.1161/circulationaha.116.026945.
Bates, G. (2019). *Supporting men who use anabolic steroids: A sequential multi-methods study.* (PhD Doctoral), Liverpool, John Moores University. Retrieved from: http://researchonline.ljmu.ac.uk/id/eprint/1101/.
Bates, G., Begley, E., Tod, D., Jones, L., Leavey, C., & McVeigh, J. (2017). A systematic review investigating the behaviour change strategies in interventions to prevent misuse of anabolic steroids. *J Health Psychol*. doi: doi:10.1177/1359105317737607.

Bates, G., & McVeigh, J. (2016). Image and performance enhancing drugs: 2015 survey results. Retrieved from Liverpool: www.ipedinfo.co.uk/resources/downloa ds/2015%20National%20IPED%20Info%20Survey%20report.pdf.

Begley, E., McVeigh, J., & Hope, V. (2017). Image and performance enhancing drugs: 2016 national survey results. Retrieved from Liverpool: www.wales.nhs.uk/sitesp lus/documents/888/IPED%20report%202017.%20FINAL.pdf.

Bell, C., Buono, A., & Rawady, T. (2009). *Bigger stronger faster: The side effects of being American*. Sandrew Metronome.

Bhasin, S., Storer, T. W., Berman, N., Callegari, C., Clevenger, B., Phillips, J., ... Casaburi, R. (1996). The effects of supraphysiologic doses of testosterone on muscle size and strength in normal men. *N Engl J Med*, 335(1), 1–7. doi: doi:10.1056/NEJM199607043350101.

Bhasin, S., Woodhouse, L., & Storer, T. W. (2001). Proof of the effect of testosterone on skeletal muscle. *J.Endocrinol.*, 170(1), 27–38. doi: doi:10.1677/joe.0.1700027.

Christiansen, A. V. (2018). *Motionsdoping: Styrketræning, identitet og kultur*. Aarhus, Denmark: Aarhus Universitetsforlag.

Cohen, J., Collins, R., Darkes, J., & Gwartney, D. (2007). A league of their own: Demographics, motivations and patterns of use of 1,955 male adult non-medical anabolic steroid users in the United States. *J.Int.Soc.Sports Nutr.*, 4, 12. doi: doi:1550-2783-4-12.

Dimeo, P. (2007). *A history of drug use in sport 1876–1976: Beyond good and evil*. London: Routledge.

Dreher, J.-C., Dunne, S., Pazderska, A., Frodl, T., Nolan, J. J., & O'Doherty, J. P. (2016). Testosterone causes both prosocial and antisocial status-enhancing behaviors in human males. *Proceedings of the National Academy of Sciences*, 113(41), 11633–11638. doi: doi:10.1073/pnas.1608085113.

Eisenegger, C., Naef, M., Snozzi, R., Heinrichs, M., & Fehr, E. (2010). Prejudice and truth about the effect of testosterone on human bargaining behaviour. *Nature*, 463 (7279), 356–359. doi: doi:10.1038/nature08711.

Evans-Brown, M., Kimergård, A., & McVeigh, J. (2009). Elephant in the room? The methodological implications for public health research of performance-enhancing drugs derived from the illicit market. *Drug Test.Anal.*, 1(7), 323–326. doi: doi:10.1002/dta.74.

Evans-Brown, M., & McVeigh, J. (2009). Anabolic steroid use in the general population of the United Kingdom. In V. Møller, M. McNamee, & P. Dimeo (Eds.), *Elite sport, doping and public health* (pp. 75–97). Odense, Denmark: University Press of Southern Denmark.

Gleaves, J., & Llewellyn, M. (2018). The "big arms" race: Doping and the cold war defense of American exceptionalism. In T. Rider & K. Witherspoon (Eds.), *Defending the American way of life* (pp. 49–66). Fayetteville, AR: University of Arkansas Press.

Graham, M. R., Ryan, P., Baker, J. S., Davies, B., Thomas, N. E., Cooper, S. M., ... Kicman, A. T. (2009). Counterfeiting in performance- and image-enhancing drugs. *Drug Test.Anal.*, 1(3), 135–142. doi: doi:10.1002/dta.30.

Guyton, A. C., & Hall, J. E. (2006). *Textbook of medical physiology* (11 ed.). Philadelphia, PA: Elsevier Saunders.

Hartgens, F., & Kuipers, H. (2004). Effects of androgenic-anabolic steroids in athletes. *Sports Med.*, 34(8), 513–554. doi: doi:10.2165/00007256-200434080-00003.

Herbert, J. (2015). *Testosterone: Sex, power, and the will to win.* Oxford: Oxford University Press.

Herman, C. W., Conlon, A. S. C., Rubenfire, M., Burghardt, A. R., & McGregor, S. J. (2014). The very high premature mortality rate among active professional wrestlers is primarily due to cardiovascular disease. *PLoS One,* 9(11), e109945. doi: doi:10.1371/journal.pone.0109945.

Hoberman, J. M. (1992). *Mortal engines: The science of performance and the dehumanization of sport.* New York: Free Press.

Hoberman, J. M. (2005). *Testosterone dreams: Rejuvenation, aphrodisia, doping.* Berkeley, CA: University of California Press.

Hoffman, J. R., & Ratamess, N. A. (2006). Medical issues associated with anabolic steroid use: Are they exaggerated? *Journal of Sports Science and Medicine,* 5(2), 182–193.

Horwitz, H., Andersen, J. T., & Dalhoff, K. P. (2019). Health consequences of androgenic anabolic steroid use. *J Intern Med,* 285(3), 333–340. doi: doi:10.1111/joim.12850.

Kanayama, G., Hudson, J. I., & Pope, H. G. (2008). Long-term psychiatric and medical consequences of anabolic-androgenic steroid abuse: A looming public health concern? *Drug Alcohol Depend.,* 98(1–2), 1–12. doi: doi:10.1016/j.drugalcdep.2008.05.004.

Kanayama, G., & Pope, H. G. (2012). Illicit use of androgens and other hormones: Recent advances. *Current Opinion in Endocrinology, Diabetes and Obesity,* 19, 1–9. doi: doi:10.1097/MED.0b013e3283524008.

Lumia, A. R., & McGinnis, M. Y. (2010). Impact of anabolic androgenic steroids on adolescent males. *Physiol Behav.,* 100(3), 199–204. doi: doi:10.1016/j.physbeh.2010.01.007.

Lundholm, L., Kall, K., Wallin, S., & Thiblin, I. (2010). Use of anabolic androgenic steroids in substance abusers arrested for crime. *Drug Alcohol Depend,* 111(3), 222–226. doi: doi:10.1016/j.drugalcdep.2010.04.020.

Mazur, A. (2005). *Biosociology of dominance and deference.* Lanham, MD: Rowman & Littlefield.

Parkinson, A. B., & Evans, N. A. (2006). Anabolic androgenic steroids: A survey of 500 users. *Medicine & Science in Sports & Exercise,* 38(4), 644–651. doi: doi:10.1249/01.mss.0000210194.56834.5d.

Pinker, S. (2002). *The blank slate: The modern denial of human nature.* New York: Penguin Books.

Pinker, S. (2011). *The better angels of our nature: A history of violence and humanity.* London: Penguin Books.

Pope, H. G., Phillips, K. A., & Olivardia, R. (2000). *The Adonis complex: How to identify, treat, and prevent body obsession in men and boys.* New York: Free Press.

Pope, H. G., Wood, R. I., Rogol, A., Nyberg, F., Bowers, L., & Bhasin, S. (2014). Adverse health consequences of performance-enhancing drugs: An Endocrine Society scientific statement. *Endocr Rev,* 35(3), 341–375. doi: doi:10.1210/er.2013-1058.

Pärssinen, M., Kujala, U., Vartiainen, E., Sarna, S., & Seppälä, T. (2000). Increased premature mortality of competitive powerlifters suspected to have used anabolic agents. *Int J Sports Med,* 21(3), 225–227. doi: doi:10.1055/s-2000-304.

Pärssinen, M., & Seppälä, T. (2002). Steroid use and long-term health risks in former athletes. *Sports Med.,* 32(2), 83–94. doi: doi:10.2165/00007256-200232020-00001.

Rasmussen, J. J., Selmer, C., Østergren, P. B., Pedersen, K. B., Schou, M., Gustafsson, F., … Kistorp, C. (2016). Former abusers of anabolic androgenic steroids exhibit decreased testosterone levels and hypogonadal symptoms years after cessation: A case-control study. *PLoS One*, 11(8), e0161208. doi: doi:10.1371/journal.pone.0161208.

Rowe, R., Berger, I., & Copeland, J. (2016). "No pain, no gainz"? Performance and image-enhancing drugs, health effects and information seeking. *Drugs: Education, Prevention and Policy*, 24(5), 1–9. doi: doi:10.1080/09687637.2016.1207752.

Smit, D. L., & de Ronde, W. (2018). Outpatient clinic for users of anabolic androgenic steroids: An overview. *Neth J Med*, 76(4), 167.

Thiblin, I., Garmo, H., Garle, M., Holmberg, L., Byberg, L., Michaelsson, K., & Gedeborg, R. (2015). Anabolic steroids and cardiovascular risk: A national population-based cohort study. *Drug Alcohol Depend*, 152, 87–92. doi: doi:10.1016/j.drugalcdep.2015.04.013.

Thiblin, I., & Petersson, A. (2005). Pharmacoepidemiology of anabolic androgenic steroids: A review. *Fundam.Clin.Pharmacol.*, 19(1), 27–44. doi: doi:10.1111/j.1472-8206.2004.00298.x.

Todd, T. (1987). Anabolic steroids: The gremlins of sport. *J.Sport Hist*, 14(1), 87–107.

Voy, R. (1991). *Drugs, sport and politics. (The inside story about drug use in sport and its political cover-up, with a prescription for reform)*. Champaign, IL: Leisure Press.

Chapter 4

Identity and recognition

Personal identity is immensely important. For those who may not have thought deeply about this before, the story of the South African runner Caster Semenya illustrates the point with searing clarity. In 2009, at the tender age of 18, Semenya won a gold medal in Berlin for her performance in the 800-meter event at the world championship in athletics, beating competitors by the biggest margin in world-championship history. Meanwhile, her stellar victory, tremendous progression over a few months and masculine appearance made the International Association of Athletics Federations (IAAF) decide to request that Semenya be gender-tested. For privacy reasons the results of the comprehensive tests were never made public, but what did leak to the press ostensibly showed that, genetically and biologically speaking, Semenya was not a female but an intersex person, with no ovaries but with internal testes that produced large amounts of testosterone (Smith, 2009).[1] The IAAF subsequently argued that her elevated testosterone levels was estimated to give her an advantage in sports. Because she had not cheated she was allowed to keep her gold medal and her prize money, but the decision then and there was that she could not take part in future athletics competitions for women.[2] It does not take much empathy to understand how traumatic this must have been for Semenya. She had grown up in a humble village where everyone had always considered her a girl, and when she returned from the championships in Berlin her compatriots aggressively defended her female identity (Tucker, 2019). In the years prior to 2009 she had made impressive progress, enjoying great success as a runner. Then suddenly there she was, deprived of two important identity markers: Semenya was not a woman, as she (and all others) had thus far identified her; and she was not an athlete, given that she was now unable to pursue her career in athletics. In terms of identity, for Semenya this was profoundly distressing, with impacts reaching far beyond some mere disagreement that would cause her to lose one or two social roles that could be replaced by other roles.

The topic of identity is widely discussed in sociology, psychology and philosophy. The framework of this book means my explanation of how I use the identity concept must, necessarily, be an abridged version of this broader discussion. Suffice it to say that what I focus on here is clarifying the identity concept for the purpose at hand, namely using it as a vital element in understanding my informants and what motivates them to work out and become bigger and stronger.

The circumstance that some people involve themselves very actively in gym life can be understood as a way to create, develop and work with their identity. At a superficial level this commitment can be seen as the person's way of interpreting and expressing values such as strength, health, dedication, youth and sex appeal. These are values rooted not only in gym culture but very broadly in the culture of the Western world. The values one identifies with and expresses through words and actions must, however, be accepted by one's surroundings before they can serve to construct identity for the individual. Identity construction is therefore a dialectic process that consists of formulating and sending signals to the surrounding world, which interprets these signals and subsequently sends back a response. These things do not take place as separate processes but are an integrated part of daily life; a factor to which we rarely dedicate much reflection (Jenkins, 2004). In keeping with this, the German-American developmental psychologist Erik Erikson talks about the "inner" or personal identity and "cultural" or group identity. Seen in this perspective, the identity concept lies in the borderlands between individual and culture, and between psychology and sociology (Jørgensen, 2008).

The identity concept

I will deal with one of this book's basic assumptions (noted in Chapter 1) — that working out and building a muscular body can be understood as a specific type of identity work — by applying an identity concept that consists of both a *malleable element* and a *stable element*. Together, these two elements explain why I can have a clear sense that I have changed over time, for instance by developing from a scrawny, insecure boy into a self-confident, muscular man while at the same time consistently feeling, despite the changes, that I have been myself all along. The Danish philosopher Erich Klawonn has made it possible to understand this seemingly paradoxical aspect of our existence by distinguishing conceptually between an "I" and an "ego" (Klawonn, 1987, 1990).[3]

My "I" is identical to my consciousness, meaning my first-person perspective, which is experienced as a permanent "I-feeling." Every experience I have, from cradle to grave, is one of *my* experiences, which are all present in my consciousness. This permanent "I-feeling" gives me an experience of being identical to, and identifiable with, myself over time. My "ego" is identical with my self-image. I compile the self-image of certain elements in my life to which I ascribe a special significance. For instance, I perceive myself as a married man in his forties who has a career as an academic and is interested in cycle sport. My "ego," in other words, is the self-image with which I identify, and which I show my surroundings through speech and actions. While my "I" first-person perspective is something I experience as stable,[4] my self-image develops over time, because it is affected by many different things. A person's self-image is affected, for instance, by whether they are biologically male or female; psychologically outgoing or solitary; and culturally raised in, say, Denmark or Afghanistan. Hence, not all elements of myself-image are equally easy to change. Imagine I admire a strong man and want to be like him. In that case, I can work to change my self-image in that direction by lifting weights, whereas it is more difficult to change the part of my self-image associated with my gender. In this way, my self-image is affected both by fundamental biological, psychological and sociocultural factors, and also by the recognition I receive in various social contexts.

This understanding of identity means, firstly, that I reject an understanding of identity as something volatile and alterable; something a person can mold and shape as they see fit; something that consists only of the various roles we have (see, for instance, Gergen, 2000). Secondly, it means that I do not agree with the school in sociology that claims the issue of identity was not actualized until the Enlightenment — as if, prior to that time, people did not think about who they were.

Two central aspects of self-image, and therefore of identity, are the many *social roles* we fulfill and participate in, and also the partly biologically anchored component that consists of our *personality traits*.

Roles and personality traits

A role can be understood as the "the behaviour expected of an individual who occupies a given social position or status" (Encyclopaedia Britannica, 1998). This means that social roles are socially contingent, and because different things are expected of us in different situations, we all have many different roles to fulfill. These roles are not necessarily linked. Depending on how important we consider it to be, an individual role can be part of our self-image. The various roles are not, each independently, decisive to our total identity or self-image. A person can have one role on the job, another role at home with their family, a third at the gym, a fourth at a high-school reunion and so on. Each individual role is socially constructed by the context of which it constitutes a part, and it is not necessarily traumatic if, at some stage, the role is no longer needed and we therefore lose it. Actually, sometimes we are relieved at not having to carry or fulfill a certain role any longer.[5]

On the other hand, we also have a biology and a number of personal traits, and unlike our roles these are not social constructions, which means they exert a more permanent influence on our self-image and our identity. Some people are generally outgoing (extroverts), whereas others are more reserved (introverts). Some people are carefree and others cautious; some meticulous and others sloppy. However, as opposed to the classical personality features from Antiquity, which were pure types (melancholy, phlegmatic, choleric or sanguine, for instance), today there is a consensus that these qualities are on a continuum and can be more or less prominent in the individual. In short no one would be only outgoing, or only reserved. All people are located somewhere along the continuum that runs between "outgoing" and "reserved." Although the various personality traits have many intersecting points, the assumption is that just five general dimensions are enough to describe the core features in most personalities. This is known as "the five-factor model" often referred to by the acronym OCEAN and representing a person's level on five parameters: (1) openness to experience, (2) conscientiousness, (3) extraversion, (4) agreeableness, and (5) neuroticism (in terms of emotional stability). The five-factor model has been translated to, and evaluated in, a wide variety of languages and cultures, and it shows a high level of internal consistency, reliability and validity across diverse population groups. Research has demonstrated, among other things, that "personality" is understood in the same way virtually everywhere, and that the five-factor structure itself is universally applicable (McCrae & Allik, 2002; McCrae & Costa, 1999).

In the context of this book, we can use the model to more precisely demonstrate that a person's identity cannot be reduced to roles and social discourses. Besides the socially constructed parts of identity, people also have a variety of personal traits that influence our thoughts, behaviors and actions, and these remain relatively stable throughout our adult lives.

Recognition

Obviously a person's identity is not fully formed at birth. This is a gradual process that takes place as we mature, influenced by our living conditions, roles, personality traits and so forth, but also influenced by the attention and recognition we receive for the things we do. That is why identity is also something we must fight for, in competition with others. Contrary to individual social roles, the elements people see as defining to their own personal identity are elements most people will fight to retain. That is why losing central parts of one's identity can be a personal tragedy, as we saw in the story of Caster Semenya. In short, identity, self-image and recognition are interlinked.

The basic thought linking identity to recognition is the idea, commonly held in sociology, that as a consequence of modernity, human beings are no longer who we are solely by virtue of our family, our property or the place we grew up. Rather, we are who we are by virtue of our actions and our efforts — wherever these efforts may be applied (Giddens, 1991). In reality, however, when it comes to education, employment, housing and health, a person's socio-economic background is still one of the best indicators of where they will end up in life (Cohen, Janicki-Deverts, Chen, & Matthews, 2010). Yet even despite this, the prevailing perception is that the recognition a person gets, which nurtures their identity, is a recognition that must be earned through their own efforts in various contexts — and which we therefore cannot take over from our parents.

The French Revolution is often considered the symbolic demarcation of the transition to modernity, but this revolution's abstract ideal of "freedom, equality and fraternity" is not unproblematic. One of the first to notice the inherent contradiction in this motto was the German philosopher G.W.F. Hegel. We cannot love all people, and if we want freedom we cannot also, simultaneously, have equality. Hegel therefore realized that if the French Revolution's motto was to be practically feasible, the three concepts had to be embedded in different institutions. The motto's internal incongruity could be canceled out if, instead of being set out as purely abstract contra-dictions, each concept was given its own separate institution. "Freedom" was to be understood in connection with the market, and it had to do with professional skills and career choices. "Equality" was to be understood in relation to the state, and it had to do with everyone being equal in the eyes of the law. "Fraternity" was to be understood as linked to the solidarity of the family's brotherhood. In this way the three concepts pointed to different types of communities: the intimate community of the family; the legal com-munity within the state; and the vocational or professional community in the workplace (Thyssen & Dahl, 2006).

Another German thinker, the sociologist and philosopher Axel Honneth, more recently added three different types of recognition to Hegel's three types of institutions: We receive emotional recognition in the family, in the form of love and care; legal recognition in the court system by virtue of our citizenship; and social recognition through the efforts we make in the con-texts where we exhibit our skills and competence (Honneth, 1995).

The important point here is that the recognition we receive within these three spheres does not contribute in equal measure to our identity. For most people in Western liberal democracies, for instance, there is little identity to be found through the legal recognition a person gets by being a citizen in a country. Conversely, most people agree that the recognition a person receives from their family, along with the elements this contributes to their identity, is one of the most valuable things anyone can have. This is partly because the family's contribution is based on bonds of blood, kinship and love, and partly because one's identity in the role of father, mother, daugh-ter, son, sister or brother is indisputable. On the other hand, this part of a person's identity is not something they can use to distinguish themselves in the social arena, genuinely setting them apart as someone special. That, however, can be done by virtue of a person's efforts, their skills and their performance on the job and in their leisure time. The social recognition one can gain in this sphere is a very strong element in identity construction, precisely because it is *conditional* upon the efforts one expends and the results one achieves, and upon the recognition of these results by one's surroundings. That is what makes it qualitatively different from the *unconditional* recognition a person receives as love from their family, or recognition in the form of legal equality for a citizen of a nation-state (Honneth, 1995). Identity elements that a person constructs by virtue of their efforts and performance are, precisely, elements for which an active effort must be made. You have to work for them. That is why losing this sort of identity element can be a tragic loss, and quite traumatic: because it entails reconstructing one's self-image.

There is one final element that should be emphasized: The reason why identity loss is experienced as so profoundly distressing is not merely because identity is linked to recognition. It is also because identity is the distant horizon we gaze at when interpreting our existence. As the Canadian philosopher Charles Taylor put it:

> To know who I am is a species of knowing where I stand. My identity is defined by the commitments and identifications which provide the frame or horizon within which I can try to determine from case to case what is good, or valuable, or what ought to be done, or what I endorse or oppose. In other words, it is the horizon within which I am capable of taking a stand.
>
> (Taylor, 1989, p. 27)

According to Taylor, a central part of our identity is based on what he calls "strong evaluations," which include our assessments of right and wrong, good and evil, important and unimportant. These are assessments of what is valuable in our lives. Hence, a well-developed identity is important when we deal with the many choices in our daily lives, since it serves as a sort of personal navigational system or GPS (Jørgensen, 2008).

All of this does not mean identity is a project isolated to the lone individual. Identity is oriented both inwards (towards the individual) and outwards (towards the world). Other people's definition of who I am, through the way they treat me and what they say about me, is a crucial part of my own self-image. Therefore it is not enough for us to claim that we have an identity, or to send out an identity signal. Such a signal must be accepted by the people in our surroundings, those we perceive as significant, before it can be considered valid (Jenkins, 2004). Our identity can only be shaped in relation to, and in distinction from, something we ourselves are not. Even though to a certain extent it is theoretically meaningful to distinguish between group identity and individual identity, it is not easy to point out the characteristics that uniquely typify each of the two. For example, a group identity does not primarily focus on similarities while individual identity focuses on differences. Similarities and differences are interwoven and can best be understood by virtue of each other. Having said that, most people find it easiest to define who they are, or which group they belong to, by pointing out what they are *not*, and which groups they definitely do *not* belong to.

This brief presentation of the identity concept aimed to show why identity is so important to us humans. The reason identity also plays an important role for the people we are going to meet in the following chapters is that identity is closely associated to the actions to which we ascribe value, and with which others associate us. In turn, the actions to which we ascribe value are actions we link to our self-image, our identity. This circularity is also a part of the inertia that generally characterizes social and cultural change. Even so, the same circularity also explains why it is illusory to think that the right kind of educational campaign will enable the authorities to find a quick fix against steroid use in non-professional gym environments.

Notes

1 Taking almost a year to reach a decision, in July 2010 the IAAF once again allowed Semenya to run. The IAAF explained they had accepted medical experts' assessment that she should be allowed to run in competitions with other women. The IAAF gave no details of Semenya's sex-verification test results, but the organization still had no firm stance on how to deal with female athletes with extraordinarily high levels of testosterone. Following a decision from the International Court for Arbitration in Sport (CAS), the IAAF was obliged in 2015 to change their rules relating to this condition, technically called "hyperandrogenism." The court referred, in its decision, to inadequate proof that testosterone had a performance-enhancing effect on women. See (Tucker, 2019).
2 In 2019 the IAAF re-opened the case, demanding that athletes with testosterone levels above 5 nmol/l who were competing in the 400 m, 800 m, 1500 m and 1 mile events should take medicine to lower their testosterone below the 5 nmol/l level. CAS confirmed the IAAF ruling, once again taking Semenya out of competition, which gave rise to further heated debate on the issue. For a thorough and unbiased introduction to the case, see South African sport scientist Ross Tucker's page: The Science of Sport: https://sportsscientists.com/ (accessed on 28 October 2019).
3 My heartfelt thanks are due to the Danish sport philosopher Rasmus Bysted Møller for drawing my attention to Klawonn's work, and for making the concepts in this section more precise.
4 The "I" or first-person perspective can, however, be affected by hallucinogenic substances as found in mushrooms, drugs, alcohol and other substances. Sometimes the experience is so strong that the affected person will use expressions like "I was not myself" or "I was beside myself." Meanwhile, someone's ability to make that assessment shows that, in their normal condition, the "I" and the first-person perspective are stable. The person "has a grip on themselves," or feels like they "have themselves under control."
5 The fact that we have different roles with different contents in different situations has motivated several sociologists, most prominently Erving Goffman, to propose that our entire lives can be understood as an analogy to the different roles in a theater production. This extends to the way the roles in our lives are also found frontstage and backstage, and to the way these roles are associated with different

expectations. In other words, according to Goffman, identity is a social construct related to the image a human being is constantly attempting to present of themselves (Goffman, 1990). Working from the same observation, others have concluded that a human being therefore has not one but multiple identities; that they are constantly shifting; and further, that we have no sort of firmly rooted core identity. Instead, they claim, our identity is plastic and always dependent on the context in which we find ourselves (Gergen, 2000).

References

Cohen, S., Janicki-Deverts, D., Chen, E., & Matthews, K. A. (2010). Childhood socioeconomic status and adult health. *Annals of the New York Academy of Sciences*, 1186(1), 37–55. doi: doi:10.1111/j.1749-6632.2009.05334.x.

Encyclopaedia Britannica. (1998). Role. *Encyclopedia Britannica*. Chicago, IL: Encyclopædia Britannica.

Gergen, K. J. (2000). *The saturated self: Dilemmas of identity in contemporary life* ([New edition] ed.). New York: Basic Books.

Giddens, A. (1991). *Modernity and self-identity: Self and society in the late modern age*. Cambridge: Polity.

Goffman, E. (1990). *The presentation of self in everyday life*. Harmondsworth, UK: Penguin.

Honneth, A. (1995). *The struggle for recognition: The moral grammar of social conflicts*. Cambridge: Polity Press.

Jenkins, R. (2004). *Social identity* (2nd ed.). London: Routledge.

Jørgensen, C. R. (2008). *Identitet: Psykologiske og kulturanalytiske perspektiver* (Identity: psychological and cultural analytical perspectives) (2 ed.). København, Denmark: Hans Reitzel.

Klawonn, E. (1987). The I: On the ontology of first personal identity. *Danish yearbook of philosophy*, 24, 43–75.

Klawonn, E. (1990). On personal identity: defence of a form of non-reductionism. *Danish yearbook of philosophy*, 25, 41–59.

McCrae, R. R., & Allik, J. (2002). *The five-factor model of personality across cultures*. New York: Kluwer Academic.

McCrae, R. R., & Costa, P. T. (1999). A five-factor theory of personality. *Handbook of personality: Theory and research*, 2, 139–153.

Smith, D. (2009, 10 September). Report claims 800m world champion Caster Semenya is a hermaphrodite. *The Guardian*. Retrieved from: www.theguardian.com/sport/2009/sep/10/caster-semenya-hermaphrodite-iaaf-test.

Taylor, C. (1989). *Sources of the self: The making of the modern identity*. Cambridge, MA: Harvard University Press.

Thyssen, O., & Dahl, H. (2006). *Krigeren, borgeren og taberen*. København, Denmark: Gyldendal.

Tucker, R. (2019). Caster Semenya. Retrieved from: https://sportsscientists.com/thread/caster-semenya.

Chapter 5

The allure of muscles, size and strength

Doing fitness training and lifting weights at the gym are not sports of the same sort as badminton, soccer or swimming. This may seem self-evident, but the observation is absolutely fundamental: If lifting weights or training for physical fitness is your primary activity — and not merely a facet of your sports training or a step in recuperating from an injury — part of the training concept is its promise of physical change, improvement or maintenance; a promise not present in other ("regular") sports. In other words, for serious gym-goers training is linked to the perception of bodily appearance, strength or health, as the word "bodybuilding" itself indicates. The intrinsic desire to build, change, improve or maintain the body means that such activities are centered around one's body image and self-image much more than activities like badminton, soccer or swimming, which focus on developing skills, potentially in a social setting. Of course, some workout enthusiasts end up going all in, in which case their original motive of improving or strengthening muscles, health or appearance can fade into the background, eclipsed by an ambition to take part in bodybuilding, fitness or powerlifting competitions. In such cases the activity's element of sport has crystallized as the primary facet of the activity, beyond the recreational level. On the other hand, for those who do not go all in, the aspiration to achieve bodily change is still deeply embedded in the activity. In this chapter we will see how these motives manifested among my informants.

The many advertisements in the public space for gyms and health-club memberships, and from manufacturers of dietary supplements and exercise equipment, contain an implicit promise that links workouts to change. These ads tell us on screens and billboards how they can help us get "ready for the swimsuit season," or "say goodbye to your old body" and "hello to the new you," which we will ultimately love so much we will have "nothing to hide." The main theme of ads for dietary supplements and exercise equipment is usually physical, bodily change. The visual language in such ads is a far cry from the Charles Atlas marketing that appeared in numerous magazines and comic books from the 1940s and onwards. Despite its stereotypical perception of gender and masculinity, as noted earlier this ad ran for decades, precisely because it played on the idea of the transformed phy-sique and personality as an elementary positive result of strength training.

I also saw this theme recur among my informants when I asked them why they had started working out. Their answers point to the way working out with weights differs, as an activity, from other types of sports, and also point to themes that are apparent in the ads for Charles Atlas and, more recently, for gyms and food supplements. These themes are: being fascinated by strength and muscles; changing one's appearance; becoming more attractive to others, and more contented with oneself; and not feeling like someone other people can push around. Several informants recalled the type of physical strength portrayed by male film and television actors, describing how this was a decisive impulse in their own decision to take up strength training. There is also a certain element of finding psychological security in one's physical form, as expressed, for instance, by Kasper, an interviewee of 21 who did intensive workouts, lived a highly disciplined life and had never used anabolic steroids:

> Ever since I was a kid, I've been fascinated by strong, muscular men. Back then there were these contests to find "the world's strongest man" and that kind of thing. And like all the other kids who sat there watch-ing those shows, I'd run around the house after the show, lifting stuff.

This fascination is recognizable in several informants in my study. It is also in line with the idea that in the classroom, muscles had the potential to make a "skinny little kid" rise in the boys' social hierarchy, keeping in mind that Kasper — now 178 cm tall — added: "As a kid I was always the wimp." Although this becomes apparent in different ways, looking up to action heroes even while feeling insecure and skinnier than your peers is a feature that recurs in a number of informants summing up what attracted them to weightlifting. Jonas, who was 187 cm tall and 27 years old, put this duality into words:

> I belong to the generation who saw the movies with Arnold Schwarzenegger, Sylvester Stallone, Jean Claude van Damme. We mirrored ourselves in that. And those guys worked out, so we did too. At the same time none of us were very good in school, so instead we found some identity and got approval for the stuff we did at the gym.

For Jonas and his friend, this fascination with the powerful, rock-solid, hypermasculine he-man, combined with the self-assurance and approval they achieved through workouts, was one reason they threw themselves into weight training rather than badminton. They both went on to use anabolic steroids and various stimulants, but as for this early fascination with strength training, as Jonas put it:

It was this thing about maybe being able to become a big, strong guy like that yourself. That's the image you got from the movies, and we thought they were just so totally awesome, those actors. Not that we really talked about *that* being why we wanted to start working out. But I've thought quite a bit about it since then, and as for us choosing to do that particular thing, I think it meant a lot.

The muscular bodies of the silver-screen heroes spurred Jonas on: He wanted to be big and strong too. Nevertheless, when it came to him and his friend starting to work out, he underscored that *"It wasn't because we were skinny or overweight that we started working out. And there was no bullying or anything in the picture either."* It was the self-image, the film heroes, the tough guys and the raw atmosphere at the gym they found appealing. Unlike school, which called for a certain type of conduct, the tone at the gym was frank and unfiltered:

They could've been, like, metalworkers, auto mechanics, something like that. Hard-talking, butch types who sounded tough. We liked their style, and we picked up some new words we could throw around and impress our buddies, so we felt like we were a part of this gym scene.

Another informant, 22-year-old Martin, who at 161 cm is rather shorter than most other men, was able to use his workouts to reinforce his self-image:

I'm not very tall, you know? So I thought: Well, if you're not tall, you've got to be wide instead. And there was this self-perception thing that came over me too. I didn't want to be lean and skinny. Plus, I've always been fascinated by people who were broad-shouldered and well-muscled.

But like Jonas, Martin refutes the claim that the fascination with strength training can be reduced to a question of low self-esteem: *"No, I've always had an easy time getting along with people and socializing, and I've never been the one who got pushed around or anything like that."* Based on these statements it could seem tempting to dismiss the issue of self-esteem as a key factor in the attraction to serious weight-lifting, but that would be unwise before we consider the role it did play for several other informants. Jesper, who is 27 years old and 172 cm tall, explains his situation like this:

I was the little red-headed kid with glasses, and with braces and freckles and a pale complexion too, and I was easy prey for bullies. I wanted to change that. I got rid of my braces and that was great, and then I wanted to do something about my size, weighing in at 58 kilos. So I starting working out when I was 18.

Jesper's motive links in with the young man from the Charles Atlas advertisement: Working out became a way for him to change his body and his self-image. Several years later he found out how anabolic steroids could help him grow even more. As he explained, his physical training did not have a functional perspective. It was all about vanity. "*It was the body aspect. I worked out for the sake of my own vanity, sure, but also, of course, because it's nice to walk around downtown and hear people say, 'Whoa, check out that good-looking guy!'*"

For Kenneth, who is 24 years old and measures 180 cm, the main object of strength training was not his looks, but the desire to achieve a sense of security through strength. He needed this to deal with his own insecurity in handling what he perceived as threatening social situations:

> My main goal has always been self-defense, and that's probably because of this basic feeling of insecurity I've always had. And that's probably the main reason why I work out at all. Let's say I'm out somewhere, partying or whatever. Then if somebody starts acting like an asshole, I have an advantage in that, hopefully, I'll be a little bit bigger and stronger than that person. So my motivation is pretty much linked to the security in that.

In my informant group, Kenneth was the one who most clearly expressed personal insecurity as a motivation for his physical training. In order to defend himself he had trained jujitsu for five years, but he discovered his techniques were inadequate if his opponent had more brute strength than he did:

> So you know, when I was just as strong as them, in terms of strength, it was pretty much equal. But as soon as somebody was a little bit stronger than me, I really had nothing much to throw into the fray. And then there were these two things I realized. One thing was, the stuff I'd spent my time training wasn't worth a thing. The second thing was, physical strength was really important. So then I started on some strength training when I was 18, and I kept that up.

Although Kenneth was focused on his ability to defend himself, this need had not arisen out of personal experience in critical situations. When asked how many times he had been in a situation where he had to defend himself, he replied: "*Not any, really. But it's more about the mental side of things. Because when I'm physically strong, I also feel mentally strong. It's probably just me, and the way it works on me.*" But Kenneth is hardly alone in such feelings. Being and feeling strong brings a feeling of calm and a sense of security that is also expressed in a person's body language. For one thing, the level of the stress hormone cortisol rises when a person feels inferior and holds a low position in the social hierarchy, whereas the level of testosterone rises when a person does well in competitions and is positioned at the top of the social hierarchy

(Mazur, 2005). Once a person has experienced that effect, this in itself can spur them to use anabolic steroids. However, Kenneth has not used steroids, even though he has studied the topic in depth and felt tempted to use them because using would enable him to more easily achieve the strength he believes he needs. The altered body image resulting from hard physical exercise is also a benefit he recognizes: "*The way I look, that in itself has also meant a lot. Trying to achieve some kind of ideal.*"

Another informant, Rasmus, also has a story where his own perception of his physique played a role. When I spoke with him he was 32 years old, 180 cm tall and strong as a bear. But years earlier, when he first began to realize what weightlifting could do, he weighed just 68 kilos. In his case, however, the influence did not come from Hollywood action heroes. Rasmus was fascinated by the extremely muscular bodybuilders he saw in American workout magazines:

> I thought I was pretty skinny, so I went over and worked out some, just for the heck of it. At the gym I met one of my friends, and he'd brought along some workout magazines that showed some seriously big guys. And that was just my source of inspiration from day one. I thought to myself, "That is just *so* insane. I'd love to look like that!" But at the time I wasn't aware it involved steroids.

Rasmus became aware of this soon enough, however, and he had availed himself of sizable doses while doing serious bodybuilding work to sculpt his imposing physique. But perhaps more interesting still, in the first analysis, is how "the extreme", in and of itself, can arouse such fascination. Anton, an athletic young man who was 22 and measured 188 cm when I spoke with him, also had personal experience with anabolic-steroid use and described his situation as follows:

> You know, I've always been fascinated by the whole workout thing. If I sat there looking at a magazine with a topless babe on one page and an über-muscular workout guy on the other page, I would look at him — not at her. Then I'd think, "Wow, that's what I want to look like!" 'Cause, well, I just think it looks totally cool!

Not everyone shares Anton's opinion, although many people do recognize in themselves the fascination with large, muscular, iron-pumping men. Still, only a tiny minority see their own bodily ideal mirrored in such bodies. Most studies show that men prefer a slim, athletic build rather than an extremely muscular, bodybuilder-type body (Barland & Tangen, 2009; Grogan, 2008; Pope, Phillips, & Olivardia, 2000), and most women find this body type distasteful or even repulsive (Gray & Ginsberg, 2007; Klein, 1993). In any case, the strength, power and brute force signaled by the bodybuilder physique exerts a fascination on some and may attract them to the activity itself.

The archaic imagery presaging the advent of the bodybuilder is the cartoon hero endowed with superpowers. The one who can beat the bad guys, save the good guys and never die himself. It is not necessarily the altruistic, self-sacrificing character of the superhero that exerts such fascination. Rather, it is the fact that the superhero transcends the human condition. That is also why advertisements for protein powders and other dietary supplements in muscle magazines still sometimes use imagery evoking "the beast" to sell their products. As 21-year-old Kasper explained this fascination, it is a feeling:

> that you're non-human. That you're Hercules. I mean, that's awesome. Everybody thinks so. There aren't many guys around who haven't read *The Hulk* or comic books with other Marvel characters. A great big ship of a man … I think at one time or another, lots of boys thought that was awesome.

At the same time Kasper realized the fascination was not about saving the world, like Superman, but probably more about saving oneself: "*You have to be as scary as possible. Also, a lot of guys do it to appear intimidating to others. That way people have to show them a certain amount of respect because they're big.*" This once again indicates a basic feeling of insecurity as an underlying motive to work out.

However, it is not only low self-esteem or a longing for hypermasculinity that make weightlifting alluring. In the long term that sort of negatively oriented motivation is hardly enough to sustain a neophyte's interest. Strength training and weightlifting also result in a well-documented feeling of general bodily satisfaction and well-being (Fussell, 1991; Klein, 1993; Monaghan, 2001). As Martin, my interviewee, explained: "*I've always liked all kinds of sports, but strength training gives you this pump. It gives you a different kind of exhaustion than ball-playing and team sports do.*" The special pumped-up feeling that weightlifting can bring to muscle tissue was something many people only became aware of after hearing Arnold Schwarzenegger explain this phenomenon in the film *Pumping Iron*:

> The greatest feeling you can get in a gym or the most satisfying feeling you can get in the gym is the pump. Let's say you train your biceps, blood is rushing in to your muscles and that's what we call "the pump." Your muscles get a really tight feeling like your skin is going to explode any minute and it's really tight and it's like someone is blowing air into your muscle and it just blows up and it feels different, it feels fantastic.

The explanation itself would hardly have garnered as much attention as it did, had Schwarzenegger not elaborated on the phenomenon in a more personal vein:

It's as satisfying to me as coming is, you know, as in having sex with a woman and coming. So can you believe how much I am in heaven? I am like getting the feeling of coming in the gym, I'm getting the feeling of coming at home, I'm getting the feeling of coming backstage, when I pump up, when I pose out in front of 5,000 people I get the same feeling, so I am coming day and night. It's terrific, right? So, I am in heaven.

(Butler & Fiore, 1977)

As Schwarzenegger's description indicates, like other strong sensations, the pump can be almost addictive. The diabolically tempting thing is that the pump is stronger when you work out on anabolic steroids. As Rasmus explained:

You get an extreme pump when your body's filled with juice. Achieving the same thing is absolutely out of the question when you're not doing a [steroid] cycle. You won't even get close. Even though you work out real hard, it disappears after 20 minutes. But when you're doing a cycle, it just stays there. Then you're pumped up constantly, and your muscles are really filled out.

Schwarzenegger has also stated that he used anabolic steroids during his bodybuilding career. Bearing this in mind, his enthusiastic description of the pump has presumably done very little to promote the success of anti-doping messages (Wikipedia, 2018).

The desire for change seems to be a basic component in the allure of strength training, but when it comes to practitioners' initial fascination with working out, this desire becomes evident in different ways. For some, anabolic steroids are part of the allure. Before exploring this issue, however, we must first take a closer look at the question of body image, insecurity and "the small man's complex" as components that can trigger an interest in muscle work and steroids. As we have seen, for several of my informants body dissatisfaction, or alternatively an idea that their body was not large enough, played a role.

Body dissatisfaction

According to an often-cited study published in *Psychology Today*, the number of men dissatisfied with their body grew from 15% in 1972, passing 34% in 1985 and reaching 43% in 1997 — the corresponding numbers for women being 25%, 38% and 56% (see for instance Garner, 1997; Gray & Ginsberg, 2007; Pope, Phillips, et al., 2000). This is a remarkable trend, suggesting that today more than half of all men are dissatisfied with their body. It also bears witness to a shift in the surrounding culture; indeed, an upheaval that has drastically affected the body image of large numbers of people. The trend in the numbers can be seen in parallel with the increased importance of the body in modern societies, in step with the growing importance of visual communication and greater focus on self-representation. This is in line with another development during the same period, where more or less nude men became increasingly frequent as eye-catchers in magazines, films, advertisements, reality-TV shows and music videos. The male body has become objectified, providing all sorts of products with sexualized ogling props in the same way the female body has done for decades. As described in Chapter 2, according to Harrison Pope and his colleagues, this development has led to a situation where many men exercise obsessively in the hopes of achieving a broader chest or a flatter six-pack. The research hypothesis was that the cultural shift had caused a number of psychologically vulnerable people to use muscle-building drugs in connection with their workouts, so they could live up to their own ideals and those of their surroundings. That is what Pope and his groups saw reflected in the remarkable numbers from *Psychology Today*, leading to the inception of their brainchild, which they named "the Adonis complex."

Although their assessment of the general cultural development is reasonable, the study from *Psychology Today* can hardly be seen as generally representing the body perception of modern males. Consequently, it is not necessarily true that only psychologically vulnerable men use steroids. First, the study cohort for 1997 consisted of just 548 American men (as compared to 3,452 women). Second, all of the study's informants were recruited among the readership of *Psychology Today*, which is about 70% female and 30% male. What is more, we must assume that this readership takes a particular interest in psychological issues, including various types of mental discomfort and dissatisfaction.

My misgivings that the respondent groups behind the surveys were not representative is supported by the failure of any other studies to reproduce its findings. On the contrary, a Norwegian study from 2009 indicates that just 20% of a representative selection of Nordic women over 15 years of age, and an even smaller percentage of men, were partly or greatly dissatisfied with their body (Breivik, Hanstad, & Loland, 2009). On top of this, another study among a good 5,000 Norwegians aged 19 showed that 22% of women and only 8% of men were either partly or greatly dissatisfied with their body (Barland & Tangen, 2009). A third explanation of the considerable discrepancies between the results from *Psychology Today* and the Norwegian studies also lies in the cultural differences between the US and Scandinavia. A fourth explanation could be the way the questions were phrased. Certain Australian research findings from 2004 are interesting in this context, as they show that when men aged 17–89 were asked directly whether they were satisfied with their muscle tone, 24% answered they were not, whereas 41% were dissatisfied with their central torso. However, when asked whether they were generally dissatisfied with their body, only 10% answered "yes." In yet another study, from 1999, as few as 6.3% of American men aged 16–48 stated that they were generally dissatisfied with their body, while inversely responding that they would feel better if they had better muscle tone (Grogan, 2008, pp. 88–89).

If you ask people about their own assessment of their distinct body parts, most people can find one or more features they are dissatisfied with, seen in isolation. And if you ask whether people would like to have a more physically fit body, most people will answer "yes, please." In the first case, the person's body parts are thought of as individual objects, separate from the person. In the second case, the person is actually being asked whether they would accept the gift of a more athletic appearance — without considering the huge effort it would actually take for them to become that physically fit. On the other hand, if you ask them how they would assess their body, all in all, most people view their body as a part of themselves, meaning that generally such a holistic assessment will show people as less critical. This interpretation also fits with studies demonstrating that general body dissatisfaction coincides with low self-esteem (Grogan, 2008, p. 87).

Other studies also confirm the input from my informants about how a big impetus for them to start working out was the desire to become more muscular. A number of studies have shown that, generally speaking, men would like to have a more muscular body than they currently have (Gray & Ginsberg, 2007). If you ask young men about the hypothetical possibility of changing their body, they answer that they would like to be more muscular than they are, and that they believe women prefer men who are more muscular than they are. Men especially want this added muscle volume on their upper body: shoulders, chest and arms (Grogan, 2008). Here it is interesting to note that the upper body is the area exhibiting the greatest difference in muscle strength between men and women, and that upper-body musculature is particularly receptive to anabolic steroids, as also discussed in Chapter 10. So when young men want a more muscular upper body, what they actually want to emphasize and strengthen are the body parts that most clearly mark gender differences (Mazur, 2005).

There are cultural differences in how much *more* muscular men want to be, and in what they think women prefer. One study asked male university students from the US, France and Austria to choose among pictures of male bodies, selecting the one they believed women would find most appealing. The men in all three countries chose a body ideal that averaged 10 kilos of muscle more than the average men in their respective countries. However, a follow-up study conducted in Taiwan found that men there had a body ideal with just 2 kilos of muscle more than the average man in their culture. The researchers concluded that ideas among Western men about what women find ideal lie further from women's actual preferences than such ideas among Taiwanese men. The study also showed that in women's magazines in the US and Western Europe, ads and images of bare-skinned, muscular men were much more frequent than in similar publications in Taiwan (Kanayama, Hudson, & Pope, 2012; Pope, Gruber, et al., 2000; Yang, Gray, & Pope, 2005).

It is plausible to assume that the media's exposure of muscular bodies contributes to the male understanding that Western women prefer a very muscular male body. However, this is not necessarily the case. Other studies have shown that women prefer men with a more "average" body. Austrian women, for instance, prefer men with about 9 to 10 kilos less muscle than Austrian men would like to have (Gray & Ginsberg, 2007). In short, when it comes to the ideal image of the opposite sex, men generally think women prefer more muscles on a man than women *actually* prefer. But laboring under such delusions is not the preserve of men. Women — and here we are talking women around the world — believe that men prefer slimmer women than men *actually* prefer (Swami et al., 2010). Our notions about, and endeavors to achieve, the ideal body therefore have to do with much more than appealing to the opposite sex. They also bear witness to a number of cultural ideals and, beyond that, to internal rivalry between men and women, and to a potential underlying insecurity about the individual's position in the social hierarchy; a position where the body, too, has a role to play.

The little big man

As noted earlier, several of my informants emphasized that the key reason they began strength training was discomfort about or dissatisfaction with their body, or a feeling of inferiority somehow caused by their body. The building of a more muscular frame and the consequent changes in one's body image were seen as a way to overcome this insecurity. Kasper, who spoke of how he was inspired by strongman competitions on television, explained:

> When I was 16, I weighed 65 kilos. Some guys were a lot bigger than me. Some guys still are. But I was also bullied a lot as a kid, so I think it's one of those inferiority complexes that first got me started.

Like the story Jesper related earlier, Kasper's account is in line with other research that shows teasing and taunting related to one's appearance can act as a prompt to begin physical training and steroid use (Gray & Ginsberg, 2007). The inspiration to lift weighs and work out at a gym is often bodybuilding. Alan Klein, clearly taking his cue from Freudian thinking, writes in his ground-breaking book *Little Big Men* (1993) about his observations among bodybuilders on the American West Coast in the 1980s. Here, under the men's impressive physique, he observed a lurking psychological insecurity. As elegantly expressed in the book's title,[1] he hinted that there might even be a correlation between physiological overdevelopment and psychological underdevelopment among these men. Taking an ethnographic approach, Klein had mapped out bodybuilding culture by participating in, observing and interviewing people at four high-profile gyms in Southern California. He stated that the impressively muscled body was a "psychologically defensive construct that looks invulnerable but really only compensates for self-perceived weakness" (1993, p. 18).

This perception has since become established as a general cliché about bodybuilders. However, there is a huge difference in culture and intensity between, on the one hand, bodybuilders in Southern California and, on the other hand, Danish youths and men who work out at their local fitness center. Caution therefore advises us to be prudent when seeking to apply Klein's conclusion to a Danish context. That said, several of my informants had also arrived at a view of bodybuilders and self-esteem that greatly resembles Klein's observations. Martin proved to be particularly aware of this link:

> There are lots of people in bodybuilding circles that really have no self-esteem, but who are trying to build it in a purely physical way. They build up their self-esteem by being big. But in reality, they might not be so hard to break, mentally speaking. But obviously you can't tell that just by looking at somebody. So, you know, you're pretty cool if you can get that 120-kilo hulk to give you a friendly nod. But is he really self-confident, or is he just a wuss?

My informant Dennis had been through the whole roller-coaster ride himself, starting with elation over his growing muscles and self-confidence, then enjoying the attention he got from men and women alike, followed by a depressive phase with serious side effects from intensive, uncontrolled steroid use. Reflecting on the "little big man" issue, he had similar comments:

> You know, lots of bodybuilders also like to wear tight clothes so they can strut their stuff. There's a hint of that: "Look at me, look at me! I'm big and strong!" And you think you are. But inside, you're actually a little boy. That's actually what you are.

I began this chapter by saying that weightlifting, with its promise of change, offers something different than badminton, soccer or swimming. Based on the input from my informants, Klein seems to have a point even in a Danish context. However, Klein further emphasized that cultivating bodybuilding as an activity was not merely an expression of psychological insecurity. It could also serve as a type of therapy:

> If not actually neurotic, bodybuilding is, at the very least, a subculture whose practitioners suffer from large doses of insecurity; hence, compensation through self-presentation of power to the outside world.

However, bodybuilding can also be seen as a form of compensatory behavior that can be therapeutic.

(Klein, 1993, p. 174)

So besides being a semi-neurotic compensatory mechanism, building one's body can help fight low self-esteem. Martin, for one, expressed this therapeutic element very concisely. Like Kasper, he took no pains to hide his motives for working out:

> It's a sport that changes your appearance. Not everybody needs to pump iron and get big to have self-esteem, but I feel like it bolsters my self-confidence to know that I do a sport that's visible, physically speaking. I needed something that could help my self-esteem. I see no reason to hide that. For me, that was important.

Martin uses the concepts "self-esteem" and "self-confidence" interchangeably. In the field of psychology, though, the two concepts are normally kept separate, with "self-esteem" denoting the basic feeling of value as a human being, which we have as part of our more or less stable core. "Self-confidence", on the other hand, is more superficial and can be affected by an experience of competence and praise from our surroundings in specific situations (e.g. Karpatschof & Katzenelson, 2011). At any rate, the thrust of Martin's statements is that being around 160 cm, he was certainly able to use weight-lifting to change his appearance and, consequently, to boost his self-confidence — and perhaps, in the longer term, his self-esteem.

With good reason Klein's thorough, well-researched book has exerted considerable influence on the academic literature about bodybuilding communities. But like all influential work, it too has raised opposition. This is perhaps most clearly expressed in the work of the British sociologist Lee Monaghan, who in many respects copied Klein's methodology. But instead of sunny Southern California, with its iconic gyms and Muscle Beach, Monaghan situated his study in the anonymous weightlifting communities of his native land, wet and windy Wales. Unlike Klein, Monaghan argues that previously experienced insecurity is neither a necessary prerequisite nor an adequate explanation for why people engage in bodybuilding (Monaghan, 2001, p. 10). Nor does he accept Klein's claim that by striving to achieve a muscular body, a person is *de facto* exposing their own insecurity, or even symbolically embodying a crisis of masculinity. Instead of taking a Freudian approach, emphasizing problems or deficits, Monaghan follows the path of the British sociologist Anthony Giddens, who emphasizes how a person's exploring and testing their identity through a multitude of potential lifestyle choices is a central element in modern human behavior (Giddens, 1991). So instead of claiming that something from the outside (culture) combines with something on the inside (a psychological deficit) and makes people work out and build muscle, Monaghan points out that bodybuilding is an elective activity that can become part of a person's identity. The mechanisms at work can only be understood if one also looks at the individual's experiences and thoughts about their training. In other words, Klein's analysis is located at a meta-level, where it tends to disregard the individual's involvement in their own physical-training activities. Although Klein's book is well-written and highly engaging, it is indeed hard to shake the feeling that right from the start the author had a particular agenda, which he pursues throughout the book. Based on this, Monaghan's critique seems reasonable. On the other hand, Monaghan's own embracing of the plastic identity concept in his Giddens-inspired approach is not without problems, as it seems to be disengaged from the bodily reality of the situation, which risks transforming our understanding of bodybuilders' motives into one of purely subjective lifestyle choices. In short, while Klein's approach involves a risk of drawing a stereotypical picture of bodybuilders as a homogeneous group of psychologically vulnerable men, Monaghan's approach, with his emphasis on individual choices and life history, involves the risk of atomizing our understanding.

Whatever a bodybuilder's motive, his or her body — its appearance, size and strength — has consequences for how that individual relates to their surroundings. And that is why changing the body can decisively influence that person's self-confidence and self-esteem.

Respect from others

The issues of self-esteem and body image were pivotal for several of my informants, not least Martin, for whom there was a huge difference between weighing 50 and 68 kilos. This was important not only for what he saw when he looked in the mirror, but also for the reactions he got from others:

> It's more about what other people do than about what they think of you. Actually, I've never really cared much about what other people think about me, as long as they treat me fair and square. But not everybody does that when you're 1.60 and you weigh 50 kilos.

Changing the body's appearance, whether because of low self-esteem or not, does more than psychologically ease the individual's preoccupations with how others see him. This circumstance is overlooked by Klein and by Monaghan in their analyses. A more muscular body has real, tangible consequences for a person's social interactions. This is how Martin described his experience of becoming stronger:

> I'm not the kind of person who exploits being stronger than other people. But there's a difference in the respect you get from people. It's

more the feeling of knowing that people aren't going to treat you like shit. Instead, they show you more respect. It's not about you being able to treat other people any way you want, but more about knowing that they're going to treat *you* fair and square.

It is worth noting Martin's use of the concept "respect." He does not talk about respect as a sort of conventional respect among citizens or as societal recognition, but rather as a sort of status he has achieved by virtue of his altered physique, which those around him take into consideration in their dealings. We are familiar with such special consideration or respect in situations where we face something potentially dangerous or fear-provoking. Good examples would be trucks on an interstate highway, a tiger at the zoo or the edge of a cliff above an abyss. These things *command respect* and must be shown special consideration because they involve a risk or hazard. The way Martin talks about respect has become quite common, and it appears in statements made by several other informants while talking about their own social hierarchies. It reflects the fact that evolution has endowed us with the ability to decode other men's positions in a hierarchy where access to resources is based on an assessment of upper-body strength (Petersen, Sznycer, Sell, Cosmides, & Tooby, 2013). The point here is that a person who emanates strength and visually exhibits muscles is sending signals both ways. The muscular body shows the person's surroundings that here is someone physically powerful, which makes others show special considerations or treat that person with respect, as Martin puts it. Such consideration makes the person relax and feel he can be comfortable in his own skin. This alters his self-image.

Anton explains that becoming stronger means you don't have to be so much on guard: *"Instead of being scared of other people and afraid of saying or doing something wrong, you relax more, 'cause you have more self-confidence and believe in yourself more."* A similar account of steroids radically changing a person's relations with others comes from a young Danish man of 23, who was interviewed for a university thesis about his own steroid use:

I have no regrets at all. Starting on 'roids is the best thing I've ever done in my entire life. Before, I felt that I looked like a little boy, on pictures and stuff. Now my face has more masculine features, and I have bigger muscles. I'm a lot better at talking with other people. I feel a lot better about myself. I just think it's awesome. People respond to me a lot better. Like, say I walk over and talk to a girl. Then I get a better response, because I'm more self-assured — and maybe because I look more appealing in terms of the kind of guy that turns her on.

(Vinther, 2016, p. 34, my translation)

Even though Anton is 188 cm tall, his experience with self-confidence and interacting with the world around him is, in many ways, reminiscent of Martin and the young man above. Here is what Anton experienced after becoming larger and more muscular:

> I've never been bullied, but it seems like I've always had low self-confidence, when it came to girls and generally speaking. But then I noticed, after I started working out, that my self-confidence just grew and grew. It's like you get stronger and stronger. And suddenly you're stronger than the people around you that you know, and suddenly you're bigger. And then people start using a different tone of voice, and respecting you. Things just changed for me. People's behavior changed. The way people talked to me changed. And then you get a whole different level of self-confidence.

Anton talks about "respect" the same way Martin does. The more respect Anton gradually noticed as he grew was not a result of what he *could actually do* with his muscles, but on what he *looked like he could do* with his muscles. This is a basic biological impulse, grounded in the fear of the consequences of violence. Humans, however, like numerous other mammals, are able to read or decode social hierarchies without first testing them, for instance in violent confrontation (Herbert, 2015). This is part of the appeal of the muscular body: It plainly signals where a person is in that sort of primitive social hierarchy, which still greatly influences our perception of social situations, even though it no longer directly relates to our survival. And the self-confidence Anton described as accompanying his new position affected him, and his perception of himself.

This also testifies to identity being variable rather than constant, and to our own ongoing preoccupation with identification processes; of *being* something and *becoming* someone, as argued by the Danish psychologist Carsten Rene Jørgensen and also by the British sociologist Richard Jenkins and the Canadian-American sociologist Erving Goffman (Goffman, 1990; Jenkins, 2004; Jørgensen, 2008). Nevertheless, Anton's description indicates an aspect that Jenkins and Jørgensen pay scant attention to, namely how important the body and body changes are to a person's identity. Jenkins sees the body as important, but in adults he only deals thematically with changes accompanying the aging process. Goffman also refers to the body's relation to a person's surroundings and its importance to identity, but he focuses above all on the face (Goffman, 1990). The significance of bodily changes for identity, as clearly evidenced in Anton's statement, are due not least to the way people in our surroundings react to the body we exhibit, thereby accepting and confirming the "new" identity, which can then take root.

Therefore, when Anton talks about the way those around him react to his bodily changes, it is not simply a misconception on his part. Experiments in

social psychology have demonstrated how people tend to be more considerate to men with stronger upper bodies, treating them with greater
respect. Two men with different physiques — say, one small and slight; the
other big and strong — will, by comparison, develop different understandings of the world around them based on their different experiences
during social interactions. Against this backdrop, they will develop different
self-images and ways of interpreting future social situations (Kenrick, Trost,
& Sundie, 2004). For instance, when men of slight build walk down a dark
alley alone at night, they rarely find that people walking towards them cross
the street to pass on the other side. Strong, tall, broad-shouldered men often
see this happen. Such differences in experiences cause people to develop
different self-images, different understandings of the world and different
learning strategies for how to act in different social contexts. Through the
prism of their various experiences, people acquire different behaviors in
various social situations. This is social learning grounded in concrete
experiences, based on one's own bodily appearance and physique, which is
consistent with what Anton said about how his surroundings reacted to him
as his physical-development project progressed.

Jesper had a similar experience with this. When asked whether only his
own perceptions had changed, or whether he also sensed changes in his
surroundings as he grew, he replied without hesitation:

> Really, really big changes, from the people around me. When I first started
> being able to wear a tank top, and … I feel kind of like: when you look at
> yourself in the mirror and you can see there's been a change, then you
> gain self-confidence, and that self-confidence is enough to make it just
> radiate out of you. And then when you've got enough of that radiation
> going, and when you've got an attitude … Just walking down the street
> with an attitude — not exaggerating, but just having an attitude — well,
> that makes people look. And just having people look at you …

This is a very accurate description of what a person who changes their body
can experience in the dialectic process with their surroundings. In terms of
identity, these experiences make a very strong impression, because the person's image of who they are, or want to be, are confirmed by their surroundings. As we have seen, Martin and Anton's stories are very similar to
Jesper's. This is how, through an ongoing dialectic process, new muscles can
change the type and the quality of a person's social interactions and thereby
also the person's body image, self-image and identity.

In her book *Body Image*, Sarah Grogan, a British professor of psychology,
health and well-being, describes body image as "a person's perceptions,
thoughts and feelings about his or her body." This description is quite
comprehensive and is also in line with the informant accounts above, as it
includes both psychological views and attitudes to the body and the person's

experience of bodily presence. However, Grogan loses sight of the bodily, physical dimension when she subsequently claims that body image is purely "socially constructed" (Grogan, 2008, pp. 3–4). Considering the discussion above, it is clear that our body image arises from the interplay with our social world. In that respect Grogan's observations are clearly right, but it is equally clear that the reactions we get from our surroundings, and the interpretations and learning strategies we develop on the basis of these reactions, are rooted in the physical, bodily reality and the range of shared conditions we have to describe and interpret our experiences with this reality. It is this reality that is the foundation of our immediate social interpretation and interaction, while the interpretations themselves are based on biologically embedded predispositions forged during the evolutionary history of humankind.

In Chapter 10, we will return to the discussion of human evolutionary history's influence on the issues of body perception and the use of anabolic steroids in gyms. So far, we can reasonably conclude that a person's body image cannot be understood as a purely social construct but is formed in a dialectic interplay between their own concrete bodily embeddedness, their self-image and the reactions from their surroundings. It is precisely because an individual's body so strongly affects the people in their environment — and these people's interpretation of and relation to the individual — that it can be so tempting to employ steroids to accelerate the muscle-building process.

Note

1 This was a loan from the 1970 film *Little Big Man*, starring Dustin Hoffman.

References

Barland, B., & Tangen, J. O. (2009). Kroppspresentasjon og andre prestasjoner: En omfangsundersøkelse om bruk av Doping (2009:3). Retrieved from Oslo: https://antidoping.no/sitefiles/1/dokumenter/pdf/omfangsundersokelsen.pdf.

Breivik, G., Hanstad, D. V., & Loland, S. (2009). Attitudes towards use of performance-enhancing substances and body modification techniques: A comparison between elite athletes and the general population. *Sport in society*, 12(6), 737–754. doi: doi:10.1080/17430430902944183.

Butler, G., & Fiore, R. (Writers). (1977). Pumping Iron. In G. Butler & J. Gary (Producer). White Mountain Films: Cinema 5.

Fussell, S. W. (1991). *Muscle: Confessions of an unlikely bodybuilder*. New York: Avon Books.

Garner, D. (1997). Survey says: body image poll results. Plagued by body image issues? The results of a national survey show you're not alone. *Psychology Today*. Retrieved from: www.psychologytoday.com/articles/199702/survey-says-body-image-poll-results.

Giddens, A. (1991). *Modernity and self-identity: Self and society in the late modern age.* Stanford, CA: Stanford University Press.

Goffman, E. (1990). *The presentation of self in everyday life.* Harmondsworth, UK: Penguin.

Gray, J., & Ginsberg, R. (2007). Muscle dissatisfaction: An overview of psychological and cultural research and theory. In K. J. Thompson & G. Cafri (Eds.), *The muscular ideal: Psychological, social, and medical perspectives* (pp. 15–39). Washington, DC: American Psychological Association.

Grogan, S. (2008). *Body image: Understanding body dissatisfaction in men, women, and children* (2nd ed.). London: Routledge.

Herbert, J. (2015). *Testosterone: Sex, power, and the will to win.* Oxford: Oxford University Press.

Jenkins, R. (2004). *Social identity* (2nd ed.). London: Routledge.

Jørgensen, C. R. (2008). *Identitet: Psykologiske og kulturanalytiske perspektiver* (Identity: psychological and cultural analytical perspectives) (2nd ed.). København, Denmark: Hans Reitzel.

Kanayama, G., Hudson, J. I., & Pope, H. G. (2012). Culture, psychosomatics and substance abuse: The example of body image drugs. *Psychother Psychosom, 81*(2), 73–78. doi: doi:10.1159/000330415.

Karpatschof, B., & Katzenelson, B. (Eds.). (2011). *Klassisk og moderne psykologisk teori* (2nd ed.). København, Denmark.: Hans Reitzel.

Kenrick, D. T., Trost, M. R., & Sundie, J. M. (2004). Sex Roles as adaptations: An evolutionary perspective on gender differences and similarities. In A. H. Eagly, A. E. Beall, & R. J. Sternberg (Eds.), *The psychology of gender* (2nd ed., pp. 65–91). New York: Guilford Press.

Klein, A. M. (1993). *Little big men: Bodybuilding subculture and gender construction.* Albany: State University of New York Press.

Mazur, A. (2005). *Biosociology of dominance and deference.* Lanham, MD: Rowman & Littlefield.

Monaghan, L. F. (2001). *Bodybuilding, drugs, and risk.* London: Routledge.

Petersen, M. B., Sznycer, D., Sell, A., Cosmides, L., & Tooby, J. (2013). The ancestral logic of politics. *Psychological Science, 24*(7), 1098–1103. doi: doi:10.1177/0956797612466415.

Pope, H. G., Gruber, A. J., Mangweth, B., Bureau, B., de Col, C., Jouvent, R., & Hudson, J. I. (2000). Body image perception among men in three countries. *Am.J. Psychiatry, 157*(8), 1297–1301.

Pope, H. G., Phillips, K. A., & Olivardia, R. (2000). *The Adonis complex: How to identify, treat, and prevent body obsession in men and boys.* New York: Free Press.

Swami, V., Frederick, D. A., Aavik, T., Alcalay, L., Allik, J., Anderson, D., … Zivcic-Becirevic, I. (2010). The attractive female body weight and female body dissatisfaction in 26 countries across 10 world regions: Results of the International Body Project I. *Personality and Social Psychology Bulletin, 36*(3), 309–325. doi: doi:10.1177/0146167209359702.

Vinther, A. S. (2016). *Steroidbrug: En kvalitativ interviewundersøgelse.* (Cand.scient kandidatspeciale), Aarhus, Denmark: Aarhus Universitet.

Wikipedia. (2018). *Arnold Schwarzenegger.* Wikipedia.

Yang, C. F., Gray, P., & Pope, H. G., Jr. (2005). Male body image in Taiwan versus the West: Yanggang Zhiqi meets the Adonis complex. *Am J Psychiatry, 162*(2), 263–269. doi: doi:10.1176/appi.ajp.162.2.263.

Chapter 6

Up close and personal with four IPED users

Based on the media's rather stereotypical representation of people who use anabolic steroids, one might expect my user-informants to have very similar experiences, motives and attitudes to their steroid use. In fact, they do not. As seen in other interview studies of anabolic-steroid users, I too found very different motivations and approaches in the stories my informants shared with me (Grogan, Shepherd, Evans, Wright, & Hunter, 2006; Kimergård, 2014; Monaghan, 2001). This chapter takes a closer look at four personal accounts, the purpose being to describe in detail their thoughts about and experiences with anabolic steroids.

Jesper: "I wanted to learn everything about how they work."

Generally, the users I interviewed in a non-career context were extremely frank and informative about their use of anabolic steroids and other drugs. This stood in stark contrast to what I had found earlier when interviewing top athletes. Although the stories of the non-career user group took different trajectories later on, initially there were certain similarities in their first meeting with image and performance enhancing drugs (IPEDs). What typically happened was that as their training developed, at a critical point they would start talking to one of the big guys at the gym, become fascinated by him and listen to his tips about how to more rapidly achieve the physique they desired.

My first example is Jesper. Responding to my opening question about why he began working out, he spoke of how he had always been *"the little red-headed kid with glasses, and with braces and freckles"* and so *"was easy prey for bullies"* (see Chapter 5). He explained that this was an essential incentive when he started working out at the age of 18:

> So then I worked out for a few years and I made progress. I started bulking up and I got the right results. And also, I was kind of interested in finding out: So, can this go any faster? Can you do something to make it go faster? Yup, you sure can: I said "hi" to the big guys over at the gym, and we started talking. And, you know, they knew — at least that

was the feeling I had at the time — they really knew what they were talking about. They'd done it themselves, see? And they invited me in and talked about the stuff. They told me: "You just have to take so many of these ones, and so many of these ones, and do this and that, and you'll get really big." And yup, I sure did. I put on 12 kilos in 10 weeks, so yeah, it worked. That's all there was to it.

Putting on more than 1 kilogram of body weight a week is a lot. Even if part of the gain is due to water retention, which is very common in those who use multiple types of anabolic steroids simultaneously, such weight increases are dramatic, testifying to the potency of the drugs. Even though, obviously, the weight increase also made him much stronger, Jesper's consistent goal was to work on his appearance and gain recognition. For him it was all about achieving a body he thought was handsome, and about boosting his self-confidence. Gradually he also developed an interest in the way the body reacts to IPEDs, and he began to advise others on steroid use.

The men Jesper met at the gym had instructed him how to proceed, and in light of the 12 kilos he gained it certainly seemed like a success. But as Jesper conceded in the interview, "it was mindless, back then. I didn't know anything about it, and I let someone else guide me. And today I know he didn't really know what he was talking about." So what looked like a success, weight-wise, was less sensible seen in a long-term perspective. That is why, after his initial experiments, Jesper tried to get a better grasp of how the drugs worked and how they interacted with the body's hormone system:

> I think I was only halfway through the first cycle when I started asking all the stupid questions. And then I found this site on the Internet where people talked openly about these things, where we could sit and guide each other. People who'd tried something out or read an article about something in a medical journal. And people took their knowledge from there, and then you could draw your own conclusions, since there really were no conclusions in this area, you know? Because there weren't. Not really, anyway.

In this way Jesper gradually accumulated knowledge he could use to select the best products, dose the drugs in the appropriate amounts and use them to compose cycles based on the criterion: greatest possible efficacy and lowest possible risk. This meant that he made an effort to understand the effects and side effects of the steroids:

> I went from being a clueless user — which I was the first time around — to start studying a little bit about it. I wanted to know things like: Is this the normal way to react? Is this the way you're supposed to do this, and will it hurt you?

Being aware that the country's official body, Anti Doping Danmark, did not share knowledge about how best to take anabolic steroids, Jesper sought information on the Internet and carefully chose what he believed he could rely on. This decision also meant he chose to ignore the warnings from what he perceived to be the three major "powers that be" on steroid use: the police, Anti Doping Danmark and his parents. These are the entities, he explained, that prohibit or condemn steroid use without being willing to discuss any angles or views except their own. In Jesper's opinion each of the three took an authoritative position, merely saying: *"It's illegal; it's dangerous; and you'll get kicked out of the house."* Instead of heeding their warnings Jesper sought out forums where his steroid use was socially acceptable: *"And so the people who accept it, you end up kind of trusting them,"* as he put it.

As mentioned in Chapter 3, one of the problems in finding knowledge about anabolic steroids is that for ethical reasons scientists cannot do studies with a "double-blinded randomized controlled trial" design to determine the effects of anabolic steroids, or of the doses and drug combinations used by some serious gym-goers. Studies have, however, been done with smaller doses, for instance when administered to healthy people and to cancer and HIV patients. Jesper examined the results of these studies and drew his own tentative conclusions: *"Since this group here has tried this out for so long with no drastic side effects, then we can step up the dose a little bit and take it over a shorter period of time, and so on."* He was well aware that one must be careful when trying to draw conclusions based on studies that got positive results on patients and animals, then applying these to the doses and cycles used in gym settings, so he also began to gather information that went beyond the effects of specific drugs:

> I've gone beyond listening to the users and started educating myself on the topic. How does it work? Why does it work? What should you take into account? That sort of thing. And this has been a process I built up through seven, maybe eight years. At this point, I think I could almost take some kind of exam in the human body's hormonal system.

Based on what he had learned, Jesper composed his own steroid cycles and put together an intensive training program and dietary regime. Unlike most others who keep their steroid use hidden from their doctor, Jesper proactively sought out a general practitioner he was able to inform. The doctor agreed to monitor Jesper's blood pressure, liver values and other key bio-markers during and after his cycles. They agreed that if the doctor said some of the values were alarming, Jesper would immediately stop his cycle. This agreement reinforced Jesper and his family in their conviction that he could minimize the existing risks. In a few cases the doctor interrupted Jesper's steroid cycle. In one instance the doctor warned him:

"There's something wrong. It shouldn't be this high." So then he tells me that either I have to put a lid on these oral steroids, or else I have to stop getting in touch with him, because he just refused to be a part of it. And then I tell him: "Fine. I'll stop now, and then we'll try to measure again in a few weeks." And that's happened a few times with some medications, when the situation has been alarming from his point of view.

During this period of his life Jesper organized his activities so he could focus on working out, eating and sleeping. Because he was in college he had ample time to exercise in the afternoon. In the evening he would prepare his food for the following day and plan his workout sessions:

But I didn't have time to work out twice a day — or else I would have. That's one hundred percent sure, because my life revolved around it. This also meant there was no room for cake, soda, alcohol and smoking. Nothing but sleep, food and workouts.

This lifestyle combined with steroids made Jesper strong and muscular, but he had no actual goal as to how large he wanted to be. Just bigger and stronger. When people he knew started telling him he was *too* big, it just made him happy:

That was the most awesome compliment I could get: "You don't mean you want to be even bigger?!" It was the best compliment I could get. And it's totally stupid, I know it is. But it was just the coolest thing, because if people were thinking that, there damn well had to be something in what they were saying. That's how I felt.

At the same time, his attitude towards the drugs changed:

Way back, I used to think of doping as kind of a no-no. You did it, but you didn't tell anybody about it. Today I'm not afraid to admit that for me, it's like lifting a dumbbell. It's a tool, like when you go to the gym and lift a barbell, or like when you drink your protein shake. It's the very same sort of thing.

Jesper's views reflect how, when a norm is overstepped often enough, and if something illicit is repeated often enough, it gradually gets normalized. This is a well-known phenomenon from the rules of social life (Ariely, 2012). In sport, this is true not only of non-competitive weightlifters and athletes but also in elite and professional sports, where a gradual breaking down of the norm leads to an altered perception of crossing the line. The American cyclist Lance Armstrong, when interviewed by show host Oprah Winfrey in

January 2013, related how over the years doping, to him, had become as routine an activity as pumping air into his tires and filling his water bottles.[1] Prominent Danish cyclists have given similar accounts of how using doping substances became normalized. One top-level cyclist interviewed for my own study of modern cycling culture related how, after feeling absolutely disgusted the first times he had to puncture his skin with a needle to inject himself, he later came to find "it became just as normal as brushing your teeth before bed-time" (Christiansen, 2005, p. 83).

So too for Jesper. IPEDs became a standard, integrated part of his life of working out and building a muscular body. Nevertheless, when he got what he referred to as his "dream job" after graduation, his intensive, targeted workouts and ascetic lifestyle were pushed into the background. But he remained part of the gym community and continued to use steroids when he felt it would fit into his life, and when he wanted to optimize the benefits of his physical training. Combining his own experiences, his self-studies and the knowledge-sharing that took place on the Internet site where he was involved, he began advising others on using steroids. He realized this was controversial, since people outside gym circles might perceive this as indirectly encouraging others to use IPEDs. But he was adamant about explaining that when advising others he would always focus on minimizing the risks they would run when using, so that people who took his advice wouldn't harm themselves one bit more than was strictly necessary. Jesper's philosophy was that if someone had decided to do something that was harmful, it would be better for them to get advice from him than from someone who didn't really know what they were talking about. When asked whether he had been involved in selling steroids himself, he immediately answered:

> No, never! I've never done that. Partly because I'm a moderator [on the Internet forum in question] and moderators aren't allowed to sell — that's the way it is. And partly because, you know, it's totally illegal. So it has to do with mutual respect, because if any of the moderators deal in there, they get taken out real fast. That's just the way it is.

To minimize the risks for the people he was advising, Jesper would elicit information about their age, training history, lifestyle and ambitions. Based on this he would decide on what approach to take in his advice:

> Should I try to stop them completely? Should I say: "Listen dude, it's not worth it. You can as easily put on those kilos without doping." Or should I advise them on how to use the drugs in a way that will be least harmful for them?

Jesper was fully aware that people who had decided to use steroids might tell him a story that fit the picture they thought he wanted to hear.

That's why oftentimes we end up with me trying to help them minimize the harm they cause. And that's the direction I try to steer most of them in. It's not hard for me to see whether they're overdosing. And it's not hard, either, to see whether they're running their cycles for too long.

Although he was mindful of the fact that lots of people did things that were just as ill-informed as when he took his first cycle, his gut-feeling was that most people in the gym world were well aware that using steroids has side effects:

Most people know that you don't just take a steroid and grow. It actually does something to your body. That's negative. No matter what people say: steroids are negative for your body. I don't try to hide that. But there are ways you can protect yourself, ways you can get beyond the side effects publicized by the media.

The perception that there are side effects associated with using steroids, and that virtually all users experience side effects, is consistent with a number of user studies. As mentioned in Chapter 3, Andrew Parkinson and Nick Evans found that in a group of 500 steroid users, 99% experienced side effects, and more than 70% experienced three side effects or more (Parkinson & Evans, 2006). Thus, there is little doubt that using anabolic androgenic steroids and doses above the therapeutic level will cause side effects. But back to Jesper's point, which was that one should focus on minimizing the side effects that will inevitably occur. Among other things, according to Jesper, people who choose to use steroids should remember to plan their cycle with an integrated after-treatment, referred to as Post-Cycle Therapy (PCT), and potentially also intermediate treatment, called Mid-Cycle Therapy (MCT). This is done to ensure that a person's hormone production is not too severely suppressed or put on hold for too long. As Jesper explained:

MCT is a mid-cycle therapy. This is what you take along the way, and you primarily take it for two reasons: one is to keep [the testosterone production in] your testicles in order. Or, well, you can't completely start up your own production, because you suppress it so much [with high doses of anabolic steroids] that the body will automatically shut it down. But you can keep it waiting in the wings. When you experience testicular atrophy [shrinking of the testes], you can keep them at an appropriate size. The other reason for MCT is psychological. Because your testicles really shrink a lot, but it's also been proved on the site [the Internet forum Jesper is involved in] that it's easier to get your production going after the cycle if you keep your testicles up and running along the way. That's why you take a few occasional shots of hCG during the cycle, as part of your MCT. You can use these AIs — aromatase inhibitors — in the same way, and they keep your estrogen level down so you don't have side effects like bitch-tits.

Jesper's explanation closely resembles what you can learn from reading a textbook or encyclopedia. Human chorionic gonadotropin (hCG) is a hormone that plays an essential role in pregnancy, closely interacting with another hormone called progesterone, among others. Some athletes use hCG in combination with anabolic steroids to prevent or reverse some of the side effects caused by steroids, such as gonad shrinkage and infertility. The mechanism is that when the male body receives a large external dose of artificial testosterone, its negative feedback loops will suppress the testicles' own production of testosterone, leading to testicular atrophy (shrinking of the testes). Using hCG during and after a steroid cycle can counteract this because, in men, hCG mimics the effects of luteinizing hormone (LH) that stimulates Leydig cells in the testicles. This results in the production of testosterone, thereby potentially helping to maintain or reestablish testicle size and testosterone and semen production (Melmed, Polonsky, & Larsen, 2015). A similar feedback mechanism can be activated by the aromatase inhibitors (AIs) Jesper mentions, which are substances that inhibit what is technically referred to as the "aromatization" effect of anabolic steroids. Certain cells in the body contain an enzyme called aromatase, which converts testosterone into estrogen. If given large doses of anabolic steroids, the body will convert some of the surplus (male) testosterone into (female) estrogen. A well-known side effect of this is gynecomastia, the development of mammary tissue in men, often called "bitch-tits" in gym circles. The formation of such tissue can be countered by using AIs such as the substance tamoxifen, often sold under the brand name Nolvadex.[2] That is also why Jesper wanted to encourage people to use a course of PCT after taking steroids:

> In strictly hormonal terms, you have to provoke the body to restart its own production. You can do this in two ways. There's one substance called hCG, which imitates the receptors. They think that hCG is the hormone LH, which promotes ... which makes you produce testosterone. So if you take it, then you'll produce some testosterone. But there's something else, too: The pituitary gland, in the brain, will still be shut down. It will still think you have too much testosterone in your body, and so it will shut down testosterone production. There's something called Nolvadex, and that's an anti-estrogen that blocks the estrogen receptor, so estrogen can't bind. Then your brain thinks: We have a lack of estrogen here, so it's time to produce some testosterone so that can be converted into estrogen, and so on. And these two drugs, working together, are what people use today. And with all that I've read, I found out that this is the best thing to do. And these are the things I tell people about on the Internet.

Jesper was clearly very interested in educating himself on the topic. As mentioned, he believed that when a person chooses to do something that is indisputably harmful for the body, then at least they ought to do it in a way that minimizes harm; something which using other medicine can help people do. The general rule he gave the people who consulted him was this: *"when they're going to go out and invest a sum of money in steroids, they ought to invest the same amount in protection. And that's what I'd really like people to understand."* The way Jesper explained it, it's not as if one PCT will have any decisive impact on that particular steroid cycle. In his experience, however, very few people stopped after taking a single cycle.[3] Most people want to try again once they've experienced the positive effects of the steroids: muscle growth, greater strength and libido, and potentially elevated feelings of well-being and self-confidence as well. According to Jesper, that's where it becomes problematic. The thing is, he explained, when people go through several cycles of steroids over a long period of time without protecting themselves with, say, a round of PCT, serious side effects can arise:

> If you're talking about the vanity phase, as I call it, meaning the four to five years of a man's life where you look in the mirror and think: "This just looks totally awful." If you look at that phase and you think: "Should I do PCT during the phase where I choose to be on juice, or should I *not* do it?" Then I think you can ultimately end up with some really bad side effects: poor sperm quality, mood swings, depression, all of that stuff. You know, it's a huge factor that if you have a testosterone level that's too low, you get depressed because you don't feel like a man. If you put enough pressure on your body, if you let it be down there in hormonal deficit for too long and you don't get it up and running again, I think ultimately you'll end up with huge side effects.

This interpretation, too, is consistent with the scientific research in the field. The positive effects of the drugs make it difficult for some people to handle the decrease in muscle volume and strength that comes in the wake of a cycle. Worse still, however, they can also feel less motivated, less decisive and less energetic. Finally, some users experience much poorer general well-being post-cycle, which may manifest as frequent bad moods or mood swings (Kanayama, Hudson, & Pope, 2008; Mangweth et al., 2001).[4]

Michael: "I wanted to be up there with the best."

Michael was an ambitious soccer player but left the game at the age of 26, dissatisfied with the levels of ambition and effort in the clubs he played for and in his teammates. They weren't passionate enough. He had always done strength training as part of his soccer-player regime, but when he left soccer he dedicated all his attention to working out, becoming obsessed with the idea of building muscle:

I just get fascinated by this muscle thing. It's the aesthetics of it that enthralls me. The fact that you can control your body in such detail, and so meticulously control your life. You have to do that if you want to get results, but it's the aesthetic aspect of it that fascinates me. The shaping; the sculpting. It rouses something inside of me.

What is more, Michael found the whole bodybuilder scene fascinating. That, combined with finding that he had a talent for this new sport, quickly got him hooked:

I've got a talent for building muscle super-fast. And it looks great. I naturally have an ultra-low body-fat percentage, and I don't have to do anything at all to keep my weight down. Nothing. So my muscles, they just build up super-quick. And without even using any kind of doping drugs whatsoever, I put on 14 kilos of pure muscle the first year, and I work out really hard.

After about a year's training without steroids, Michael increased his weight by roughly the same amount (14 kilos) as Jesper did in ten weeks on steroids (gaining 12 kilos). However, after a year with constant, rapid progression Michael's physical development started to plateau. This came as no big surprise to him, and along with his training partner, who had several years of experience using performance-enhancing drugs, Michael decided to continue developing his physique by means of anabolic steroids. He started out using "Thai pills," an oral product with the brand name Dianabol, which has been a starting point for many steroid users — perhaps because they are known in gym culture as "Arnold's breakfast" or "the breakfast of champions" with reference to Arnold Schwarzenegger (Fussell, 1991). But Michael quickly replaced these tablets with another anabolic steroid: Winstrol depot (stanozolol), which he had to inject instead. He actually liked the new product much better, as it seemed more effective and did not have the tablets' side effect of retaining water or depositing extra subcutaneous fat. Michael describes the years that followed as some of the best years of his life:

I enjoyed it. I was just one big smile. I was in the best mood in the world when I was working out, and after I'd worked out. I was so happy. So happy. I was doing something good for myself. The whole time I'm on steroids, I'm just the happiest man in the world. The happiest in the world.

His elated state was also associated with a certain amount of self-absorption:

I'm high. I can hardly get enough of myself. I get really narcissistic. Whenever I get the chance I look at myself in the mirror; look at the muscle tone and the striations. Then I stand there and flex my arms and my chest. A lot of times I just walk around at home in my apartment, bare-chested, or in just my shorts, and then walk over to the mirror to find out: How do I look? What about my thighs? How do I need to build? Do I need to work out more laterally for a while? I'm going around constantly assessing how I can get the whole picture to fit.

Gradually as Michael developed his physique, he also gained greater recognition in the gym community. His life became structured around his workouts, meals, restitution and drugs. He concentrated on his own personal project, but he was also honest about his priorities. Later, when he met a girl, he made a deal with her and spelled out his terms:

> "If we're going to be together, I can't have you freaking out the day you look into the vegetable drawer in the fridge and see that it's full of insulin and growth hormone. Or if you see 500 vials of something in my sports bag. Because if that's going to happen, were not going to be together." And then she said: "Okay. I'm all right with you using steroids, as long as you don't start on the nose candy." 'Cause that's part of the scene too. People don't drink, but to party to the max at weekends they do cocaine instead.

These were the conditions for their relationship, which they both accepted and respected. Michael's use of steroids, combined with his rapid physical development and his acceptance into and recognition from a community that worked out hard and seriously, gave him an obvious air of self-confidence, which he enjoyed: *"It gives you an extreme perception of self. A sharpness. An edge. I thought I was really handsome. When I stood there alone, I felt like: 'Holy crap, this looks amazing. Like totally insane, man!'"* At one point, Michael harbored ambitions of competing, but his intense drive meant that he was not content with starting at the bottom, in the lighter categories, and working his way up. He decided that if he was going to compete in the Danish championships in bodybuilding, he was going to go for the "90+ kilo" class — the most prestigious in the sport. Within bodybuilding circles this heavy category commands far more respect than the others. *"There's this whole different kind of status around it,"* he said, using a motor-sports analogy to explain the difference:

> So, which would you rather win: GP2 or Formula 1? Of course you can always go for GP2 to qualify for a Formula 1 seat later. But I'm going to skip that, 'cause I know I'm good enough to stand up there. In competition terms, I want to go right into the big category, because I can get there. I've got the talent, the genetics and the mentality.

His own approach and the complements he received meant he was not competing in the heavy category to be part of the scene. He wanted to win.

This was his impetus. He constantly wanted to get just a little bit bigger. To "*stand up there with the gods, with the greatest,*" as he put it. I clearly sensed during the interview with Michael that this combination of ambition, mental stamina and his approach to the sport added up to what the sports world often refers to as "a natural" or "a born winner." In Michael's case this also meant he had no illusions about what it would take for him to achieve his goals: large amounts of performance-enhancing drugs.

Michael related how the members in his local gym community got their knowledge about how to use and combine drugs from previous and current users in the bodybuilding world, based in Denmark and in the US. "*And we also know a couple of doctors who are part of the inner circle, but who aren't users themselves. But they do work out, and they know how this stuff works, so they can advise us.*" However, even though through these channels Michael and the others were advised of certain limits they needed to be aware of, health-wise, they exceeded these limits. When I asked Michael about his thoughts on health, his own health in particular, he replied:

At that point I've probably gone beyond the whole thing about this stuff hurting your health, or being dangerous. I've left that behind. I leave it behind the moment I start using Winstrol, and start to use lots of it. I use a whole lot.

This did not make him oblivious to the side effects. That would have been unwise, given that his focus was on competing at the Danish championships.

So I also take drugs that are supposed to make sure I don't get this aromatization effect — you know, the testo-tits and all that — and don't become a wild animal, mentally. I keep that in mind all the time. I'm afraid of overstepping some limit where I get crazy, 'cause I've seen so many people who get crazy when they're on steroids.

All in all, the efficacy of his drug regime was so good that he was not affected by the negative aggressiveness he had seen in others: "*Not at all. I'm in an amazingly good mood. And I have an amazing sex drive.*" Not long after this, Michael supplemented his steroids with cycles of growth hormone and insulin to build even more muscle, working towards the competition:

Where you get the biggest effect, I think, is when you pair growth hormone with insulin, and you pair that with testosterone or Winstrol. If you pair it with Winstrol, you're still razor-sharp and you just keep building muscle. You know, when I'd be sitting there in the sofa, I'd feel this tingling sensation in my body, like I could feel myself growing. I'd just sit there thinking, like: "Whoa! This is totally insane!"

Yet at the same time at this juncture the ambition had taken hold of him, beginning to gnaw away at his sense of reality. He gradually lost his sense of perspective, giving no thought to aspects of life that lay outside his sport; no consideration to his body, other than his purely aesthetic thoughts and doing what was necessary to keep from becoming "a wild animal, mentally":

> I'd reached the point where I would normally say: "No, now I'm going to take a break," say, four months off steroids. But I didn't. Now I was just on one cycle, and it was one long cycle. I didn't take any breaks in between.

Initially that did not worry him, as he believed he had seen others who could apparently handle such regimes with no adverse health consequences. But Michael's gradual shift away from alternating on and off steroids cycles, which eventually landed him on one long steroid cycle, was also fueled by a fear that had crept up on him:

> The fear that when I hit the point when I wasn't on a cycle, then I'd lose weight. That I'd get smaller. That this desire to be voluminous, big, strong, invincible, beautiful; that it would fade. That I'd go into a dive. So I just used some other products. Then I'd go with those for a few months, then I'd go with something else after that, and then a third product after that. So instead of taking a break, I'd just alternate the various products.

With his continuous need to become larger and stronger, and with his focus on the competition ahead, Michael could not mentally deal with the muscle loss he knew would be unavoidable when he stopped his cycles. He felt he would become less of a man when he lost muscle, so instead he increased the doses.

> And I start going overboard. Doses that are way too big. At this stage it's slipped over into abuse, 'cause I'm also mentally dependent on the stuff. 'Cause of the fact that if I stop now, things will start going the wrong way. I'd look forward to getting home and filling myself with steroids.

Meanwhile, his body began to react to the continuous treatment and the high doses of different types of drugs, and after almost two years with no breaks between cycles he became seriously ill. At this time, three weeks before he was scheduled to take part in his first competition — as one of the front runners in the heavy, 90+ kilo class — his body collapsed. He had become seriously big: "*I'm really heavy at this point. I weigh 108.5 kilos. And I'm ripped, cut down to a body-fat percentage of 6.2.*" Dizzy and with blurred vision, high fever and low blood sugar, Michael was able to contact his general practitioner and was immediately hospitalized. His dream of success at the Danish championships was shattered. In the weeks and months that followed, while convalescing he began to comprehend the severity of his condition, slipping into a depressed state:

> And those three months, when I'm staying at home, when I'm detoxing, I just have one long slide downhill, mentally speaking. I go from walking around being the happiest man in the world for four years in a row, to just being so glum. I'm just so sad. It's a very depressive state. I'm so incredibly sad. And I lose weight really, really fast, also because my mental state is so bad. So after just a week, I can't stand to look at myself in a mirror. And then I go through a long spell where I don't want to look at myself, even though obviously I'm still pretty huge.

After a detox period at home, Michael was readmitted to the hospital for a planned follow-up. During this stay he had a conversation with the senior specialist on the ward; a conversation he vividly recalls:

> Then the doctor comes in. She shuts the door and sits down on my bed, and she starts talking with me. Then I break down. I actually just sit there bawling my eyes out like a little kid. She says to me: "The next time you come out here to me, Michael, you'll be arriving in a plastic bag. Next time, you're not going to survive." That was a real slap in the face.

Here, Michael paused for quite a while. He was still, looked away, took a moment to regain control of his voice. Then he went on: "*It wasn't so much the fear of me kicking the bucket. It was just my entire dream of standing up there on the stage, sharp as a razor. It just disappeared. Everything had caved in.*" Learning of his brush with death made an impression, of course. But it was not the fact that he had been in a life-threatening situation that caused his despair. It was the feeling that something had been taken away from him. He felt it was deeply unfair that his body had not been able to handle the regime, and that he had not been allowed to compete and see his project through. At that time, however, he was incapable of accepting responsibility for his unfortunate situation. Instead, he blamed the doctor sitting at his bedside, having "the talk" with him:

> I was furious with her. I had to lay the responsibility on someone, and I laid it on her. It was her fault that things didn't turn out the way I wanted them to. It damn well wasn't my fault — 'cause I couldn't bear if it was. To have this whole entire world around it all ... just crumble, just cave in. And then if I had to carry that responsibility, at the same time as I had to stop this steroid abuse, which I was deeply, deeply mentally dependent on. I couldn't bear that. So my world falls apart.

At the time of his interview with me, clearly Michael was fully aware that his feelings of anger towards the doctor were a result of projection. Afterwards, he was grateful for their talk:

> I really appreciated the things she told me, afterwards. I've had this feeling a lot, like I want to go out there and visit her, just to say to her, you know: "I owe you one." I've felt like that lots of times. Just to show her that everything's okay.

Michael made it through his health-threatening ordeal. He left the body-building community altogether and said goodbye to many old friends, made new friends and got a new job. Even so, during the interview he did not act like some repentant sinner who was disgusted with steroids. He could still feel the fascination:

> I sometimes find myself thinking: "Wouldn't it just be cool to put the pedal to the metal again, and go full throttle?" To be back there again. Not for competition. Just because it's awesome. It's totally awesome. The whole entire experience. I sometimes find myself thinking that. And that's one of those abuse thoughts. It's a dependency thought. The mental dimension of it — like: Whoa! It's just awesome! And God, does it ever work on you. You just know what an impact it'd have, the next time you go work out. "Damn, this is good. And a month from now, man, I'll be so ripped."

But Michael steered clear and instead poured his passion into his job and spending time with his sons. In his training regime, progression and goals Michael had been dedicated and ambitious, endowed with the mindset of a top-level competitive athlete. Nevertheless, he found himself abusing steroids in a situation he could not control.

Jonas: "It was mainly about what other people were thinking."

As described elsewhere, Jonas began training based on his fascination with action-film stars. Along with the masculine atmosphere at the gym, these figures were a stimulating contrast to school and homework. He started lifting weights with a friend at the age of 15 or 16. But working out requires discipline and can be tough, so it was hard for Jonas to keep up his motivation. Meanwhile, his friend was an avid gym-goer and met a man who made a difference to both young men:

> But my buddy kept going. Then he was introduced to this slightly older friend, an acquaintance, who was much bigger. We thought he was ... "a man of the world," as you might say. Somebody who'd been around.

And, well, this guy was on steroids, and my friend found out. And then my friend wanted to start taking this miracle drug too. We're 19 at the time.

Without telling Jonas, this friend procured products for a steroid cycle, and even though he grew rapidly in size and Jonas couldn't understand what was going on, his friend staunchly maintained *"that it was just because he'd started eating right."* Jonas knew it was naïve to believe that explanation, because *"his head looked like a basketball."* At the time, Jonas could not make the logical connection between his friend's physical changes and bloating, a side effect of using synthetic testosterone. As he explained in the interview: *"I didn't know the first thing about it. I thought steroids were something professional cyclists took."* But while visiting his friend Jonas came across some hypodermic needles, prompting his friend to admit that his optimizing regime over the last few months had gone beyond just eating more oats and tuna. Having been revealed, the friend enthusiastically talked about how effective steroids were. *"And I kind of let my judgment be dazzled by the fantastic potential, by what you could achieve. He'd put on at least 15 kilos in those two to three months."* Jonas, convinced by his friend's apparent expertise, was persuaded to try steroids himself:

> He told me about how you did the deed, and I pretty much thought he was some kind of professor on the topic. All I had to do was buy about 600 dollars' worth and there'd be more than enough stuff for me to grow. I just thought it over real quick, and then I said: "Yeah, I'm gonna try this out. Yeah, this is what I'm gonna do. Heck yeah: This is what I wanna do with my life!" So despite the fact that I was 19 years old, again, I was dazzled by the film-star-hero thing. So I got a hold of the 600 dollars, which I gave him, and then I got a bag with some stuff.

After Jonas took his first dose the two friends went straight to the gym. Euphoric at getting started, Jonas immediately felt like the steroids were taking effect:

> And then we worked out like crazy! Just the feeling I got, knowing that, dammit, now I was on 'roids! So I stepped up maybe twenty percent or more on all the exercises. It was insane. You know: I was on steroids! I was ready for action!

Although the two young men had only limited knowledge, the effect of the drugs was clear, as Jonas explained: *"I went from 78 kilos to 92 on that first cycle, so it must've worked. But of course my face looked like a beach ball because of all the water you retain when you're taking that junk."*

At the time of his interview Jonas was quite obviously reflecting, from some distance, on his former steroid use. However, he still vividly recalled the experience of being on steroids and his own initial thoughts about it. At first Jonas set up a system and planned his cycles with help from his friend, who, with one cycle behind him, was the more experienced of the pair:

> We sat ourselves down with a calendar and laid out these substances in front of us. Then he told me to take it all over a two-month period: First, I was supposed to increase the doses a little, then take the highest dose for three weeks, then gradually reduce, nice and easy. And that sounded pretty reasonable; thinking a little bit about taking care of yourself by regulating the doses. To me, it almost seemed to have a doctorish feel to it.

This last comment is typical. Many steroid users have no more confidence in doctors' knowledge about anabolic steroids than they do in websites, or their friends. One survey found that when it came to the effects of steroids, a full 40% of users had more faith in their dealer than in their doctor (Pope, Kanayama, Ionescu-Pioggia, & Hudson, 2004). Unlike Michael, Jonas and his friend were not part of a gym environment that focused on pursuing the aesthetic norms of the bodybuilding sport. Their training was less structured, and it had no specific, objective goals. Generally speaking, Jonas didn't know what he wanted to get out of using steroids. It was just something he wanted to try out, so there was no long-term planning.

The way Jonas presented his story, at the outset he was probably more a follower than an initiator. When the products from the first cycle were gone, he talked with his friend about what to do next: "*But my friend, he kept going. When he could see that everything he had bought was running out, he just bought another batch. He just kept at it.*" Jonas had to decide what to do. His thoughts revolved around how he would maintain his motivation to work out with his friend and also continue to be part of their social circle if he wasn't on the bandwagon:

> I stood there and was like: "What's up with this? Do we just keep going, or what?" It wasn't like I was shedding muscle or anything. It was more the fact that I wasn't on 'roids anymore, so working out just got kind of dull. The others just kept going. "Well then," I thought, "I'd better order another batch." If nothing else, I'd be keeping up with the crowd. Plus, I could kind of identify with the others because I'd be on steroids too.

These brief misgivings and questioning the situation did not mean Jonas was trying to place responsibility for his actions elsewhere. No one forced or pressured him to do what he did, and he was not a tentative participant on the fringes of the group. He made a decision and obtained more drugs, and with his second cycle he abandoned calendar planning:

I ordered twice as big a batch and dropped the calendar. Now I just jabbed it in however I wanted, or whatever I felt like doing that day. I also got some pills the second time around, which I hadn't had the first time.

Just like Jesper and Michael, Jonas also altered his perception of what was normal. Even though his account about that period of his life was characterized by an ironic distance and by reflection, he spoke candidly about the gym environment and his own circle there, and about how he quickly increased his doses to

around 1,000 milligrams a week. That's so totally wrong. But you know, we didn't think of it as anything special. I was a twenty-year-old kid who maybe hadn't even topped out on his own testosterone production. So we're like: "Let's do some of these 'roids, man." And we sat there and took it before we went over to the gym. And it hardly mattered where we sat; we'd just jab the stuff in. The most bizarre thing is that it'd become just as natural as you and me sitting here drinking coffee. It became a completely normal part of us hanging out together. That's what it was all about. And I don't think there was anybody in our circle who didn't work out, or wasn't doing it. So from having a planned schedule at the beginning, it came down to me just having whole pile of stuff at home, and then I'd just keep going until it was all used up. And then I'd buy another batch. That's the way all the other guys did it too.

Instead of primarily concentrating on aesthetic and athletic goals and striving to meticulously, symmetrically build the body's muscles — like Michael and others did — Jonas focused on the recognition his larger body earned from his friends, and from their wider social and party circle. They also enjoyed the attention from the ladies:

When we'd go out, people would say stuff like: "Whoa dude, did you start working out or what!?" Yes! Suddenly people can see you're working out. It was just fabulous, you know? We'd been working out for years and years, but now suddenly people could see it. To me, this was clearly a positive thing. And you know, we thought this was something all women would fall for. So: time for a tight T-shirt, or a slim-fit shirt. It was mainly about what other people were thinking.

As noted, there were no athletic goals behind their physical training, so they had no focus on developing their bodies in a balanced way. *"There was no leg training. It was just total ice-cream cone — perfect for the beach."* There was no focus on diet either:

Not at all. None whatsoever. I ate a can of tuna a day. There were no vegetables in the picture, or any knowledge about how much protein you can absorb. Vegetables were for rabbits and fitness babes. And I had no problem at all eating a pizza right after a workout. We were about as half-assed as you can get. There was some talk about what you were supposed to eat, but nobody ever got seriously into that. It was just too much work, so we didn't feel like going into it. It was easier to just jab some juice into your thigh, instead of juggling pots and pans and all that.

At the same time, partying to the max, often at bars and clubs downtown, was part of their lifestyle; a part that was just as integral as the workouts and the steroids. Life in the fast lane called for a cocktail of booze, cocaine and amphetamine:

So, on weekdays it was the steroids that ran the show. We would rarely go out on Thursdays or Fridays. It was almost always on Saturdays. Then we'd get together after we'd been at the gym. First we'd eat a whole bunch of food, and maybe we'd put on a new, tight T-shirt or shirt. Then we start drinking, a few beers or whatever. And then somebody would put some amphetamine on the table. It was mostly amphetamine, which meant we could drink a lot and stay alert and awake. And sometimes, somebody would also bring some cocaine. And of course, we drank like crazy. When you've taken amphetamine, you can drink a lot more than you normally can, so we had maybe a whole bottle of booze, each one of us, before we went out. And then maybe somebody would take a shot of Winstrol before we left, just to get that little bit more ripped. Yeah, we had that whole thing going. There were six or ten of us guys, and only one guy who didn't work out and didn't take steroids. But then he'd take some of the other drugs, like amphetamine, instead.

This account from Jonas illustrates how initial experiments with steroids, prompted by young men's fascination with "big guys" and the tough tone at the gym, can gradually change to a situation where steroids become an integral part of an uninhibited "fast and furious" lifestyle. This is a far cry from the lifestyles described by Michael and Jesper, but the three narratives also show commonalities. One is that the doses they took were not very different; another, that their circle of friends changed. Because Jonas directed his daily life and his attention towards workouts and partying, his circle of friends and acquaintances also gradually changed: "As you get bigger, start using steroids, and work out with other people, you get other friends." And like Jonas himself had been persuaded by his friend to use steroids, he too persuaded others to begin using:

The good friends you've got from school or from your neighborhood, either they disappear or you drag them down with you. Fortunately, I didn't do that to too many people. But I did introduce a few people to the stuff. And I told them how fabulous it was. So it was *me* who was their professor, and *me* who had everything under control — even though I didn't have a damn thing under control. But you felt like you did, you know? So I think that I probably dragged two buddies down with me.

Jonas was clearly not proud of this role. However, his attempts to convince his friends of the blessings of steroids is understandable: At the same time as his circle of friends is gradually changing, he wishes to legitimize his actions by convincing old friends that what he was doing was right — by making them do it too. Presumably, this gave him a sense of psychological security and confidence in his identity, allowing him to assure himself that when the people around him were doing and thinking the same things as he was, it couldn't be so wrong.

As discussed in Chapter 4, identity has what we can think of as an internal and an external component. Other people's external definitions of who we are, shown as the way they treat us and what they say about us, is a decisive part of our own self-image and thoughts about ourselves. That is why it is not enough to claim an identity, or to send signals about an identity. The signal has to be accepted by the people around you, whom you perceived as significant, before it has any real importance. The ongoing dialectic process of integrating other people's views of oneself, and of communicating one's own perspective to one's surroundings obviously goes more smoothly if the views of others roughly match one's own view. In this light it is understandable that Jonas persuaded some of his friends to follow his example. Gaining recognition for what we do, say, and claim in relation to our self-image is a key factor, not least in the early phases of a person's adult life, when their identity is less firmly rooted.

What is interesting about Jonas, however, is that he could not reconcile himself with the self-image he had built. He became more and more uncomfortable with the lifestyle and values that dominated the environment he was in. He began to feel a hollowness in the camaraderie of his friendship circle's workouts and partying. After a couple of years the excitement and glamor were wearing thin. At the same time he had noticed there was easy money to be made on the gym scene, which began to interest him more. He set up shop as a dealer in steroids, amphetamine and cocaine. This career change was paired with a growing conviction that a life built primarily on workouts, muscles, drugs, ladies and partying was too superficial, so while he was dealing he slowly withdrew into the background of his circle:

I'd started selling lots of the stuff myself: amphetamine and cocaine. It had really taken off. I knew people who sold to some other people, and my name became known, and so people knew "he's the go-to guy." And it was, like, 50 grams at a time. As it ended up, though, the police had been tapping my phone for more than six months. And all of a sudden: "Gotcha!"

Based on the police's telephone surveillance and his subsequent arrest, Jonas found himself in a very serious situation. In spite of that, by his own account he had stopped selling amphetamine, cocaine and steroids and had pulled out of the gym scene when the police apprehended him, so he did not go to prison. Also, since he had gotten rid of the drugs, the police found nothing in his possession. Based on all this, the judge found that Jonas had left the scene of his own free will, and that consequently he would not benefit from a prison sentence. Instead he ended up with a suspended sentence and community service. His own explanation of why he had stopped using and dealing at the time of his arrest was mainly that he could no longer see himself continuing to be part of that scene:

I had actually stopped before the police moved in. Because I'd found out how ridiculous that entire scene is. Because drugs and steroids, they go hand in hand, and it's like that everywhere. Of course, not when we're talking super-high-level athletes. It's probably rare for them to take amphetamine. But in the world I know, everyone who's done steroids has also done drugs.

One thing Jonas realized was that one of the people he had looked up to was not as epically cool as Jonas had imagined. The man had been bullied in his youth, and his strategy to get away from that life had been to take steroids, get tattoos, become big and strong and beat up anyone who got in his way:

And then this bell started ringing in my head. About how the only thing they have in their lives is workouts and steroids, and that they're addicted to it. They're addicted to that drive; the way it has to keep getting more and more wild. That was probably it. I found out it really is a putrid scene. And that probably speaks to my credit: I found out how stereotypical that world is, how mediocre it really is. So it wasn't because the police hauled my ass in that my eyes were opened to this. It was more like, little by little, the pieces of the puzzle fell into place.

This is quite a momentous insight, and almost certainly a difficult one for others in a similar situation to reach, given that it also requires them to confront and refute the image and role they have constructed for themselves. In conventional thinking, people who end up in such a criminal environment are stuck there until some external party — a social worker, a police officer, a new partner — helps them reach new insights and can pull them out of their setting. This common belief, which is somewhat deterministic, comes partly from sociologists who have thematically uncovered how the labeling and stigmatization of people as "criminal deviants" or "delinquents" gives them an identity as precisely that, which they then assume and thereby confirm (see, for instance, Becker, 1991; Goffman, 1990). The story we have from Jonas tells us that people have the ability to reflect on external identification and go against it. We must therefore be more aware of the decision-making processes at work in those identified as "deviant." The role as a socially deviant drug dealer was not just something Jonas passively received, from the outside, and took upon himself. Initially it was a role he actively sought out and could use for his own self-image, one reason being that it was precisely that: deviant. He was conscious about this role, knew of its privileges and had a fairly good idea of how deviant he was, but he grew out of the role. According to Jonas himself, the insight that he was no longer able or willing to identify with life as a steroid user and party animal was something that only gradually crystallized. Although his social circle remained in that setting, he successfully rebutted their attempts to pull him back. He did not replace all his gym friends at once, but simply steered clear of steroids, drugs and partying. He was able to handle the opposition this gave him because he was certain of his decision to stop, and gradually his friends accepted the situation:

> It was only the first few months when they'd be like: "Boy, you sure got skinny!" For all the positive input you get around town when you got big, you get just as much negative input when you're not big anymore: "Whoa, what's up bro? Did you stop working out?" That kind of thing. That's what it was like for the first three months. So you just had to get over that hurdle. All the comments you'd shot off yourself, well, there they were, comin' right back at you. But I have to say, I felt so much better not doing it anymore that it was okay. Well, true, at the very start I thought, like: "I wonder if I could just …?" But the more time that went by, the more I could just let it slide.

It takes a good measure of mental fortitude to make it through the process Jonas described to me. He was well aware that he had not always had that strength. For instance, his insecurity in school was one of the reasons he originally felt drawn to gym culture: "*I think I became sure of myself. I wasn't always like that. Looking back at my insecure school years, it wasn't like that. You see, my inner scaffolding wasn't too great. But I built it up.*" The security and the internal "scaffolding" enabled him, among other things, to distance himself from the gym circle and the customers to whom he had started selling drugs:

Finally, I just couldn't see myself as a "drug gangsta" type. From then on, it was just business. "You're the stupid ones. You're the ones sitting there taking that shit; the shit you buy off of me. I'm the one making big bucks off you." I think that was the way I found out. I could look at the situation and say: "Who are the smart guys here, and who are the stupid guys?" That's why I could see it was *not* a scene I wanted to be a part of.

Eight months after Jonas had stopped using drugs himself, and largely stopped dealing as well, the police came knocking. As mentioned, he was fortunate enough to end up with a suspended sentence and community service.

Since then, he has neither used nor dealt in steroids or other drugs. At the time of the interview he was still seeing four or five of his old friends who were still using steroids. He had tried telling them it was not a good life choice, but on the other hand he didn't want to play the repentant sinner:

I've told them: "Don't do it!" But that doesn't get me anywhere. Anyway, it's people's own business. I've been there myself, so who am I to say: "Now I see it all so clearly." That's really stupid, too. Of course it's stupid to do steroids, but if they want to do it, then do it. It's none of my business.

Jonas also made new friends, some at college, where he earned his degree as a social educator, and some at the fitness center where he later started exercising. He got a steady girlfriend and a job, and he began strength training again, realizing how important it was to eat right to achieve good outcomes from one's training. When I spoke to him he felt stronger and in better physical shape than when he was on steroids. In that sense his narrative is a success story. He went through a phase with unbridled use of steroids and other drugs, then a phase of dealing and being sentenced, then recognized that was not what he wanted to do with his life. I can hardly imagine him agreeing to give an interview while he was in the thick of it. But because he had moved on, taking a new direction, he reacted to the notice I posted and he saw the interview as an opportunity for him to tell his story — to me and to himself. When I posed my final question about how he was doing at this point, he replied: "*Really good! I'm so sure of my own identity and my own life now that whatever my old friends do, it doesn't matter to me. Not one bit.*"

Adam: "I just want to feel really good"

Among my informants, Adam, who was 36 years old when I spoke to him, had been the youngest anabolic steroid user in the group. After his initial, unpremeditated encounter with steroids as a teenager he stayed away from the drugs for several years before starting up again. Originally, however, he had no desire to compete (like Michael) and felt no need to work on his self-esteem after being bullied (like Jesper). He explained that his motivation to start lifting weights had two elements to it: *"I think it was a masculine thing, and of course some vanity too."* When he tried anabolic steroids for the first time as a teenager there was also an element of rebellion, a need to test boundaries:

> I think I was 15, maybe 16 years old when I fooled around with steroids for the first time. Back then nobody knew what it can mean for the body. It can stop your bones growing and that sort of thing. There was no Internet where you could find information, the way you can today.

While the belief that anabolic steroids can hamper bone growth is widespread it is not thoroughly documented (Hoffman & Ratamess, 2006), and it is not the key message here. The point is that Adam was not particularly worried about his health when he began using steroids. At the time of the interview he had become more aware of the side effects and of his own health in general, wishing to avoid too many side effects. But when he went back to using steroids in his twenties, he did so with a new motive that went beyond size and strength. He decided to change his life: *"For quite a while there I'd just been vegging out, not socializing much, and not really taking very good care of myself."* Adam changed his situation, partly by starting to work out again: *"Pretty soon after that, it struck me there was something from the old days that could give you that little boost."* Then he began using again, doing what he described as careful little steroid cycles: *"I started out kind of nice and easy with some Primobolan, which isn't so heavy."* Here, he emphasized that in his case the aspect of body, looks and steroids definitely had a social dimension. It had to do with self-confidence and leaving the "vegging out" rut where his social life and health had been stuck: *"Yes it did, a lot. And part of why I use them was also to get started again, with my social life, and to boost my self-confidence. All of a sudden there were lots of girls who thought you were cute."* He immediately felt an improvement on just sitting at home alone, playing computer games.

Health was not a decisive factor for Adam. He was more preoccupied with his general well-being, although made a conscious effort to use in a way that — in his own estimation — would cause as little harm as possible while allowing him to reap the greatest possible benefits. I asked him what he got out of using steroids:

> Well, again, you know, it's about vanity, respect, well-being. I don't know whether I could have those things without steroids. Maybe I could, but I know it's easier to get them *with* anabolic steroids. And I'm willing to accept the potential risk in taking this stuff. But I don't think the risk is that big. And also, my goal isn't to work my way up to 120 kilos. So in that sense it's easier for me to maintain the level I have, or

to reach the goals I set, than it is for a real bouncer type who has to weigh 120.

This approach is well known from other studies of steroid users. Many users believe that as long as you know what you're doing, the risks are manageable (Bates, 2019; Kimergård, 2014; Monaghan, 2001). Adam knew, however, that anabolic steroids are not innocent candy, and that choosing to use them has consequences. Acknowledging this, he based his decision to use steroids on an assessment that the advantages of using outweighed the disadvantages. For him, it was a question of striking the right balance between pros and cons:

> As far as possible I try to listen to my body, and I take the different stuff you can take to minimize the side effects. This can be various things. If I'm doing something that causes aromatization in the body and makes estrogen I always take some kind of estrogen blocker, maybe Arimidex, Femara or Nolvadex, or something like that.[5]

Adam's ambition of trying to avoid serious side effects also meant he was very clear on which substances he was prepared to use, and which not: *"It's the health risk that draws the line. Getting into insulin; that's something I'm not going to do, because I know it can kill you."* I asked him whether he didn't see a paradox in talking about health even while using many different products:

> Oh yeah, I'm aware of the double-standards aspect in this. But that's just the way it is. I'm well aware that it's not healthy for the body, filling yourself with all kinds of stuff. But that's a choice I make, and I'm aware it can have certain consequences. But at the same time I feel like what I'm getting out of it weighs heavier than the potential harmful effects it may cause. So I try not to lie to myself or other people about that. I don't say: "No, no, it's really not that dangerous!" I accept the risks that exist.

One of the other products Adam used, besides his periodic steroid cycles, was growth hormone, which he took in small daily doses. But that had nothing to do with maximizing his bulk, he explained:

> I think it just keeps you young, you know? It makes you feel that little bit better. And I also feel more fully rested in the morning. Your skin starts to look younger, and generally I get more energy. I see it kind of like a dietary supplement for physical well-being. So it's not to achieve any particular muscle growth, but mainly just for well-being.

Adam's reference to human growth hormone as a "dietary supplement" is something of an understatement, but it does tell us about how he regards well-being: as the keyword in his personal equation. His choices are based on maximizing benefit, even though he refuses to gamble with his health. For Adam, the morally questionable aspect of using illegal substances plays no role at all:

> Morally speaking, I don't have many qualms. I believe in personal freedom. And I believe that heck yeah, people should be allowed to do whatever they want, as long as they're not hurting anybody else. That's the way I see it.

At the time of the interview steroids were part of his lifestyle, and he had no plans to stop using them. He was extremely frank about his aim with the substances and dietary supplements he was taking: "*It's not a question of getting huge and muscle-bound. At this point, I just want to feel really good.*" He had no plans to change the feeling this gave him, or the lifestyle he had chosen, in which physical training was a key component:

> I imagine I'll probably use this for the rest of my life. At least for as long as I'm capable of taking care of myself and getting my workouts done. But I think I'm more selective about the drugs I use, and the doses I take. And as time goes by, it also becomes more a question of feeling good and of maintaining a certain level, rather than setting unrealistic goals you can only reach by taking massive doses of something incredibly toxic.

Adam used anabolic steroids and other substances as part of a certain lifestyle in which well-being — physical, mental and social — was paramount. He had consciously reflected on his use, educated himself about the effects of the products he was using, and attempted to avoid side effects, of which he actually had very few.

In this, Adam resembled Jesper, but they also differed on two points. First, Jesper was much more focused on muscles and strength than on well-being, and second, Jesper focused much more explicitly on knowledge and information-sharing. But even though Jesper aimed to become big and strong, he was much more in control of himself and his steroid use than Michael was. Michael had become totally immersed in the values of bodybuilding as a sport — growth and aesthetics — and he completely lost control of his substance use. So much so that it almost cost him his life. Jonas, too, had little control over his substance use. He maxed out at the gym and on the party scene, caring little for tomorrow. His motives for using steroids lay in the recognition he gained from his peer group, and in the pulse-quickening training and partying that came with it. He spent little time contemplating questions like break times, diet and exercise principles, and he mixed IPEDs with alcohol and amphetamine when he was out on the town, until he realized the lifestyle was too hollow and superficial for him and gradually withdrew.

This chapter with its four narratives focusing, respectively, on minimizing harm; performance; fast and furious party life; and well-being, serves a dual purpose. Firstly, it illustrates the huge variety and the many shades of gray in the thoughts and experiences of anabolic steroid users. Secondly, it can give us a basic framework for generally describing the different approaches to steroid use. When we compare the stories of these four IPED users with other research done in the field, we can actually elevate them to a general level, which enables us to point out certain shared features among those who use anabolic steroids. In other words, these four narratives can provide a backdrop against which to sketch out an ideal typology for anabolic steroid use in gym settings, which I do in the next chapter.

Notes

1   "Yes. But — and I'm not sure that this is an acceptable answer — but that's like saying we have to have air in our tires or we have to have water in our bottles. That was, in my view, part of the job." [...] "And again I don't want this issue of performance enhancers to … again to me that was, 'We're going to pump up our tires, we're going to put water in our bottles, and oh yeah that too is going to happen.' That was it." Lance Armstrong's interview with Oprah Winfrey (Mahon, 2013).
2   See note 5.
3   Research in the field also shows that many users who start on anabolic steroids are firmly convinced they will only try it once, as in: run through one steroid cycle. See, for instance (Christiansen & Bojsen-Møller, 2012; Cohen, Collins, Darkes, & Gwartney, 2007; Parkinson & Evans, 2006).
4   In certain users a depression-like condition occurs after a steroid cycle is over (Hartgens & Kuipers, 2004; Sjöqvist, Garle, & Rane, 2008; Thiblin & Petersson, 2005). This is due to the powerful influence of testosterone, not just on muscle volume and strength but also on a man's general well-being (see Chapter 3). Following a cycle, the body is in a state of testosterone deficiency, after the large external doses of synthetic testosterone have put the body's own testosterone production on hold. Typically, a cycle gives the body 500–1,500 mg of testosterone a week (with some competitive bodybuilders taking upwards of 3–5,000 mg per week or more). When a cycle ends, this level can drop to almost zero, as the body's own production may have shut down completely. Compare this with normal levels in healthy men of 30–60 mg of testosterone weekly, stemming from internal hormone production (Hartgens & Kuipers, 2004). Deficiency can cause intense discomfort, so some users find it hard to adhere to the planned break between cycles, made all the more difficult by the memory of how good it felt to be on the drug. But by shortening the break and starting on a new cycle, users risk ending up in a vicious circle with ever-shorter breaks that ultimately disappear, effectively going on one long steroid cycle. The side effects of this situation can be extremely serious. This is the type of negative spiral Jesper wanted to prevent by integrating MCT and PCT when planning steroid cycles for himself and others. This approach, attempting to alleviate side effects of one drug by using another, leads users into "polypharmacy," the simultaneous use of many different types of medicine. This makes it even harder to transfer results from well-established, evidence-based research on steroids to the non-professional usage patterns seen in gym environments. Despite Jesper's good grasp of hormonal mechanisms, this means the knowledge on which he is basing his advice cannot be described as

scientifically based. It does not build on any predefined, systematic approach, nor does it stipulate any clear criteria as to which results are includable and non-includable. It is, instead, based on a subjective range of information from personal study of relevant Internet forums and magazines, and on knowledge-sharing with peers. The British sociologist Lee Monaghan has referred to this as "ethno-pharmacological knowledge," a concept that originally denoted an independent scientific research area concerned with documenting the medical knowledge of native peoples and the medicinal substances they use (Viljoen, 2019). An interesting point Monaghan implicitly makes by adopting this concept in his book is that one does not have to visit a remote Pacific island to examine the unconventional use of medicines among subcultural groups. The gym just around the corner may be an equally excellent object of study. In this context the concept "ethno-pharmacological knowledge" denotes the detailed understanding among laypeople in fitness, gym and bodybuilder culture of the pharmacological properties of certain drugs. This knowledge includes a certain taxonomic classification of various types of steroids; how to dose them; how to take them; and how to compose a cycle appropriate to one's goals (Monaghan, 2001, p. 95).

5 Both Arimidex (anastrozole) and Femara (letrozole) are anti-estrogen drugs (estrogen antagonists) developed to treat breast cancer in women. Some bodybuilders use these drugs to lower their estrogen levels in order to counter side effects (such as the formation of mammary tissue in men) that arise when the body converts excess testosterone into estrogen. Bodybuilders have also used Nolvadex (Tamoxifen) for this purpose for many years. The effect became well known after the "steroid guru" Dan Duchaine first recommended it in his *Underground Steroid Handbook* in the early 1980s. Nowadays, Nolvadex has lost ground to Arimidex, Femara and other drugs, because it also has an estrogen agonist effect, which causes it to act like estrogen in certain parts of the body.

References

Ariely, D. (2012). *The (honest) truth about dishonesty. How we lie to everyone – especially ourselves*. New York: Harper Collins Publishers.

Bates, G. (2019). Supporting men who use anabolic steroids: A sequential multi-methods study. (PhD Doctoral), Liverpool, UK: Liverpool John Moores University. Retrieved from: http://researchonline.ljmu.ac.uk/id/eprint/11012/.

Becker, H. S. (1991). *Outsiders: Studies in the sociology of deviance*. New York: Free.

Christiansen, A. V. (2005). *Ikke for pengenes skyld: Et indblik i moderne cykelsport* (Not for the money: An insight into modern cycling) (1st ed.). Odense, Denmark: Syddansk Universitetsforlag.

Christiansen, A. V., & Bojsen-Møller, J. (2012). "Will steroids kill me if I use them once?" A qualitative analysis of inquiries submitted to the Danish anti-doping authorities. *Performance Enhancement & Health*, 1(1), 39–47. doi: doi:10.1016/j.peh.2012.05.002.

Cohen, J., Collins, R., Darkes, J., & Gwartney, D. (2007). A league of their own: demographics, motivations and patterns of use of 1,955 male adult non-medical anabolic steroid users in the United States. *J.Int.Soc.Sports Nutr.*, 4, 12. doi: doi:1550-2783-4-12.

Fussell, S. W. (1991). *Muscle: Confessions of an unlikely bodybuilder*. New York: Avon Books.

Goffman, E. (1990). *Stigma: Notes on the management of spoiled identity*. London: Penguin Books.

Grogan, S., Shepherd, S., Evans, R., Wright, S., & Hunter, G. (2006). Experiences of anabolic steroid use: In-depth interviews with men and women body builders. *J Health Psychol*, 11(6), 845–856. doi: doi:10.1177/1359105306069080.

Hartgens, F., & Kuipers, H. (2004). Effects of androgenic-anabolic steroids in athletes. *Sports Med.*, 34(8), 513–554. doi: doi:10.2165/00007256-200434080-00003.

Hoffman, J. R., & Ratamess, N. A. (2006). Medical issues associated with anabolic steroid use: Are they exaggerated? *Journal of Sports Science and Medicine*, 5(2), 182–193.

Kanayama, G., Hudson, J. I., & Pope, H. G. (2008). Long-term psychiatric and medical consequences of anabolic-androgenic steroid abuse: A looming public health concern? *Drug Alcohol Depend.*, 98(1–2), 1–12. doi: doi:0376–8716(08)00191–00199.

Kimergård, A. (2014). A qualitative study of anabolic steroid use amongst gym users in the United Kingdom: Motives, beliefs and experiences. *Journal of Substance Use*, 20(4), 288–294. doi: doi:10.3109/14659891.2014.911977.

Mahon, D. (2013). Full transcript: Lance Armstrong on Oprah. Retrieved from: https://armchairspectator.wordpress.com/2013/01/23/full-transcript-lance-armstrong-on-oprah.

Mangweth, B., Pope, H. G., Jr., Kemmler, G., Ebenbichler, C., Hausmann, A., De, C. C., … Biebl, W. (2001). Body image and psychopathology in male bodybuilders. *Psychotherapy and Psychosomatics*, 70(1), 38–43. doi: doi:10.1159/000056223.

Melmed, S., Polonsky, K. S., & Larsen, P. R. (2015). Williams textbook of endocrinology Retrieved from: www.statsbiblioteket.dk/au/#/search?query=recordID%3A%22summon_FETCH-LOGICAL-a30872-42fa576401a0e013881ff98332f3158bb1362cb2ff176a0c6aa2322e137cb2ed3%22.

Monaghan, L. F. (2001). *Bodybuilding, drugs, and risk*. London: Routledge.

Parkinson, A. B., & Evans, N. A. (2006). Anabolic androgenic steroids: A survey of 500 users. *Medicine & Science in Sports & Exercise*, 38(4), 644–651. doi: doi:10.1249/01.mss.0000210194.56834.5d.

Pope, H. G., Kanayama, G., Ionescu-Pioggia, M., & Hudson, J. I. (2004). Anabolic steroid users' attitudes towards physicians. *Addiction*, 99(9), 1189–1194. doi: doi:10.1111/j.1360-0443.2004.00781.x.

Sjöqvist, F., Garle, M., & Rane, A. (2008). Use of doping agents, particularly anabolic steroids, in sports and society. *Lancet*, 371(9627), 1872–1882. doi: doi:0140–6736(08)60801–60806.

Thiblin, I., & Petersson, A. (2005). Pharmacoepidemiology of anabolic androgenic steroids: A review. *Fundam.Clin.Pharmacol.*, 19(1), 27–44. doi: doi:10.1111/j.1472-8206.2004.

Viljoen, A. M. (2019). Journal of ethnopharmacology. An interdisciplinary journal devoted to indigenous drugs. Retrieved from: www.journals.elsevier.com/journal-of-ethnopharmacology.

Chapter 7

Ideal types in IPED use

While media representations of steroid users are often very one-dimensional, the four accounts in the preceding chapter show great variation. This diversity can make it seem tempting to draw the diametrically opposite conclusion and claim that the variations are much too great to justify any general pronouncements about steroid use and users. However, that conclusion is also too categorical — and not very productive if we want to try to understand what is going on. Consequently, based on the four accounts, I propose a model that can explain people's approach to steroid use within the framework of four general "ideal types" of male anabolic-steroid users in gym settings. This will enable us to see a number of shared traits, as patterns based on user approach begin to take shape. The object of my ideal typology is not to place specific people in stereotypical boxes that disregard the individual's personal history, experiences and life trajectory. On the other hand, the typology does enable us to distinguish certain general features that can help us understand the differences and similarities among users.

We saw in the four personal IPED-user stories how Jesper built a sizable body of expertise and detailed knowledge about steroids, cycles and the body's hormonal system, focusing on maximizing drug efficacy and minimizing harmful effects. Michael was not concerned with his health but instead took a purely athletic approach, becoming totally preoccupied with building his body and channeling all his resources into maximizing his competitive edge in anticipation of the Danish bodybuilding championships. Jonas used steroids as part of a wild-child lifestyle that included workouts, party nights and other drugs without any sports-related performance goals or concern for his health. Finally, Adam was focused on well-being and developed a lifestyle-oriented approach to steroid use, mainly aimed at optimizing his own physical and social well-being without risking too much. While Jonas lived a risky life, Michael was the only one of the four who actually lost control as a user, ending in steroid abuse before he finally stopped using altogether.

Now, if we draw the personal elements out of these narratives, take the stories up to a general level and compare them with the international literature, we can set up a model to explain how steroid use is distributed over a framework of four general user types: *the Expert type, the Athlete type, the YOLO type* and *the Well-being type.*[1] Their respective positions in the framework are based on their understanding of, and approach to, risks and effectiveness — two issues or dimensions that recur wherever workouts and steroids are discussed, be it academic journals and books, popular magazines or Internet forums and blogs. The typology takes into account not only users' own subjective understanding of risks and effectiveness, but also what users have told me (and other scholars) about their substance use and other lifestyle aspects. The "risk" dimension focuses on how users themselves experience their health and the risks they run, and on assessments from expert health professionals. These issues are seen in light of the descriptions of which substances the person uses, which doses, and for which periods, as well as their overall lifestyle. The "effectiveness" dimension is assessed based on the user's aspirations and goals — from moderate to more extreme — based on the role they believe steroids play in reaching these goals, and based on their statements about how important effectiveness is to them. These issues are then correlated with the person's use of steroids and general training and diet patterns. Based on all this, we can begin by positioning the four types within the framework matrices shown in Figure 7.1.

Ideal types

We know that the most frequent reasons by far for using steroids are the wish to become stronger; increase muscle bulk; improve appearance; and thereby move closer to having the kind of body one covets as "ideal" (Cohen, Collins, Darkes, & Gwartney, 2007; Gray & Ginsberg, 2007; McVeigh, Bates, & Chandler, 2015).[2] The model sets out these general goals and motives, and the ways people pursue them, in a highly concrete way within the framework of the four ideal types.

In developing these ideal types I have drawn upon the thinking of the German sociologist Max Weber and his ideal-type methodology (Weber, 1970, 2013). Weber held that the social-science researcher's most important tool is what he termed "the ideal type" (rather than the individual concept), and that this analytical tool holds the potential to overcome the notorious boundaries in the social sciences between subjective meaning on the one hand and structural forms on the other. According to Weber, in order to establish an ideal type one must, in the first instance, be aware of the "social facts" — the things or phenomena to which the social actors attribute meaning. In our context here, the social facts are the values, norms, views and actions that steroid users express, specifically concerning their use of steroids, and more generally concerning workouts and the gym scene. The next step is to pay due respect to one's research question and synthesize the most relevant aspects of the social facts into an ideal type (Hekman, 1983). This exercise simultaneously points towards the two main aims of establishing a typology. The first is to combine people's subjective perspectives, behavior and meanings with more structural circumstances; the second, to assess on more than one dimension at a time (in this case, the dimensions of risk and effectiveness). The latter aim is what distinguishes a typology from a classification, which only operates on one dimension (Weber, 1970). The interviews were analyzed to clarify salient features in the informants' accounts of their IPED use, after which the key elements were synthesized relative to the two dimensions: risk and effectiveness (Christiansen et al., 2017). What an ideal typology does is not to describe a specific person, but rather to identify general features that apply to people with certain motives and a particular behavior. It should thus be viewed as a heuristic device that does not necessarily describe real-world people but is a way of learning about the real world (Hekman, 1983). Then, when comparing actual individuals with the ideal types, the point is not to make the person precisely match or mirror an ideal type, but to see whether particular features in that person, or their entire personality, approximates the type, thereby setting up a baseline or finding a way to explain potential discrepancies. Put differently, the core element in this ideal typology is not a specific user, but rather the characteristics of a certain type of user behavior. By now it will also have become clear that in this context the word "ideal" does not refer to something normative, nor does it describe features that are particularly desirable or worth emulating. As mentioned, the typology is inspired by the stories that Jesper, Michael, Jonas and Adam shared with me. In this typology, however, the personal aspects have been culled out and the narratives raised up to an "ideal" level, which was also in accordance with my reading of other interviews from my study and other international studies of comparable design. It is against this backdrop I venture the claim that the typology reaches beyond a purely Danish or Scandinavian perspective.[3]

The Expert type, the Well-being type, the YOLO type and the Athlete type

The two figures (see Figure 7.1 and 7.2) position the four ideal types in a matrix with "effectiveness" marked on the horizontal axis and "risks" on the vertical axis. Obviously the form is stylized, so a word of caution is fitting: Any attempts to devise a formula and precisely calculate a person's use or approach are futile. This is also why the axes have no numerical values. What their "low" to "high" ranges do offer, however, is an opportunity for us to understand the two dimensions as more or less prominent in a given person.

Beginning in the lower right-hand corner, an *Expert type* user is intent on exploiting the steroids he takes as efficiently and safely as possible, seeking to obtain the muscularity, size and strength he desires while not taking too many risks. He has considerable knowledge about drug groups, doses and

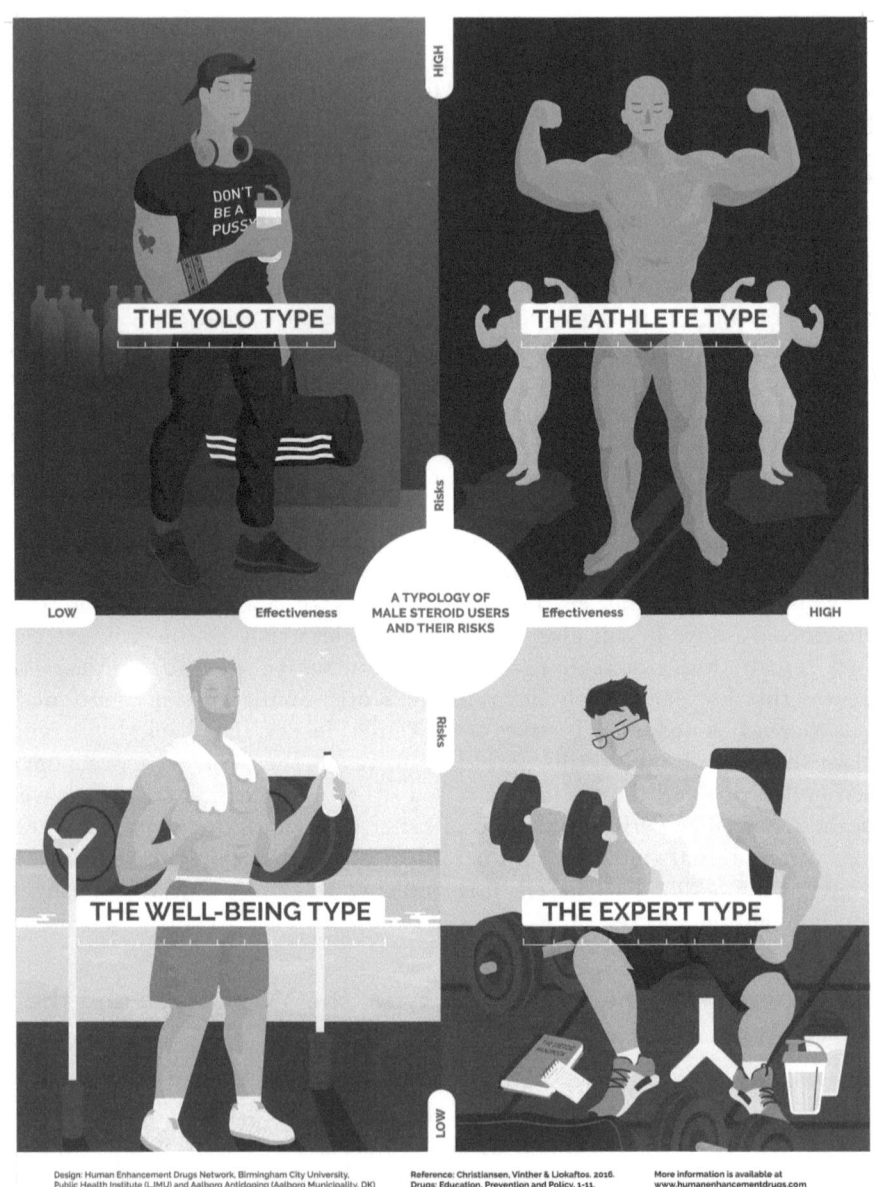

Figures 7.1 A typology of male steroid users and their risks

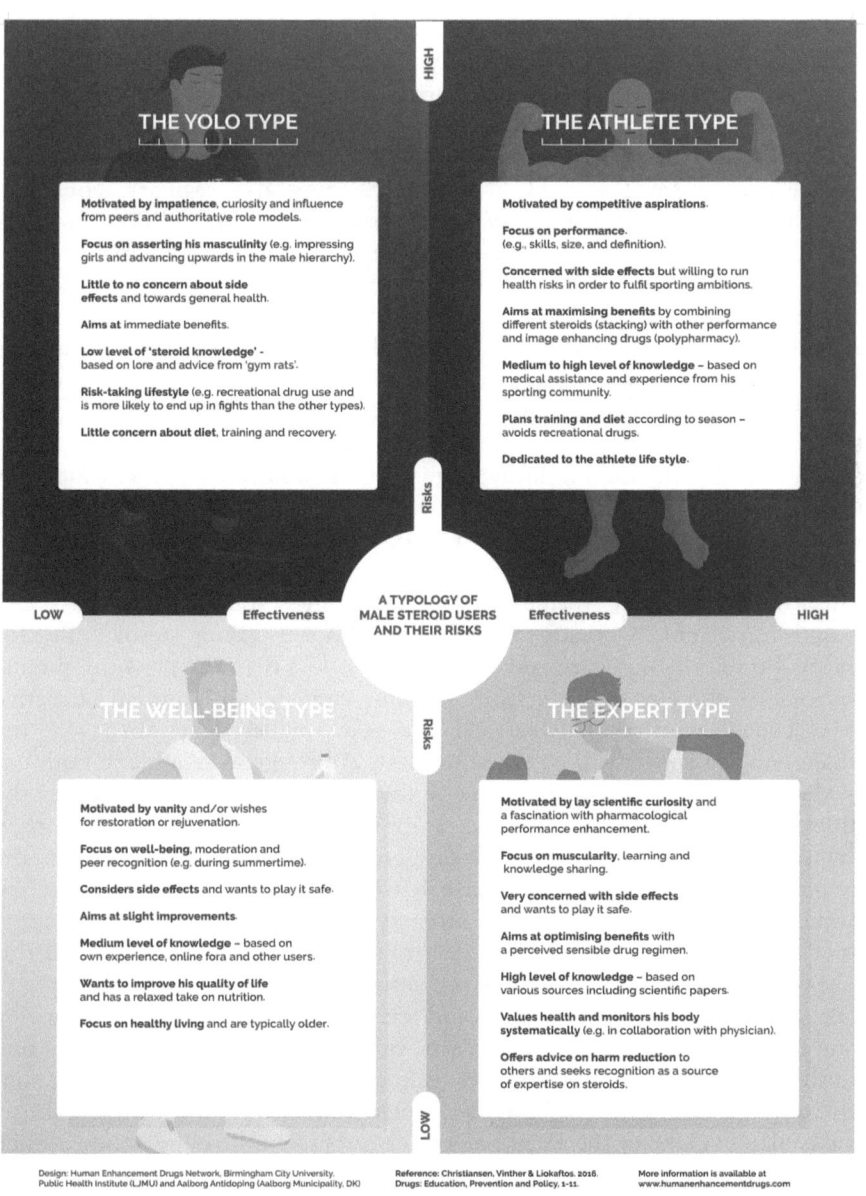

Figure 7.2 A typology of male steroid users and their risks
Design: Human Enhancement Drugs Network, Bir mingham City University, Public Health Institute (LJMU) and Aalborg Antidoping (Aalborg Municipality, DK). https://humanenha ncementdrugs.com/info-for-healthcare-providers/infographics/

cycle durations, and he also knows about the advantages and disadvantages of different combinations. He is highly risk-conscious and focused on minimizing risks, which is why he familiarizes himself with available literature, studying articles, blogs and websites on the topic. Using this knowledge he combines the drugs in various cycles and includes other medication, for instance during MCT and PCT phases. He may also regularly consult a physician who monitors his key health parameters. In addition to other medication he also spaces his cycles and varies doses to counteract the side effects he knows anabolic steroids can cause. He endeavors to make his knowledge base as solid as possible, because he believes that everyone who avails themselves of something as potentially hazardous as steroids ought to be conscious of the risks involved. Also, he believes that people generally know too little about the drugs and the risks of using them, and so he feels obliged to share his knowledge while at the same time taking pleasure in the recognition he gets for his knowledge and his ability to advise others. A number of other studies have also described users with the features this matrix attributes to the Expert (Christiansen & Bojsen-Møller, 2012; Hoff, 2016; Monaghan, 2001).[4]

At lower left is the *Well-being type*, who finds total muscle mass and strength important — obviously, or he would not be taking steroids. But for this ideal type, absolute size and strength mean less than the physical, mental and social well-being he gets from working out and building an attractive body. That is why typically he will also take smaller doses than, say, the Athlete, and his goals will be more modest. Although "the athletic body" is his ideal, he does not have the same ambitions for building his body as the Athlete type. Instead he aims for a more mainstream look, as seen in Olympic athletes like sprinters, decathletes or swimmers. Very often the Well-being type will previously have lived like one of the other types, so normally he is also older than the other types. He is conscious, and happy, about the social benefits associated with having an attractive body, and this makes him feel younger and more self-assured. He thinks about the risks of using steroids, does his homework and takes his precautions, for instance by using medication to counter side effects, but he is not a facts-and-figures buff like the Expert. The Well-being type exemplifies how in some respects steroid use is becoming part of a more mainstream health and fitness culture. This is also evident in the Well-being type's focus on "feeling good," which stands in stark contrast to the constant struggle for improvement that typifies the Athlete's approach. Often those in the Well-being quadrant have a liberal approach to steroid use, believing that people must assume responsibility for what they do to their own bodies. The Well-being type strongly resembles the users described in the study by Cohen and his colleagues (2007), but the approach and values this ideal type represents also figure prominently in several other studies (Hoberman, 2005; Kimergård, 2014; Walker & Joubert, 2011).[5]

Further up the axis, on the left, the *YOLO type* is prepared to run risks to experience life intensely. The whole YOLO attitude ("you only live once") implies living in the fast lane, going to the edge or beyond, despite the risks — since who knows whether you'll ever get the chance again? The YOLO type is largely uncritical and unstructured in his use of steroids. A lifestyle of partying, booze and narcotic substances means his cycles and workout sessions are less effective than they could be. He takes steroids because a muscular, well-trained body brings status and recognition among friends and peers and can also be a way to advance in the social hierarchy.

Typically this ideal type will have his steroid debut at a younger age than the other three, and more often he will have social-background issues. Of the four ideal types, the YOLO type is the least disciplined, and also the least aware of the nature and effects of the various types of steroids, doses and cycle planning and breaks. His unpremeditated "yeah, whatever" approach can seem naïve and reckless. He jumps head first into risky cycles and sees no problem in combining steroids with intoxicating substances like alcohol, marijuana, amphetamine and cocaine. The knowledge he has is mainly based on his own experience and tips from his peers or dealer, and his cycles are more likely to be based on what he has at hand, or feels like using, rather than following a planned schedule. He is aware of the risks associated with steroids but does not worry much about them, seeing them more as part of the package, a bit like a hangover after a night on the town. He has the same careless, happy-go-lucky approach to his health in general, and to his food intake in particular. All in all, his lifestyle causes him to end up in arguments or even brawls more often than the other three ideal types. In this context, the contested question of whether steroids lead to aggressive, violent behavior is irrelevant. The point is that a YOLO type more often gets into fights because of his lifestyle in general, which cultivates masculine group activities involving a variety of risk behaviors that may include violence. Describing the YOLO ideal type actually gives us a new and more comprehensive understanding of the correlation between steroids and violence; an understanding that can flesh out descriptions given elsewhere in the literature (for instance in Christoffersen, Andersen, Dalhoff, & Horwitz, 2019; Jenssen & Johannessen, 2015; Kanayama, Hudson, & Pope, 2010; Lundholm, Kall, Wallin, & Thiblin, 2010). The media often portray "typical" steroid users as YOLO types, and the features in his profile are well known from a number of other studies (Christiansen & Bojsen-Møller, 2012; Maycock & Howat, 2005; Monaghan, 2001).[6]

Finally, at the high end on both dimensions, in the top right corner we find the *Athlete type*, who is motivated by competing and performing well. He may be a bodybuilder, but he could also be a powerlifter or a crossfit or fitness athlete. He consistently focuses on progression, efficacy and effectiveness, not unlike an Olympic swimmer or a competitive cyclist who is constantly reflecting on all the parameters that are relevant to optimizing his performance. Each day he reflects on how he can improve; what to optimize. He also gathers knowledge that can help him become even better — tweaking workouts, increasing bulk, burning fat — as he works towards his ultimate goals. He is performance-oriented and competitive, perceiving himself on a par with other top athletes, and his physical-training regime is extensive, exacting and highly disciplined. Unlike the Well-being type, the Athlete is not motivated by what people outside the world of gym culture think of his body or his build. His approach to workouts, food, restitution and steroids is all about reaping the maximum yield on his investment. That is why he staunchly steers clear of parties, alcohol and drugs that may impair his physical condition. This dedicated, uncompromising approach is what tends to make him increase his steroid dose if his judgment tells him it will yield better results, or if he finds out his competitors are using higher doses than he is. So despite considerable knowledge about the drugs, he is more willing than the Expert to run health risks if he beliefs it is necessary in order for him to reach his goals. Several studies also provide good insight into the lifestyle of the Athlete ideal type (Klein, 1993; Liokaftos, 2017; Probert, Palmer, & Leberman, 2007)[7].

Clearly, YOLO and Athlete types tend to run greater risks than Expert and Well-being types. Similarly, the Expert and the Athlete focus more on effectiveness than the YOLO and the Well-being types. Further, although the four ideal types express different kinds of masculinity and are associated with different subcultures, our two dimensions — risks and effectiveness — are key to understanding their attitudes, approaches and behaviors regarding steroids and other drugs. As stressed earlier, no individuals in the real world live as an ideal type. Everyone will have overlaps, and at any given time a person will exhibit traits from more than one ideal type, just as a given trait can be seen in more than one ideal type. For instance, one trait shared by all four types is their conviction that as long as steroids are used wisely, side effects can be kept at a minimum (Grogan et al., 2006; Kimergård, 2014; Petrocelli, Oberweis, & Petrocelli, 2008).[8]

As we saw in the previous chapter, people who take more than one cycle of steroids will develop and change their approach and views over time. Moving from one type to another is not uncommon, and such shifts can be triggered by special events in a person's life: a change of environment, new knowledge or a new phase of life. The fact that such shifts occur does not undermine the quality of the typology or its potential to help us identify and understand certain people's approach to steroid use. A clear advantage in this typology is that it includes elements that are both structural and subjective. This means, on the one hand, that it can act as a bulwark against the waves of purely theoretical abstraction and, on the other hand, that it can serve as the life-vest that keeps us afloat, preventing us from drowning in the multiplicity of the social world.

Since the typology applies ranges that go from "less" to "more," and so is without numerical scales, those who use it must specifically assess each steroid user they know, or know of, to position them as deemed appropriate, relative to the ideal types and the two dimensions. Likewise, it is up to those using the typology to assess whether a person moves over time from, say, primarily being in the Athlete quadrant towards the Well-being quadrant. Beyond that, as we saw in Michael's case, some steroid users can also lose control of their doses and cycles and go from a user scenario to being an abuser.

The abuser

In this light, some readers might ask why the typology does not include a fifth type: "the abuser". The type who becomes dependent on steroids and on his physical size; who becomes unable to make it through off-periods and ends up letting one cycle of steroids blend into the next. I would argue that there are good reasons *not* to include the abusive steroid user as an ideal type. Foremost is the argument that each of the four types has an intention behind using steroids: achieving the ideal body, which involves a calculated and rational risk mindset (Expert); climbing up in the sport's hierarchy and competing (Athlete); achieving fast results and gaining social recognition (YOLO); or increasing one's general levels of mental and physical contentment in life (Well-being). No one aspires to become "an abuser" when they start using anabolic steroids. On the contrary, abuse is a situation a person will gradually slip or deteriorate into because there is a risk in using such drugs. Considering their overall risk profiles, the YOLO and Athlete types are in greater danger of developing abuse than the other two ideal types. Abuse situations can arise when a person's discipline in using the drugs weakens, when use of the substances spirals out of control and the person ends up in a situation that requires treatment, as we heard of in Michael's story in Chapter 6. Consequently, "the abuser" cannot be regarded as an independent ideal type on a par with the four others but is, instead, a deteriorated form into which any of the other four types might degenerate.[9]

The typology's usefulness and limitations

Looking at an individual IPED user over time, one can hardly expect to understand him based on a single ideal type. As the four stories in Chapter 6 demonstrated, users undergo personal development and phases overlap, which means any assessment is a snapshot of the here-and-now. As a steroid user gradually gains experience, his approach changes. Just as a real-life user may more or less closely match a certain ideal type — some Athlete types may be more dedicated than others, for instance — his approach and use patterns may also change. At one point he may fit best into the YOLO quadrant, but later a modified pattern of use may more appropriately reflect the features in the Well-being quadrant, as in Adam's case. Obviously, a person may even stop using, as Jonas did. An altered course in life may result from any number of circumstances: important life events, new knowledge, a change of scene, transitioning from one phase of life to another. Such circumstances must naturally be considered when looking at a person's steroid use over time. Nevertheless, in understanding the bigger picture of steroid use at a generalized level, this typology is a useful heuristic tool for shedding light on the individual user's approach.

So firstly the framework of the four ideal types enables us to identify general traits, and secondly it enables us to position specific users within a framework after assessing their positions on the two dimensions: risks and effectiveness. In this way the typology can also inform counseling and community-education campaigns to reach certain types of users (Vinther & Christiansen, 2019). What is more, although the ideal types occur in the same general environment, the typology shows the existing range of differences in personal experience and lifestyles, and it bears witness to the differences in the choices steroid users make. An important factor here, discussed in the next chapter, is how users feel and perceive the effects of their practice on their own body, and how they handle the side effects that almost invariably arise.

Notes

1 This typology is described in greater detail in an article I published with my colleagues Dimitris Liokaftos and Anders Schmidt Vinther; see (Christiansen, Vinther, & Liokaftos, 2017).
2 See also (Backhouse, McKenna, Robinson, & Atkin, 2007; Barland & Tangen, 2009; Kimergård, 2014; Pedersen, Ingholt, & Tjørnhøj-Thomsen, 2014; Pope, Phillips, & Olivardia, 2000; Sagoe, Andreassen, & Pallesen, 2014).
3 This view has been confirmed by the typology's reception at several international conferences, where it has been presented by myself and my co-authors Anders Schmidt Vinther and Dimitris Liokaftos. Feedback we have received from many sides — professionals in workout and gym communities, anti-doping organizations and professionals working with a wide range of substance use and abuse issues — shows that the traits described for the four ideal types are recurrently observable in gym environments in Denmark and elsewhere. The typology has also reached the wider workout community, as it was described over four pages in the Dutch edition of *Muscle and Fitness* (in the April 2017 issue) and also served as the theoretical framework of a study that described the motivating factors for 660 British users of anabolic steroids and other muscle-building drugs (Zahnow et al., 2018).
4 See also (Barland, Tangen, & Johannesen, 2010; Bilgrei, 2013; Grogan, Shepherd, Evans, Wright, & Hunter, 2006; Maycock & Howat, 2007; Walker & Joubert, 2011).
5 See also (Barland et al., 2010; Bilgrei, 2013; Pedersen et al., 2014).
6 See also (Barland & Tangen, 2009; Hoff, 2016; Khorrami & Franklin, 2002).
7 See also (Andreasson & Johansson, 2014; Fussell, 1991; Grogan et al., 2006; Hoff, 2016; Maycock & Howat, 2005; Monaghan, 2001).
8 See also (Barland et al., 2010; Walker & Joubert, 2011).
9 Generally speaking, the concept of "abuse" is hotly contested and difficult to define in any precise, practically useful way (Hernandez & Nelson, 2010; WHO,

2019). Some researchers have instead begun to talk about a sort of dependency on anabolic steroids that develops in some users. Although "dependency" is not an unambiguous concept either, it is easier to classify scientifically (Hildebrandt et al., 2011; Ip et al., 2012; Kanayama, Hudson, & Pope, 2009). Having said that, internally in gym communities the term "abuser" is often employed by steroid users who, perceiving themselves as serious, speak about others who have YOLO-type features or the like. In their eyes, "abuse" signifies the type of use that is not sufficiently well-planned, rests on inadequate knowledge of physiology, diet, training and hormones, or is simply unstructured (Grogan et al., 2006; Monaghan, 2001, 2002). To this group, then, "abuse" is what others do when using steroids wrongly, so when such users employ the term "abuse," they do so because others are breaking a norm that they (the self-perceived serious users) regard as right or appropriate. Among serious gym goers, speaking of "abuse" is therefore often an identity marker that is part of building social boundaries and defining those who are "right" as opposed to those who are "wrong." Hence, the self-perceived serious users apply "abuse" and similar language to users they consider inadequate at living up to their norms, values and rules for steroid use.

References

Andreasson, J., & Johansson, T. (2014). *The global gym: Gender, health and pedagogies.* Houndsmills, Basingstoke, UK & New York: Palgrave Macmillan.

Backhouse, S., McKenna, J., Robinson, S., & Atkin, M. (2007). International literature review: attitudes, behaviours, knowledge and education – drugs in sport: Past, present and future. Retrieved from: www.wada-ama.org/rtecontent/document/Backhouse_et_al_Full_Report.pdf.

Barland, B., & Tangen, J. O. (2009). Kroppspresentasjon og andre prestasjoner – en omfangsundersøkelse om bruk av Doping (2009:3). Retrieved from Oslo: https://antidoping.no/sitefiles/1/dokumenter/pdf/omfangsundersokelsen.pdf.

Barland, B., Tangen, J. O., & Johannesen, C. A. (2010). Doping, muskler, mestring og mening. En kvalitativ studie av unge menns bruk av muskelbyggende medikamenter. Retrieved from Oslo: https://brage.bibsys.no/xmlui/handle/11250/175072.

Bilgrei, O. R. (2013). Symbolske kropper – en kvalitativ studie av menn som bruker anabole steroider. Retrieved from Oslo: www.fhi.no/globalassets/dokumenterfiler/rapporter/symbolske-kropper-studie-om-anabole-steroider.

Christiansen, A. V., & Bojsen-Møller, J. (2012). "Will steroids kill me if I use them once?" A qualitative analysis of inquiries submitted to the Danish anti-doping authorities. *Performance Enhancement & Health*, 1(1), 39–47. doi: doi:10.1016/j.peh.2012.05.002.

Christiansen, A. V., Vinther, A. S., & Liokaftos, D. (2017). Outline of a typology of men's use of anabolic androgenic steroids in fitness and strength training environments. *Drugs: Education, Prevention and Policy*, 24(3), 295–305. doi: doi:10.1080/09687637.2016.1231173.

Christoffersen, T., Andersen, J. T., Dalhoff, K. P., & Horwitz, H. (2019). Anabolic-androgenic steroids and the risk of imprisonment. *Drug Alcohol Depend*, 203, 92–97. doi: doi:10.1016/j.drugalcdep.2019.04.041.

Cohen, J., Collins, R., Darkes, J., & Gwartney, D. (2007). A league of their own: Demographics, motivations and patterns of use of 1,955 male adult non-medical anabolic steroid users in the United States. *J.Int.Soc.Sports Nutr.*, 4, 12. doi: doi:10.1186/1550-2783-4-12.

Fussell, S. W. (1991). *Muscle: Confessions of an unlikely bodybuilder.* New York: Avon Books.

Gray, J., & Ginsberg, R. (2007). Muscle dissatisfaction: An overview of psychological and cultural research and theory. In K. J. Thompson & G. Cafri (Eds.), *The muscular ideal: Psychological, social, and medical perspectives* (1st ed., pp. 15–39). Washington, DC: American Psychological Association.

Grogan, S., Shepherd, S., Evans, R., Wright, S., & Hunter, G. (2006). Experiences of anabolic steroid use: In-depth interviews with men and women body builders. *J Health Psychol*, 11(6), 845–856. doi: doi:10.1177/1359105306069080.

Hekman, S. J. (1983). Weber's ideal type: A contemporary reassessment. *Polity*, 16(1), 119–137. doi: doi:10.2307/3234525.

Hernandez, S. H., & Nelson, L. S. (2010). Prescription drug abuse: Insight into the epidemic. *Clinical Pharmacology & Therapeutics*, 88(3), 307–317. doi: doi:10.1038/clpt.2010.154.

Hildebrandt, T., Lai, J. K., Langenbucher, J. W., Schneider, M., Yehuda, R., & Pfaff, D. W. (2011). The diagnostic dilemma of pathological appearance and performance enhancing drug use. *Drug Alcohol Depend*, 114(1), 1–11. doi: doi:10.1016/j.drugalcdep.2010.09.018.

Hoberman, J. M. (2005). *Testosterone dreams: Rejuvenation, aphrodisia, doping.* Berkeley, CA: University of California Press.

Hoff, D. (2016). *Dopningens olika ansikten. En kvalitativ studie av AAS användning på gym.* Retrieved from Lund: http://lup.lub.lu.se/luur/download?func=downloadFile&recordOId=8519176&fileOId=8520230.

Ip, E. J., Lu, D. H., Barnett, M. J., Tenerowicz, M. J., Vo, J. C., & Perry, P. J. (2012). Psychological and physical impact of anabolic-androgenic steroid dependence. *Pharmacotherapy*, 32(10), 910–919. doi: doi:10.1002/j.1875-9114.2012.01123.

Jenssen, I. H., & Johannessen, K. B. (2015). Aggression and body image concerns among anabolic androgenic steroid users, contemplators, and controls in Norway. *Body Image*, 12, 6–13. doi: doi:10.1016/j.bodyim.2014.08.009.

Kanayama, G., Hudson, J. I., & Pope, H. G. (2009). Features of men with anabolic-androgenic steroid dependence: A comparison with nondependent AAS users and with AAS nonusers. *Drug Alcohol Depend*, 102(1–3), 130–137. doi: doi:10.1016/j.drugalcdep.2009.02.008.

Kanayama, G., Hudson, J. I., & Pope, H. G. (2010). Illicit anabolic-androgenic steroid use. *Horm.Behav.*, 58(1), 111–121. doi: doi:1016/j.yhbeh.2009.09.006.

Khorrami, S., & Franklin, J. T. (2002). The Influence of competition and lack of emotional expression in perpetuating steroid abuse and dependence among male weightlifters. *International Journal of Men's Health*, 1(1), 119–133.

Kimergård, A. (2014). A qualitative study of anabolic steroid use amongst gym users in the United Kingdom: motives, beliefs and experiences. *Journal of Substance Use*, 20(4), 288–294. doi: doi:10.3109/14659891.2014.911977.

Klein, A. M. (1993). *Little big men: Bodybuilding subculture and gender construction.* Albany, NY: State University of New York Press.

Liokaftos, D. (2017). *A Genealogy of male bodybuilding: From classical to freaky.* New York & Oxon, UK: Routledge.

Lundholm, L., Kall, K., Wallin, S., & Thiblin, I. (2010). Use of anabolic androgenic steroids in substance abusers arrested for crime. *Drug Alcohol Depend*, 111(3), 222–226. doi: doi:10.1016/j.drugalcdep.2010.04.020.

Maycock, B. R., & Howat, P. (2005). Overcoming the barriers to initiating illegal anabolic steroid use. *Drug Educ Prev Policy*, 14, 317–325. doi: doi:10.1080/09687630500103622.

Maycock, B. R., & Howat, P. (2007). Social capital: Implications from an investigation of illegal anabolic steroid networks. *Health Education Research*, 22(6), 854–863. doi: doi:10.1093/her/cym022.

McVeigh, J., Bates, G., & Chandler, M. (2015). Steroids and image enhancing drugs: 2014 survey results. Retrieved from Liverpool: www.ipedinfo.co.uk/resources/downloads/SIEDs%20Survey%20report%202014%20FINAL.pdf.

Monaghan, L. F. (2001). *Bodybuilding, drugs, and risk*. London: Routledge.

Monaghan, L. F. (2002). Vocabularies of motive for illicit steroid use among bodybuilders. *Soc.Sci.Med.*, 55(5), 695–708.

Pedersen, P. V., Ingholt, L., & Tjørnhøj-Thomsen, T. (2014). Disciplin og dedikation: Unges perspektiver på træning, kost og brug af muskelopbyggende og præstationsfremmende midler. Retrieved from Odense: http://si-folkesundhed.dk/upload/disciplin_og_dedikation.pdf.

Petrocelli, M., Oberweis, T., & Petrocelli, J. (2008). Getting huge, getting ripped: A qualitative exploration of recreational steroid use. *J Drug Issues*, 38, 1187–1205. doi: doi:10.1177/002204260803800412.

Pope, H. G., Phillips, K. A., & Olivardia, R. (2000). *The Adonis complex. How to identify, treat, and prevent body obsession in men and boys*. New York: Free Press.

Probert, A., Palmer, F., & Leberman, S. (2007). The fine line: An insight into "risky" practices of male and female competitive bodybuilders. *Annals of Leisure Research*, 10(3–4), 272–290. doi: doi:10.1080/11745398.2007.9686767.

Sagoe, D., Andreassen, C. S., & Pallesen, S. (2014). The aetiology and trajectory of anabolic-androgenic steroid use initiation: A systematic review and synthesis of qualitative research. *Substance Abuse Treatment, Prevention, and Policy*, 9(1), 1–14. doi: doi:10.1186/1747-597x-9-27.

Vinther, A. S., & Christiansen, A. V. (2019). Different users, different interventions. On the ideal typology of anabolic-androgenic steroid use and its implications for prevention and harm reduction. In K. van de Ven, K. Mulrooney, & J. McVeigh (Eds.), *Human Enhancement Drugs* (pp. 249–263). London: Routledge.

Walker, D. M., & Joubert, H. E. (2011). Attitudes of injecting male anabolic androgenic steroid users to media influence, health messages and gender constructs. *Drugs and Alcohol Today*, 11(2), 56–70. doi: doi:10.1108/17459261111174019.

Weber, M. (1970). *From Max Weber: Essays in sociology*. Oxon, UK: Routledge & Kegan Paul.

Weber, M. (2013). *Economy and society: An outline of interpretive sociology* (G. Roth & C. Wittich (Eds.)). Berkeley, CA: University of California Press.

WHO. (2019). Lexicon of alcohol and drug terms published by the World Health Organization. Retrieved from WHO: www.who.int/substance_abuse/terminology/who_lexicon/en.

Zahnow, R., McVeigh, J., Bates, G., Hope, V., Kean, J., Campbell, J., & Smith, J. (2018). Identifying a typology of men who use anabolic androgenic steroids (AAS). *International Journal of Drug Policy*, 55, 105–112. doi: doi:10.1016/j.drugpo.2018.02.022.

Chapter 8

Side effects as perceived by IPED users

Practically everyone who takes significant doses of anabolic steroids will experience side effects of some sort. However, the way people approach and perceive side effects varies greatly, partly because of each person's ideal-type traits and partly because of their history of side effects. Some users take an Expert-type approach, thoroughly contemplating their situation, studying the topic and taking the precautions they believe are relevant. Others reflect less on what the drugs may do to them. Bearing in mind the diversity of approaches and perceptions, it is understandable that a one-pronged anti-doping strategy is not very effective for countering problems with anabolic steroid use.

In this chapter we look at how users experience and deal with the side effects of steroid use. Beginning with the superficial effects, notably pimples and hair loss, we move on to the more serious somatic effects on the heart, blood pressure and blood sugar, followed by the mental side effects. Another important aspect directly affected by anabolic steroids is the libido, which is why I round off the chapter with observations from the users about their sex lives and drives.

Very few people who go through a prolonged period of using more than 300–500 mg of anabolic steroids per week can avoid side effects altogether. Most of my informants had personal experience with water retention, pimples and shrinking testicles. In some instances this was combined with suppressed libido, particularly after a steroid cycle was over. Several informants described having high blood pressure, and some also spoke of being more irritable and having a "shorter fuse" during a cycle. Users often perceive and explain serious, long-term side effects (such as cardiovascular problems) as something seen in those who don't know what they are doing, or as something you just have to accept. As for the less serious, often temporary side effects, these are often perceived as part of one's lifestyle; as something that, to a certain extent, one can and should take precautions to avoid.

By way of example, Oskar, who was 41 when I interviewed him, had never held back, and he had been through the whole gamut of muscle-building substances. His original interest in such drugs was not based on a wish to compete, but rather on *"youthful curiosity"* and, further down the road, on an ambition to become bigger and stronger:

It was just something I had to try out. I think a lot of people feel that way. Well, of course I can only speak for myself, but I think it's a general thing. That you always just want to be able to run a tad faster, or lift a tad more. You'd always like just a tad more bulk. You want to press yourself a little bit. That was probably the driving force.

In terms of the ideal typology, during his interview Oskar most strongly resembled the Well-being type. Prior to that, however, during the period he refers to in the quote, he lived like an Athlete, albeit with a somewhat undisciplined approach. Others who knew Oskar have told stories about him with distinctly YOLO-type traits, so at the time of the interview he had changed quite a bit. He began using steroids to satisfy his curiosity and his desire to get bigger and stronger and test himself. A couple of times he started working towards a competition, but that was not the main goal of his training. At times his steroid use had been extreme, but in his own view it never got out of hand. Even though competing was not his main motivation for working out, in describing his approach he still compared his dedicated efforts to those of a top-level athlete:

You know, generally it's like that in all top sports: you go all-in and train every day. It's tough on your body, and on the people around you. You have to load up on food, you know, and that's where your mental focus is, constantly. And you also get little injuries here and there. And you may get kind of touchy if you're taking a little bit of juice. So yeah, you do get kind of annoying to the people around you. That's something I think most athletes would recognize.

Oskar did not make much of a fuss about doses or harmful effects. He had taken sizable doses of anabolic steroids — for long periods he was taking more than 2,000 mg a week — so "a little bit of juice" is a gross understatement. A healthy man produces an average 30–60 mg of testosterone weekly, so the 2,000 mg weekly put Oskar at roughly 40 times the normal level (Herbert, 2015). In keeping with his low-key, laid-back attitude he brushed off the side effects he had experienced and said:

My blood pressure probably rose, and I may have been just a tad aggressive. But it's never been like my liver started hurting, or my kidneys started hurting, like some people say they can feel. I haven't had my heart take any double beats either. Fortunately, I've never felt like that.

Q What about your sex drive?

Yeah, well, it rises when you rig up your body with extra testosterone, so it's easier to get your rocks off. But I don't really think it affected me that much.

On the other hand, he was aware that with the doses he had taken the steroids might have some long-term effects he just had not felt yet: "*Of course, it may be that I've caused some kind of damage to my liver or kidneys so that when I turn 60 I'll need a kidney transplant.*" As for the less severe side effects, Oskar said he did not have any experience with "*bitch tits*"; only that his nipples had been "*just a tad tender*" after a cycle. Nor had he suffered from pimples or acne. As mentioned earlier, Oskar had never reached a point where he lost control and tipped over into abuse. One difference between Oskar and Michael (who was an Athlete type) is that Oskar consulted his doctor and took a break when warning signs appeared:

> At one point I had high blood pressure — just as I was at my peak — and then my doctor said it would be a good idea if we took a break off the steroids. So then I got some blood-pressure medicine, and after that I took a long, long break.

During his interview Oskar ended up mentioning most of the side effects that can occur in connection with steroid use: those that are more or less temporary (like pimples, hair loss and male mammary tissue) as well as the potentially more serious long-term effects on the heart, liver and kidneys. He also mentioned mental side effects, including mood swings and altered libido.

Experiencing physical side effects

Pimples, breasts and hair growth

The YOLO-type user Jonas, whom we met in Chapter 6, is one example of temporary or "reversible" side effects like hair loss and pimples not occurring in all steroid users. If anything, his life was unhealthy and involved not just unstructured steroid intake but also parties, junk food, booze and amphetamine. Although Jonas did have pimples, he said it was "*not a total pain for me. It was like other teenagers. It's not like I was filled with zits on my back or my face. I didn't feel like I was.*" In the typology, Anton, whom we met in Chapter 5, belongs somewhere between Athlete and YOLO, although he was nowhere near as dedicated as Michael or Rasmus. Anton wanted to give the impression that part of the time he had been a dedicated athlete, and he actually had taken part in powerlifting competitions. Nevertheless, his goals were aesthetic and his knowledge about the effects of steroids was limited. At the same time he enjoyed going out and getting attention from peers and women. Like Jonas, Anton reported that he had not had any major problems with breast tissue or pimply skin:

> So what happens is that when you take "test" [testosterone], you get those little nodules behind your nipple. But they disappear again after a

while, once you're done. Zits haven't really bugged me either. I might've gotten, like, a pimple on my shoulder, on my bicep, or on my chest — maybe four pimples in all. But that was it. Otherwise I had nothing. Nothing.

Rasmus, who was almost a pure Athlete type, described his personal experience with short-term, visible side effects: *"I've had pimply skin, but that was just in the beginning. I don't get that anymore."* Meanwhile, he mentioned another side effect that was highly visible: *"Yes, I have had more hair growth. All over my body. Except up here,"* he grinned, pointing at his bald head, then continued: *"But I just trim my body with a hair trimmer."* Kasper, who had never used steroids but had followed a devoted training regime with the mindset of an Athlete, pointed out that pimpling is not necessarily caused by the steroids. Skin problems can also arise from the use of protein powder, normal but unhealthy foodstuffs and, not least importantly, the huge amounts of food that he and other serious gym-goers must consume while they are gaining weight:

> There are some protein powders which, when I eat them, I can see I get bumps on my back. I get pimples, too, when I eat potato chips. Let's say I "sin," for once, eating potato chips to make my parents or somebody else happy. The next day my forehead looks like I got the plague. I think there's something called an "overload pimple" as in: you're overloaded with food. Because I can see it. When I start losing weight, right away my skin gets cleaner. Because your body isn't constantly being punished in the same way. It's like when we get stressed out, that gives us pimples too.

This is probably a fair point. Steroid users put a strain on their system, and if at the same time you eat enormous amounts of food, breaking out in pimples is no surprising outcome. This does not mean steroids do *not* cause pimples — a side effect that is thoroughly documented. It simply means diet and food intake may also be a contributory factor.

Heart and blood pressure

Although Jonas did not have to deal with pimples, he did not escape side effects altogether: *"I got more aggressive. And I had trouble sleeping too. One reason was that my blood pressure was way too high. So sometimes I had a hard time falling asleep."* However unpleasant this may sound, it was not the side effects that ultimately got Jonas to quit steroids. What made him stop was a personal rebuttal of his previous life of partying, drugs and a scene that revolved around vacuous masculine values.

Among my other informants, only those who took very high doses talked about heart problems. Dennis, a textbook YOLO type, had experienced the most serious health consequences of years-long and largely uncontrolled steroid use:

> My heart. It's not like it's supposed to be these days. It's not. It's a little bit enlarged. The doctor told me so. And I can actually feel it. Especially right before I go to sleep. I get this really bad pain. Also, my heart kind of skips a beat sometimes. It hurts.

Irregular heartbeat (cardiac arrhythmia) resulting from high steroid intake has been described in a number of case reports (including Christiansen & Bojsen-Møller, 2012; Pope, Wood, et al., 2014), but thoroughly substantiated studies of such heart problems have only recently been published (Baggish et al., 2017; Rasmussen et al., 2018). At any rate, given that nearly all types of anabolic steroids cause elevated blood pressure, and given that quite a few steroids also increase the proportion of red blood cells and therefore make the blood thicker, using steroids undeniably puts a strain on the body's circulatory system. Some researchers have suggested a possible explanation for why premature mortality resulting from cardiovascular problems is not more prominent in the literature about steroid side effects: The large user groups only began to appear in the 1980s and so are still relatively young, whereas heart problems typically do not manifest until later in life. With this in mind, experts in the field expect the coming years to show a significant rise in the number of cardiovascular problems attributable to steroid use (Pope, Wood, et al., 2014).

Of my informants, Rasmus, the consummate Athlete type, was taking the highest doses at the time of his interview, and he spoke of his experiences with high blood pressure:

> I've occasionally had an elevated pulse. And my blood pressure was high when I was dieting and doing trenbolone, because that increases your blood pressure. I had some episodes where I had to drop by the emergency room, because my blood pressure was 200 over 90. You could see it, visually, and my pulse was around 160 when I was lying completely still. Obviously it was pretty horrible. I didn't really know what was going on, or what to do. But it fell as soon as I made it to the emergency room.

This experience did not get Rasmus to stop using steroids, however. He had ambitions of competing and, as he explained, the problem disappeared as quickly as it had arisen. Consequently, he simply adjusted his cycles and afterwards avoided trenbolone. The drug trenbolone, originally developed to increase appetite and muscle growth in cattle, is not used for medical purposes on humans. As one of the most potent anabolic steroids it is often referred to among bodybuilders as "the King of Steroids," but it is also high on side effects. The drug effectively increases muscle growth, fat-burning and muscle strength without too much water retention. Many case studies report augmented sex drive in trenbolone users, although paradoxically the drug can also adversely affect virility as it increases the level of the female sex hormone progesterone — an effect many bodybuilders counteract with Viagra or similar drugs (McVeigh, Bates, & Chandler, 2015). As reflected in what Rasmus stated, trenbolone puts more strain on the heart than most other steroids, so it is not uncommon for its users to have a higher resting heart rate, higher blood pressure and larger amounts of unhealthy fat in their blood (a poor blood-lipid profile). All the more surprising, then, that an American study reported that half of its 1,955 respondents used trenbolone, and that users of the drug rated it as the second-best of 20, based on their perceived effectiveness-to-side-effect ratio (Cohen, Collins, Darkes, & Gwartney, 2007).

Michael and Rasmus were the only two informants in my group with any insulin experience. Although insulin can result in acute and dangerous side effects — extremely low blood-sugar levels and potentially even diabetes in the longer term — Rasmus was very relaxed about these risks, believing that the drug works fine as long as you take precautions. He also spoke about his own use of insulin:

> I've had a couple incidents where I almost went into low-sugar-shock [hypoglycemia – low blood glucose]. But I could feel it myself: "Now I'm just about to stall!" And then I've just grabbed a bunch of stuff and shoved it into my face. Quick carbohydrates like, say, honey on a rice-puff cake, or sugar water, or whatever. Then a couple minutes later you're stable again. And that's just something you have to be okay with before you start playing around with it. You have to have something [sugary] close at hand, just in case things go wrong.

This sort of training scenario sounds incredibly risky, to a degree that only a dedicated athlete would accept, yet Rasmus was very pragmatic when it came to his side effects, and he was prepared to endure great hardship to attain the goals he had set. In that light I asked him where his own limits were, and what might make him stop using anabolic steroids:

> Impotence, for example. But only if it was permanent. As long as it only lasts three months, that's okay. And stuff like dizziness, vomiting and nausea. I really don't want to go around feeling sick. Nope, no way. I have to be able to live a normal life. And do the things I like doing.

He was aware that what he was doing was not healthy, but he also said he wasn't currently concerned about it. His carefree approach with a high acceptance of risks in the interest of great gains only went as far as his own health, however. When asked, hypothetically, what he would do if he had a son who around age 20 or 22 started to ask Dad about how to use steroids, Rasmus would definitely not recommend that his son use them. Taking my cue from the double standards inherent in this response, I asked him to explain why. *"Heck, I don't know. That's kind of hard to answer,"* he replied. *"Maybe if he ... Nope, I wouldn't recommend him to do it, no way, no how. Because it's, you know ... It's back to his running a risk of getting addicted to it."* A person does not become physically dependent on steroids in the same was as you can become addicted to nicotine, alcohol or crack cocaine. It has none-theless become increasingly clear over the past decade that a psychological state can arise where a person becomes dependent on the body and muscles they can obtain with steroids (Ip et al., 2012; Kanayama, Hudson, & Pope, 2009; Pope, Kanayama, et al., 2014). But when Rasmus argued against his hypothetical son's potential steroid use, he was hardly contemplating the latest research. His observation that the question was "hard to answer" may have resulted from his discovery of a potential inconsistency in his own views. He believed that what he was doing himself was okay, under control, and he felt he was taking adequate care of himself. That is why he came close to saying that it might be all right if such a son, with sufficient guidance and advice, gave it a shot (*"Maybe if he ..."*). Yet at the same time he knew enough about steroids and the attendant problems that, in his role as a father, he would not be prepared to accept seeing his son run a similar risk. Perhaps Rasmus also had an inkling that the way he was managing his own life was not entirely rational; a deficiency he would prefer not to see repe-ated by any future son of his.

This situation — that we don't think our children ought to run the same risks *we* ran, almost as a matter of course, in our own youth — is one most parents of adolescents will recognize. It is caused by a change in perspective. Even while we feel in control of ourselves, we are not sure others will be capable of exerting the same degree of control in their lives. In other words, we generally trust our own judgment more than we trust the judgment of others. As an extension of this trend of thought, it is common knowledge that when experiencing success ourselves, we are more likely to explain this by referring to our own skills, talents and qualities. Inversely, when others are successful, we believe it is more attributable to fortuitous circumstances, or to good luck or chance. By the same token we tend to explain our own failure or misfortune as a consequence of unforeseeable bad luck or the adverse effects of external circumstances, whereas inversely we explain other peoples' failures or misfortune as a result of their own lack of skills or qualities. Psychology refers to this phenomenon as "the fundamental attribution error," and it is reflected in the lack of faith Rasmus has in his hypothetical future son's potential use of steroids (Jones & Harris, 1967; Ross, 1977).

His views are also colored by the fact that although he knew people who had used large amounts of steroids for many years without health problems, he had also seen one of his friends die young:

> Then again, he did drugs on the weekends too, and he ate hot dogs and all kinds of crap on a daily basis. And you could see from the way he looked that he was unhealthy. He had high blood pressure, and he always had bad skin; was kind of chubby ... always coughing, and huffing and puffing, and on top of that he smoked a lot. It was bound to go wrong, you know? One morning he died of a heart attack. He was thirty-two.

Because Rasmus had extensive, routine experience with the various ways of dealing with steroids, effects and side effects, like several other informants in my group he did not feel confident that other people would be able to handle the same risks he believed he had under control.

Martin had much the same views as Rasmus. Just as we saw in Anton, Martin was fascinated by sportspeople and would have liked to demonstrate a disciplined lifestyle, but he also enjoyed going out and getting attention from the ladies. Typology-wise he would probably describe himself as an Athlete, but my overall impression was that he was very close to the center of the typology matrix. And like Rasmus, he did not feel at risk of becoming a steroid abuser due to his awareness of the side effects. I asked him what might make him stop using steroids, considering that the side effects he had experienced so far had not done so:

> Even though a cycle might've been expensive, I'd always stop if it turns out my body starts to quit on me. Then I'd call it off. Definitely. Training means so much to me, and my highest aspiration in life at this point in time is to work out and do bodybuilding. But I'd still be ready to break off a cycle if it turns out to be harmful.

Martin did not feel he had experienced any harmful effects yet. Still, it was difficult to know whether he really would stop if his "body starts to quit" on him. The question is, what level of harm would that imply? Michael also stopped using steroids after his body began to give up — but not until the very last moment, by which time it was almost too late. However, Martin did not have the same Athlete-type traits as Michael did. He was less dedicated than the typical Athlete, and he thought much more about risks, healthy food and restitution than the ideal-typical YOLO. So although we cannot use Martin's statements to make any kind of precise calibration of how far he would be prepared to go, he clearly knew about side effects, and although he was going to use steroids, he would be doing so with a modicum of caution. In addition, Martin argued that steroid users ought to have access to medical monitoring of their pharmacological experiments so they don't have to make their own assessment of when their "body starts to quit" on them.

Anton also believed he would be able to break off a cycle if he started to feel serious side effects. To underscore that he was attentive to his body's signals and would stop a cycle if needed, Anton gave this example:

> One time I also took those Oxy-pills[1] — some of the toughest stuff you can lay on your liver. And then I started getting these pains in my side and around the back. But then I started drinking, like, four liters of water a day, and I said to myself that if it didn't go away within a week, then I'd stop. But then it went away after three days.

Based on the symptoms Anton described, his entire system must have been on overdrive. The probable rationale behind his self-treatment was that if only he drank a lot of water, his organs would be able to cope with the strain. Just as in Martin's case, here we cannot determine whether Anton would stop if his symptoms became worse. But even though he was more of an Athlete type than Martin, his life was not quite so focused on workouts, performance, competition and progress as we saw in Michael, Rasmus and certain others. Using the knowledge he possessed, Anton attempted to balance risks with advantages and effectiveness. He was aware that steroids could be harmful, and his approach was that a person must listen to their body's signals and act accordingly.

Experiencing mental side effects

Rasmus, with his clear-cut Athlete profile, had tried out most of what is available, in heavy doses, but he never had anything negative happen with substances affecting his psyche. I asked him about his mental state during a steroid cycle:

> I'm on the top of the world. Basically, no worries at all. And the things I do worry about, I get over really fast. You're always in a good mood; always. You've got energy to spare, for everything, see? And for me there's no aggression and stuff. None at all. Me, I don't even get that with the really heavy-duty stuff like trenbolone and Winstrol.

Not so for everyone. Two other informants in my group, Anton and Martin, had also used trenbolone — the substance Rasmus was on when he ended up in the emergency room with extremely high blood pressure. Anton did not mention elevated blood pressure in connection with the drug, but he did relate how, during a cycle with trenbolone, he would often "be steaming hot. I could easily wake up three, four times a night bathed in sweat. That's the only thing that was really aggravating." In Anton the drug effectively promoted muscle growth, an aspect that pleased him, but it also affected his mood. He could go from feeling elated while doing the things he loved, to being aggressive and short-tempered when things were not going his way. Anton's story testifies to the enormous potency of such substances and how they can affect a person's physical and mental state. He spoke of how a group of "immigrant guys" would sometimes provoke him, trying to elicit a reaction. Such provocations affected him most when he was on trenbolone:

> I was hot-headed. Really hot-headed. I don't know how to describe it. It's like these little stories kept running through my head. About what might happen if, say, a group of ten immigrant kids came walking towards me and we started fighting. See, I've been on the receiving end of so much hassle from them over the years that I actually just walk around waiting for the next time it happens. So if I run into a bunch of guys like that in the big shopping street downtown, and if I have my pretty girlfriend with me, I sometimes catch myself thinking: "Which one should I hammer first?" They think it'd be fun to get into a fight with a guy like me. See, it's cool for them to be able to say they took down a guy like me, even though there would be 10 or 15 guys on their side. But if I ran into a bunch of guys like that, I'd think: "Who should I take first?" It was just an automatic thing. I was really hot-headed. Constantly had my hands balled up into a fist, and my teeth clenched.

He felt the same aggressive energy during workouts, but there it would affect his mood positively:

> When I'd work out I didn't want anyone talking to me. It was really grunting, just lifting all the heaviest of the heaviest equipment. It couldn't get too heavy for me, or too crazy. But even though, to put it mildly, I turned into a real beast, it was pretty cool too. I just got *so* much attention it was insane. People were like: "Hey man, what *are* you eating for breakfast?!" But obviously, you know, given that I put on almost 13 kilos in just three and a half weeks, I was really truckin'. So I got a whole lot of attention, and I was constantly walking around with this big grin on my face. I was really happy that whole time. Then again, if I got into situations where I was being provoked, things would turn around real fast for me.

Anton's description of how his mood could swing from one extreme to the other is noteworthy; particularly the aggression, with envisioned fights and violence relating to groups of immigrant youths, which he imagines and braces himself to meet. This tells us something of how such drugs can affect the mental state of some users.

Martin also shared his personal experience of drastically affected mood and self-image during a trenbolone cycle:

> I had a girlfriend at the time and she didn't dare to tell me this until after the cycle was over. But she said that I was just so cocky, mouthing off. And actually we knew each other pretty well and had always been good together. But during that time I got so self-confident I almost thought I was a god. I just felt like: "Screw 'em all." Nobody was a match for me, and I was just Superman, yeah. And she said it just basically made her want to puke. But I didn't even notice it myself. You always get a kick when you're on a cycle, but that particular time with trenbolone, that made me weird. Hugely self-centered, which I've never liked being, because that's not like me at all.

So besides effectively boosting muscle growth and strength, "the King of Steroids" clearly affected Anton and Martin mentally, which Martin described as undesirable (although Anton did not expressly say the same). Martin therefore intended to stay away from the drug in future, as he believed there were alternatives that worked almost as well for him. Anton, on the other hand, did not categorically deny potentially revisiting the drug, although both he and Martin believed it had to be handled with care. Along with the input from Rasmus, these descriptions tell us that the same active substance (in this case trenbolone) can affect different users in very different ways.

Jonas did not recall any particular physical side effects from using steroids. Once a consummate YOLO type, Jonas was a party animal who would use other drugs along with steroids, and he did describe the aggregated effects of this on his mental state:

> The side effects I had were mostly mental and were probably caused by the weekend amphetamine. You could really feel it on a Sunday, that you weren't doin' too good; hadn't slept much or eaten right. So I wasn't feeling good on Sundays, and not always on Mondays either. But then you'd slowly start to get back into gear.

Besides feeling physically ill, Jonas became more aggressive during and after his weekend partying and nights out: "*I could actually feel myself getting somewhat more aggressive. A lot more. It didn't take much. Especially if you'd been downtown partying and hadn't slept much, and you were kind of bickering with each other.*" This also meant he would end up in fights more often:

> Yes, I did. All because of the doping. Otherwise I'm usually like: "Hey, take it easy dude!" But my fuse was a lot shorter. I was more aggressive, and then of course, combine that with the drugs we took when we went out. That's just a totally lethal cocktail. And sometimes you were just

itching for something to happen, and so you went looking for it. You didn't want anyone to even look sideways at one of your buddies. "Hey you, what's up? Are you eyeballing this guy?!" Stuff like that. And you felt like you had to assert yourself. After all, you were working out, and you were on steroids, and you thought you were one hell of a he-man.

This account from Jonas fits the YOLO description like hand in glove. What is more, it plainly shows that when seeking to understand the links between anabolic steroids, aggression and violence, looking at a person's total lifestyle is a more fruitful approach to take than attempting to identify any causal biochemical relation between steroids and aggression or violence.

All in all, Jonas did not experience the physical side effects as significant or remarkable and, as noted earlier, the mental and physical side effects were not what prompted him to quit steroids. He quit so he could break free from the predominantly YOLO-type lifestyle in his social circle.

It is obvious that Jesper, the Expert type who worked out and also spent time advising others, was aware that the steroids were affecting his psyche. However, as with the physical side effects he also attempted to take a pragmatic approach to his mental state, with similar precautions:

It really helps if you're aware of how steroids can affect your mood. So you see, if you take this substance, certain things might start to irritate you, so then you have to learn to count to ten, and you have to *not* go looking for trouble. All that partying and taking drugs and drinking while you're on steroids, and needling other people just a little bit too hard, that really contributes to lots of the bad things about steroids. You know, the way people go looking for problems. You shouldn't do that.

Because he was consciously aware of the effects of the drugs, Jesper — unlike Jonas — did not party when he was on a steroid cycle. He also took precautions at home, telling his girlfriend about the situation so she would know that his mentality might be different during the cycle:

One of the positive things in my relationship with my girlfriend is that we sat down and dug deep; we had a good, long talk about all this. She knows what I take, and she's tried to educate herself about it. So much, in fact, that she knows more about steroids than a lot of my buddies do. And this means that, just like I have to watch myself around her once a month, she's been able to watch herself and think about what she says to me during the times I've been on a cycle. We've done a good job on this together, being considerate towards each other.

This is the Expert's pragmatic approach to hormonal mood swings. Jesper and his girlfriend both knew their mood could be affected by the hormonal fluctuations of natural cycles and drug cycles, so they deliberately took the necessary precautions to address these situations. Just as we saw with physical side effects, here we see how different informants had very different experiences of the mental and psychological effects of steroid use. It is very likely that some of the perceived changes in their aggressiveness while on steroids springs from the very knowledge that such an effect can arise, causing them to react according to that knowledge. As described in Chapter 3, one study has demonstrated that test subjects show more selfish and antisocial behavior when taking a placebo but *believing* they have been taking testosterone (Eisenegger, Naef, Snozzi, Heinrichs, & Fehr, 2010). The explanation is that they are familiar with the popular preconception that testosterone makes people more aggressive and egotistical, and so they act accordingly. Testosterone plays a crucial role not just for muscle growth but also at a general level for male behavior and well-being. Steroid-cycle effects on the mental state, as described by my informants, is therefore undoubtedly rooted in the pharmacodynamics of the substances used — how the drugs act in and on the body. However, as evidenced here and in Chapter 7, the expression of these effects in each individual is also influenced by that person's general typology-based approach, so it cannot solely be explained by the biochemical effects of the drugs.

More sex

So far we have mainly looked at the increase in strength and muscle volume that results from combining physical training and steroids. Beyond that, none of the informants had any doubt that the sexual attraction of having a handsome body is also an important part of their fascination.[2] Dennis phrased this very bluntly: "*Bodybuilding and workouts equal sex. Sex is what it's all about. It's that simple.*" Anton was also very conscious of what he gained from working out, taking IPEDs and growing larger and more muscular. It facilitated contact with the opposite sex, which was actually part of his original intent: "*Yeah, back then it was kind of a motivation,*" he said, explaining:

> I'd say, before, it would take a lot for me to be able to pick up a girl. That's certainly not a problem any more. Quite the opposite, actually. Back then it could take years for me to just start talking to a girl, but now, to be quite honest, it's almost like they won't leave me alone. But most girls just want me for my body.

This last comment was accompanied by a smile that clearly showed he knew the classic feminist accusation that men only see women as sex objects. Then he elaborated:

You know, it's so plain to see what they're interested in. I know it wouldn't have been like that if I hadn't worked out. Everybody says "it's not your looks that count," but you're lying if you say looks aren't important.

Anton clearly felt that getting more muscular had made him more attractive and got women to notice him more. He offered a simple explanation:

I think it's sexual. Of course that's something that ups your self-confidence. And I sense this everywhere. Just having this profile on Facebook, I have lots of girls who write to me out of the blue. Or if I go out, or just go for a coffee, or if I go dancing, some of them start talking to me. I have girls come on to me all the time. That's really a blast, always having a new girl who wants to get to know me. Or wants to have a good time. And yeah, that's totally cool when you're not used to it. It's just in the past two years things've really started picking up. It really is a blast, yeah. But I *do* know what their motive is. Because I know that if I hadn't worked out, they wouldn't have approached me. So I can see through it, too. I know what's going on. I know from personal experience what it's like to try to get talking to a girl for months, just to have even the remotest chance of picking her up, and her having to get to know my personality. The girls who approach me now aren't interested in my personality. They're only interested in the car I'm driving, or the body I've built.

Anton's new situation with lots of attention had made him very selective about who he wanted to be with. In that sense he was no better than the girls he criticized for only thinking about physical appearance: Anton also sounded like he was more interested in looks than personality. He had actually come to focus on appearance so much that he found his own statements almost immoderate:

I used to have no problem hooking up with a girl who was maybe a little bit heavy, or who didn't look that great. But now I can go out and get maybe a dozen offers and I don't even give them a second glance, so it almost has to be picture-perfect before I even feel like making an effort. So I've become really, really picky. If they have just a little bit of belly fat, or … Gosh, this is almost embarrassing; I can hear that myself. But I've become really picky in that department.

It is easy to take exception to such superficial comments that only go skin-deep, but if we want to understand the attraction of combining workouts and steroids we must try to put ourselves in the user's shoes. In Chapter 5 several of my informants mentioned how, as teens, they had felt small and in some cases lacked self-confidence, and how this had been the impetus for them to start physical training. They wanted to change their situation and get even with those who had belittled them (Hoff, 2016). Anton, too, spoke of social difficulties and awkwardness, which he later overcame.

Combined, workouts and steroids offer a great potential for changing how an individual relates to their surroundings. Compared to such a convincing proposition, anti-doping authorities clearly face a huge challenge when trying to convince steroid users that such drugs are harmful and unnecessary, and that the best thing users can do is to stop using. To the young men on the receiving end of anti-doping campaigns, the message can easily sound something like this:

> You should go back to the life you had, back to the time when you lacked self-confidence and had a hard time talking to girls. That was better than the life you have now, with self-confidence to spare, more friends, and girls galore.

To a slightly insecure young man who has experienced changes in his physique and self-image similar to Anton's, no wonder the establishment's "say no to steroids" message seems unappealing.

Not all users undergo a transformation like Anton's or enjoy the same attention from the opposite sex. Meanwhile, the idea that change is achievable, and that muscles equal sex, is so well-established that for over half a century it has been used to sell physical fitness and a wide variety of dietary supplements. Consider a case in point from the monthly magazine *Muscle and Fitness* — for decades a leading publication in its class with a circulation of over 320 thousand. Over several issues this magazine ran an ad featuring the American professional bodybuilder Mark Dugdale, dressed in tiny swimming trunks and flexing his abundantly muscled body. Next to him is a scantily clad, seductively posed, large-bosomed woman whose damp body almost seems to be sliding down over the enormous pill container she is sitting on, with "Vitrix — maximum impact" on the label. The adjacent text reads "More Muscle & Better Sex."

The basic idea is, of course, to sell a dietary supplement (referred to as "a testosterone stimulator") which according to the advertising text is "The only product proven to build more muscle AND enhance your sex drive" (emphasis as in the source). It is easy to smile at the blatant symbolism in the ad, or to assume it is designed to be intentionally ironic — which is rarely the case for dietary supplement ads.

There does, however, seem to be a touch of irony in a pair of advertisements for the Danish alcoholic energy drink *Cult Shaker*, which features two buff, well-proportion, nude bronzed bodies, both set against a black background. One is a woman, the other a man (see the male version in Figure 8.1). No faces. Both posters enthusiastically urge readers to "Shake it baby!" The woman holds her beverage bottle between her breasts while the man's bottle

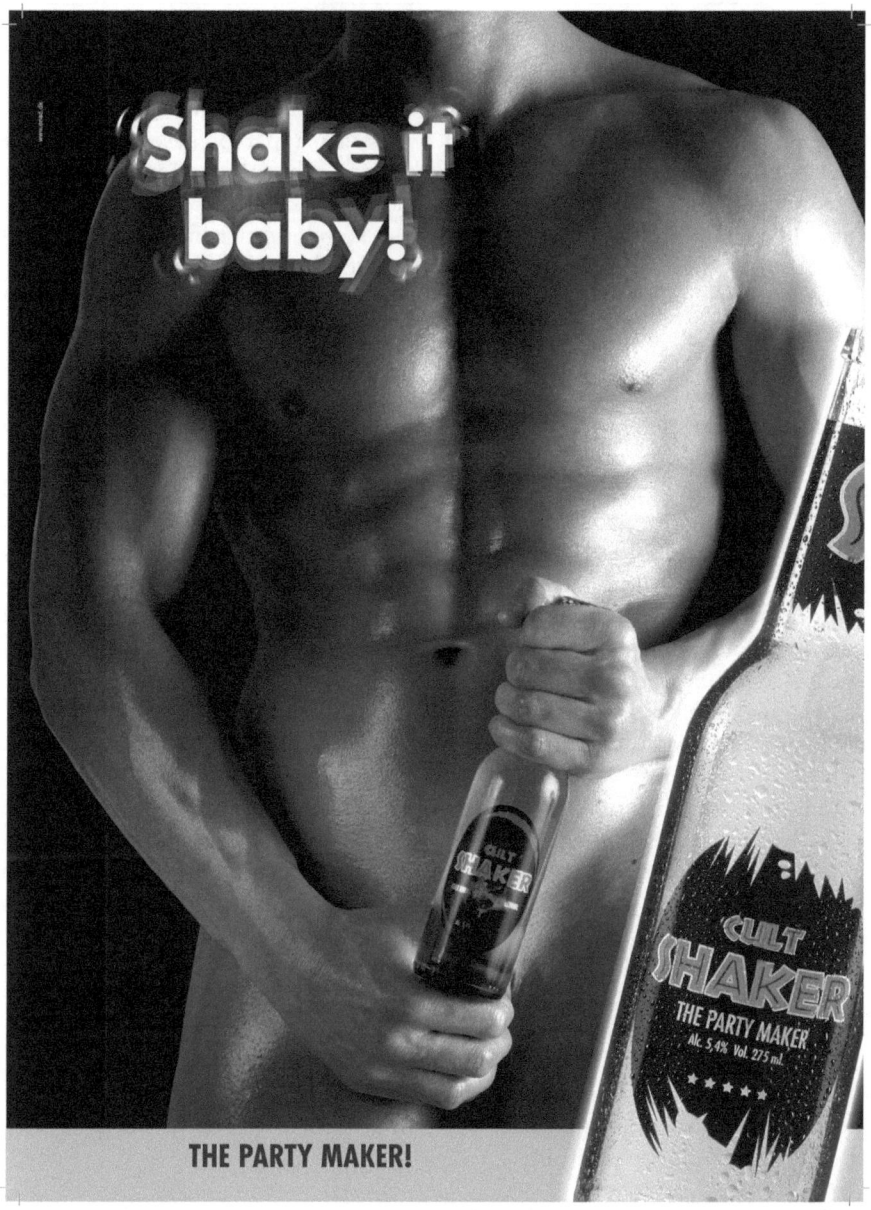

Figure 8.1 "Bodybuilding and workouts equal sex. Sex is what it's all about. It's that simple" (Dennis). The advertising industry also knows that sex and muscles are linked, and you don't need a PhD in image analysis to decode the message in these ads for the Danish alcoholic energy drink SHAKER: A muscular, shapely body gives you access to sex. But the paradox is that although steroids can help pave the way to a toned body and more sex, there is a risk that users will be uninclined — or unable — to have sex when the opportunity arises. © Unibrew/CULT Danmark

is placed in front of his genitals. It doesn't take a PhD in advertising to decode the posters: a muscular, well-trained body, (alcohol) and sex go together. They convey a message that is in direct contrast to many educational campaigns, which state that steroids (or alcohol) will *lessen* a person's sex drive. The muscle–sex link is crystal clear in such advertising, but the real irony is that if a person gets really big, like Mark Dugdale and his peers, part of the sexual attraction of muscularity disappears because many women find hypermuscularity repulsive (Thompson & Cafri, 2007). Despite this, some anabolic steroids users maintain that one reason they use the drugs is to increase their sex drive (Bates & McVeigh, 2016; McVeigh et al., 2015).

It is only in more recent studies that informants have begun directly citing heightened sex drive as a motive for using steroids, but this does not mean the motivational element is new. To researchers it is old news that many users experience a reinforced sense of masculinity when their level of the male sex hormone is augmented with anabolic steroids. Also, the medical community has known for almost a century that testosterone plays an important role for libido (Herbert, 2015; Hoberman, 2005). One indicator is that when men with low testosterone levels receive therapeutic doses of testosterone, they experience an increase in spontaneous sexual thoughts and fantasies, more intense sexual desire, more (potent) erections and increased sexual activity (Hoffman et al., 2009).

In keeping with Oskar's description earlier in this chapter, several other informants similarly described how steroids increased their sex drive. Michael had a sense of condensed masculinity when he was on cycles, working out, and having sex with his girlfriend. Putting his experience into words, he enthused: *"It's just totally awesome! It's just the best. You're totally on a roll! Just imagine how much man you are when you're cut to the bone and you can screw your brains out for eight hours!"* This sounds enticing, but there is a downside: *"The only problem is, you can have a hard time coming. So it can take a long time."* Michael knows that testosterone-induced sex drive gives you a false picture of who you are, and of what you can do. As he rationalizes: *"Of course, that's a delusional picture too. 'Cause reality's not like that. 'Cause you're not some kind of porn stud. Not a lot of people can perform that way, in real life. People who can do that, they make movies."* Martin also talked about feeling more sexual desire during a cycle, but paradoxically this was combined with difficulty achieving an erection:

> Well, especially Deca[3] can make it hard during that time to get a hard-on. Lots of people think it's the other way around: that the more "test" [testosterone] you get, the hornier you get, and that you just turn into a randy goat. It's certainly true that you do get hornier. But when you're on juice it can be kind of hard to get it up sometimes. And that's where it comes from, this whole myth about steroids making you impotent.

The problem of Deca causing impotence is well-known among steroid users, to the point that the phenomenon is known in gym lingo as "Deca dick." But Martin did not believe the drug causes permanent impotence, maintaining it is only an issue during use and will disappear again, provided the user remembers to stick to his breaks:

> It's just an effect that's there while the steroids are in your body. So it's only if you've been on it for two years in a row, with no breaks, that you can become impotent. I've had that happen to me, having a hard time. In other words, my ability to get a hard-on was a little bit lower, but I was a lot hornier. You don't become completely impotent. It just takes a little more to keep it up, but you think a lot more about sex when you're doing a cycle.

Evidently, steroids are not necessarily the aphrodisiacs some people make them out to be. Dennis, who is clearly in the YOLO quadrant of the typology, recalled several episodes with women that he thought would develop into real sexual adventures, but which ended up as embarrassing no-go scenarios:

> The whole sex thing, it's kind of a strange deal. Because your equipment doesn't always work. One time I brought home this incredibly gorgeous babe. But my tool didn't work. And so there you are, apologizing to this girl: "Listen, I'm kinda tired, you know. I really want you, but ..." And then the girl goes: "What do you want me to do for you, 'cause your thing's not in gear." "You know, I'm just so tired ... so tired. That's why. It's not like you're not hot. You're totally gorgeous, but I'm just so tired."

This sort of experience is definitely not conducive to a person's self-confidence, which is undoubtedly why Viagra is widely used among steroid users (McVeigh et al., 2015; Sagoe et al., 2015). Anton was also familiar with this problem, although he believed it only arises when Deca is combined with testosterone. He described the experience on testosterone alone as very different indeed:

> If you only take "test," it works like Viagra. At least it did for me. This one time, it'd been a while since I'd felt like having sex with my girlfriend. I just felt no desire whatsoever. I could've been looking at the hottest girl around and it just did nothing for me. Nothing at all. Then I started on my "test" cycle, which I'd been waiting to do for several months. Then all my girlfriend had to do was kiss me and I'd get an epic hard-on. And I was up for it four times a day, and I'm talking every day, all the time. It was so insane that if I was sitting at school and I heard

some girl walk by in a pair of high-heeled shoes, I'd sometimes call my girlfriend and ask if she was home from school yet, so I could drop by her place. That's all it took.

The point here is not whether scientific evidence substantiates the effect of testosterone Anton described in this quote. Rather, the point is that Michael, Martin and Anton all experienced a significant effect on their sex drive from taking steroids. Conversely, Rasmus, who was 32 at the time of his interview, confirmed what Dennis described: that steroids can also have a negative effect, beyond mere erectile dysfunction. For Rasmus, after one of his cycles his own body's production of testosterone took a very long time to resume, and at the same time his testicles shrunk and he had severe virility problems. This made him decide to take a six-month break:

And for those six months, I took nothing. But I had three months with no sexual activity at all. I was just finished, bombed out. Very frustrating for my girlfriend — of course it was. I had told her about it, so I'd warned her that it might turn out that way, because I knew it might, you know? But still: I felt really bad, and it does put a mental strain on you when you can't satisfy your girlfriend.

This was clearly very frustrating for Rasmus, whose high spirits during cycles we heard about earlier. For him, being "bombed out" for the first three months of a six-month break was a stark contrast to feeling good. As discussed earlier, this type of experience may cause some users to return to steroids earlier than planned, and that exact choice may be the riskiest element of steroid use: A user may not adhere to the breaks in his plan, because even while the mental strain during a break is considerable, the memory of the steroid-induced high spirits, strong biceps and untamed virility is still agonizingly vivid.

Notes

1 The active substance is oxymetholone — sold under that name and other drug brand names, including Anadrol and Anapolon.
2 As noted in Chapter 1, all the men I interviewed identified as heterosexual. I am aware of the growing body of literature on gym culture, homoeroticism and homosexuality (see for instance Halkitis et al., 2008; Lanzieri & Hildebrandt, 2011), and the relationship between gym culture and homosexuality was already discussed by Klein in his seminal work (1993). However, it did not surface as a topic in my interviews, so I have not addressed it here.
3 The substance nandrolone, sold under the drug brand name Deca Durabolin, among others.

References

Baggish, A. L., Weiner, R. B., Kanayama, G., Hudson, J. I., Lu, M. T., Hoffmann, U., & Pope, H. G., Jr. (2017). Cardiovascular toxicity of illicit anabolic-androgenic steroid use. *Circulation*, 135(21), 1991–2002. doi: doi:10.1161/circulationaha.116.026945.

Bates, G., & McVeigh, J. (2016). Image and performance enhancing drugs: 2015 survey results. Retrieved from Liverpool: www.ipedinfo.co.uk/resources/downloads/2015%20National%20IPED%20Info%20Survey%20report.pdf.

Christiansen, A. V., & Bojsen-Møller, J. (2012). "Will steroids kill me if I use them once?" A qualitative analysis of inquiries submitted to the Danish anti-doping authorities. *Performance Enhancement & Health*, 1(1), 39–47. doi: doi:10.1016/j.peh.2012.05.002.

Cohen, J., Collins, R., Darkes, J., & Gwartney, D. (2007). A league of their own: Demographics, motivations and patterns of use of 1,955 male adult non-medical anabolic steroid users in the United States. *J.Int.Soc.Sports Nutr.*, 4, 12. doi: doi:10.1186/1550-2783-4-12.

Eisenegger, C., Naef, M., Snozzi, R., Heinrichs, M., & Fehr, E. (2010). Prejudice and truth about the effect of testosterone on human bargaining behaviour. *Nature*, 463 (7279), 356–359. doi: doi:10.1038/nature08711 .

Halkitis, P. N., Moeller, R. W., & DeRaleau, L. B. (2008). Steroid use in gay, bisexual, and nonidentified men-who-have-sex-with-men: Relations to masculinity, physical, and mental health. *Psychology of Men & Masculinities*, 9(2), 106–115. doi: doi:2048/10.1037/1524-9220.9.2.106.

Herbert, J. (2015). *Testosterone: Sex, power, and the will to win.* Oxford: Oxford University Press.

Hoberman, J. M. (2005). *Testosterone dreams: Rejuvenation, aphrodisia, doping.* Berkeley, CA: University of California Press.

Hoff, D. (2016). *Dopningens olika ansikten. En kvalitativ studie av AAS användning på gym.* Retrieved from Lund: http://lup.lub.lu.se/luur/download?func=downloadFile&recordOId=8519176&fileOId=8520230.

Hoffman, J. R., Kraemer, W. J., Bhasin, S., Storer, T., Ratamess, N. A., Haff, G. G., ... Rogol, A. D. (2009). Position stand on androgen and human growth hormone use. *Journal of Strength and Conditioning Research*, 23(5 Suppl), S1-S59. doi: doi:10.1519/JSC.0b013e31819df2e6.

Ip, E. J., Lu, D. H., Barnett, M. J., Tenerowicz, M. J., Vo, J. C., & Perry, P. J. (2012). Psychological and physical impact of anabolic-androgenic steroid dependence. *Pharmacotherapy*, 32(10), 910–919. doi: doi:10.1002/j.1875-9114.2012.01123.

Jones, E. E., & Harris, V. A. (1967). The attribution of attitudes. *Journal of Experimental Social Psychology*, 3(1), 1–24. doi: doi:10.1016/0022-1031(67)90034-0.

Kanayama, G., Hudson, J. I., & Pope, H. G. (2009). Features of men with anabolic-androgenic steroid dependence: A comparison with nondependent AAS users and with AAS nonusers. *Drug Alcohol Depend*, 102(1–3),130–137. doi: doi:10.1016/j.drugalcdep.2009.02.008.

Klein, A. M. (1993). *Little big men: Bodybuilding subculture and gender construction.* Albany, NY: State University of New York Press.

Lanzieri, N., & Hildebrandt, T. (2011). Using hegemonic masculinity to explain gay male attraction to muscular and athletic men. *Journal of Homosexuality*, 58(2), 275–293. doi: doi:10.1080/00918369.2011.540184.

McVeigh, J., Bates, G., & Chandler, M. (2015). Steroids and image enhancing drugs – 2014 survey results. Retrieved from Liverpool: www.ipedinfo.co.uk/resources/downloads/SIEDs%20Survey%20report%202014%20FINAL.pdf.

Pope, H. G., Kanayama, G., Athey, A., Ryan, E., Hudson, J. I., & Baggish, A. (2014). The lifetime prevalence of anabolic-androgenic steroid use and dependence in Americans: Current best estimates. *Am J Addict*, 23(4), 371–377. doi: doi:10.1111/j.1521-0391.2013.12118.x.

Pope, H. G., Wood, R. I., Rogol, A., Nyberg, F., Bowers, L., & Bhasin, S. (2014). Adverse health consequences of performance-enhancing drugs: An Endocrine Society scientific statement. *Endocr Rev*, 35(3), 341–375. doi: doi:10.1210/er.2013-1058.

Rasmussen, J. J., Schou, M., Madsen, P. L., Selmer, C., Johansen, M. L., Hovind, P., … Kistorp, C. (2018). Increased blood pressure and aortic stiffness among abusers of anabolic androgenic steroids: Potential effect of suppressed natriuretic peptides in plasma? *J Hypertens*, 36(2), 277–285. doi: doi:10.1097/hjh.0000000000001546.

Ross, L. (1977). The intuitive psychologist and his shortcomings: Distortions in the attribution process 1. In B. Leonard (Ed.), *Advances in Experimental Social Psychology* (Vol. 10, pp. 173–220). Cambridge, MA: Academic Press.

Sagoe, D., McVeigh, J., Bjørnebekk, A., Essilfie, M.-S., Andreassen, C. S., & Pallesen, S. (2015). Polypharmacy among anabolic-androgenic steroid users: A descriptive metasynthesis. *Substance Abuse Treatment, Prevention, and Policy*, 10(1), 1–19. doi: doi:10.1186/s13011-015-0006-5.

Thompson, J. K., & Cafri, G. (Eds.). (2007). *The muscular ideal: Psychological, social, and medical perspectives* (1st ed.). Washington, DC: American Psychological Association.

Chapter 9

Diet and lifestyle choices

One paradox in the general stigmatization of androgenic-anabolic-steroid users is that a good deal of them lead lives which — steroidal drugs aside — are aligned with the recommendations of many health experts. If we think back on the stories of the four IPED users in Chapter 6, this was not true of Michael and Jonas (an Athlete and YOLO type, respectively), whereas it was largely true of Jesper and Adam (an Expert and Well-being type, respectively). So far only a single study has looked at how users of anabolic steroids are distributed among the four ideal types. Based on a cluster analysis of the motives of 660 male anabolic-steroid users in the UK, aged 30 on average, the Australian researcher Renee Zahnow and her British colleagues found that 39% of these users primarily exhibited features from the typology's Well-being quadrant; 25% in the Expert quadrant; another 25% in the Athlete quadrant; and 11% in the YOLO quadrant (Zahnow et al., 2018). Based on these findings, and on general literature in this field, there is good reason to assume that a large proportion of user profiles would be located at the bottom or middle area of the risk scale (see the typology graphics in Chapter 7). If the object of the exercise were to develop more precisely targeted prevention and education initiatives, it would, of course, be relevant to conduct similar studies of this sort to get a better picture of user distribution within the typology framework (Vinther & Christiansen, 2019).

At any rate, it is clear that not all steroid users lead YOLO-type lives, an impression confirmed in a Danish study from the National Institute of Public Health. This study, conducted on behalf of Anti Doping Danmark, investigated young people's views on their body, physical training, diet and steroid use. The findings showed that young Danish users were very conscious of their diet, avoiding fast food and largely staying away from alcohol; that they took care to get adequate sleep; and that they worked out regularly (Pedersen, Ingholt, & Tjørnhøj-Thomsen, 2014). Similar features were found in a study done among young Norwegian men (Barland, Tangen, & Johannesen, 2010). These Danish and Norwegian youths did everything the authorities and their parents wanted young people to do, and avoided everything the same authorities wanted them to avoid — with the notable exception of steroids, obviously. But better still, positive secondary effects were found to occur as a result of their behavior. Their intense workout regimes demanded such disciplined planning of their food intake, training sessions, school and other leisure activities that the youths themselves believed they had acquired skills in terms of hard work and self-discipline when striving towards an established goal; skills they would carry with them into later studies or workplaces. These youths were not simply ascetics, flogging themselves to reach an unachievable ideal, nor was their disciplined lifestyle merely meant to improve their physique. Their workouts also gave them a sense of "physical and mental satisfaction, increased well-being, and increased self-esteem and recognition" (Pedersen et al., 2014, p. 14).

This characterization underscores yet again the danger of misunderstanding the whole phenomenon if we categorize anabolic steroids and other IPEDs alongside the narcotic drugs, alcohol and tobacco that are also prevalent features in youth culture. The latter substances impair one's ability to function and work; their desired effects are immediate; and they are not believed to have any positive secondary effects on users' school or work life. On the contrary, anabolic steroids, which build up the body, are taken to increase strength, and they must be used for weeks or months along with rigorous dieting and physical training for the user to achieve the desired effect. Add to this the apparently positive secondary effects for some users and it is easy to see why people who take performance-enhancing drugs object to automatically being referred to as "abusers." For them, a life that focuses on physical training and a strict diet, potentially combined with steroids, is by no means comparable to the life led by alcoholics and drug addicts. At the same time it is worth repeating that this lifestyle, food and workouts included, will vary depending on one's personal approach and ambitions.

Dieting, discipline and steroids

People who are zealously dedicated to workouts, physical fitness and bodybuilding often relate to their diet in a way that seems odd and mechanistic to those who live outside the gym community. They think of food as calories and macronutrients rather than meals associated with enjoyment and socializing. When I spoke to Kasper, whom we met in Chapter 5, he was in a phase where, having bulked up on muscle for several months, it was time for him to lose weight and become more "ripped" and well defined. He had never used steroids, but he was a dedicated gym-goer, which was also reflected in his approach to his diet. His approach is illustrated in this description of the typical day at that point in time:

> I get up at 5 a.m., then I go for a half-hour walk. Got to get rid of some of that fat. When I get back I take 200 grams of rolled oats[1] and half a liter of milk, plus a scoop of protein, then run that through the blender

and drink it. Then I go to work, and at 9 o'clock I eat a protein bar and two pieces of fruit. Later, around 12 or 1, I eat 100 grams of pasta, 400 grams of vegetables, and 250 grams of turkey. Somewhere between 3 and 4 p.m., in the car on my way home from work, I have a protein shake with 50 grams of protein, plus two pieces of fruit. Then I get home, and at 6 o'clock I have 100 grams of rice[2] and 300 grams of vegetables and 300 grams of chicken. And then I have something called Super Charge, as I'm changing before my workout. It's a kind of creatine–caffeine–taurine product that I drink. It gives you a whole bunch of energy, and you get a good pump going in your body. Then I work out for an hour, maybe an hour and a half, and around 9 p.m. I have a weight-gainer — that's protein and carbohydrates mixed. Then, when I get home, I have one or two pieces of heavy pumpernickel — just the bread, nothing on top — just to get something in my belly, and then I go to bed.

After hearing Kasper's routine I felt obliged to ask him the somewhat rhetorical question of whether he regarded his strength training and weightlifting as a sport. "No," he replied without hesitation. "It's a lifestyle." He had the following thoughts on the difference:

Sport is something you do when you're there, on location. When you play soccer, then you play when you're out there with your teammates and that's that. But when the alarm rings in the morning, we eat because we're going to work out. And we do it again at 9, and at 12, and at 3, and at 6. And then we work out, and then we eat again at 9, and then we go to bed, because we know we need eight hours of sleep to get maximum growth out of all this. The people who play soccer can get away with sleeping five hours and still go to soccer practice. So I think the dividing line goes between whether you're focused on it 24–7 or not.

A good many soccer players would probably disagree with this description, but the message is unmistakable. What Kasper does is not a hobby. It is a dedicated lifestyle. This means it commands his focus every waking hour, which includes meticulously following a detailed dietary regime. However, when I spoke to Kasper, then 21, he actually told me that his current diet wasn't hard to follow, since he had cut down on the calories in order to lose weight. A few months earlier he had been eating a lot more food; something of an ordeal. His actual transformation took place when he moved away from home, following a dedicated training and nutrition program and successfully putting on 20 kilos in eight months. Twenty kilos!? I looked at him, astonished, and asked if he had done this without using steroids. This he confirmed, explaining it was not impossible at all:

Everybody can do it. It's a question of wanting it bad enough. It's all about eating more than you metabolize, and getting enough protein — so that's what I did. But I will say this: I often had to lie on my back to force down that last piece of chicken.

Kasper laughed at the incredulous expression on my face, then explained that this was a technique he had taught himself so he wouldn't vomit. The supine position seemed to give him just a bit more room, even though he felt fit to burst:

Obviously when you've eaten a kilogram of potatoes and 300 grams of meat, sure you're full. At least you're full if it's the first time you're doing it. It's no problem any more, but it was back then. Yeah, back then it was really a chore to eat that much. But you know, I'd decided I wanted to get bigger, and so I had to do it.

I was quite surprised to hear of techniques like his, where food had become a fuel that had to be swallowed using special tricks. As it turned out, several other informants spoke of similar techniques. Some had even, although briefly, taken eating one step further, as Anton described doing based on a mixture of gym lore, science and guidelines from gym and fitness magazines:

I've taken it to extremes at times, getting up at night to eat every three hours. You've got to get your 30 grams of protein every three hours. You have these gateways that open, and then you just have to consume all you can.

Anton's comments illustrate the widespread interest in bringing more or less well-founded principles into play to make the most of combining one's training, dietary intake and steroids. This strategy even runs through the entire matrix of ideal-typical approaches to steroid use. Nevertheless, when it comes to actual, factual knowledge, the same goes for nutrition, physical training and diets as for steroidal drugs: The level of expertise among informants is hugely varied. Anton is, however, aware of the sometimes limited applicability of the theories that circulate in gym circles:

Well, bodies are different, and there are different theories. Some say you have to ingest the 30 grams every three hours. Then again, others say it varies from person to person. Some people can absorb more, others less. If you eat more than you can absorb, then you just piss it out again, and then it doesn't matter how much protein you eat, and you risk damaging your liver and your kidneys. So what you have to do is find the ideal balance.

At this point Anton, a big guy who stood almost 190 cm and weighed 90 kilos, had stopped getting up at night to eat, but his total caloric intake was still massive and he followed what resembled a well-ordered system:

> I make a protein shake in the morning. And as soon as I wake up, before I even yawn, I gulp it down. Then about half an hour later I eat 200 grams of rolled oats and a muesli bar — which is packed with calories and carbohydrates. Let's see: Then I have some scrambled eggs and bacon around 11, and then around 1 or 2 o'clock I cook up 250 to 300 grams of beef along with rice, and then I have a protein shake half an hour before my workout, and I have another one right after my workout. And after that, it's straight home to eat again. I might have, say, 300 grams of steak or chicken and rice. So when it comes to protein, I'm getting those 500 grams of beef and 300 grams of chicken a day. Plus six to eight eggs and one, maybe two cans of tuna and some bacon, and about three shakes a day. And then a lot of times I'll eat another 200 grams of rolled oats again before I go to bed, because that has slow-absorption proteins and lots of carbohydrates. And even though my metabolism is really high, I don't have time to burn that before I go to bed, and so it lies there storing up in my body all night long. It's best if I make it to 6,000 calories in the course of a day.

I have no way of knowing whether Anton really ate this much, and he was somewhat imprecise in the concepts he used several times during our conversation. But assuming he did consume 6,000 kilocalories (corresponding to 25,200 kilojoules) daily, he would be ingesting at the same level as Tour de France cyclists and Olympic athletes in endurance disciplines, which ought to result in a caloric surplus he could use to grow.[3]

Eating such quantities of food is not cheap. Martin, who was living on an apprentice's wages, had financial constraints that made it hard for him to live up to his goal of staying in charge of his food intake and being able to afford his steroids. He felt that with having to buy so much food on a tight budget, he wasn't able to get all the proteins and steroid cycles he would have liked:

> It's tough for me. That's also why I haven't been through as many cycles as my training buddy. Otherwise I would've been through them — definitely. But it's really hard for me to finance. I have about 600 *kroner* [about 100 US dollars] I can spend on myself every two weeks, after I've paid my food and all that. But I could easily spend more money on food, so that I could have some more meat and more vegetables, and the stuff I need. And at the same time I spend money on protein powder so I get three shakes a day. So saving up to buy juice besides, that's really difficult. But if I could afford it I would definitely do some more cycles.

Martin's frustration over his financial situation is not least a result of his knowing that you have to be extremely disciplined about your diet when making such a big deal of your physical training. Otherwise you just won't get enough out of it: "*A lot of it's about control. You get that 'bad conscience' feeling when you don't get the right things done.*" Despite having to skimp and save Martin tries hard to follow the guidelines, having taken to heart the professional experts' insights into the link between nutrition and training:

> What you eat and your physical training, those two things kind of go hand in hand. If you eat well but don't get your workouts done, your food is all in vain. And if you work out well but you eat poorly, then your workouts are all in vain. So the two things are linked pretty closely, and that's *so* demanding. So even though you do your best, it's not easy to get big.

When Martin finally has enough to afford steroids, he has to pay extra attention to his nutrition and diet, because everything has to be in sync so he can maximize the benefits:

> Also, when you're on juice you know the time is now, and you really have to eat, so you eat that extra helping too. Everyone knows what it's like when you've had a really big dinner and feel exhausted. Imagine feeling like that all the time — five times a day. And you know, there's no "breakfast" or "supper." Nope, you eat according to time: every two and a half to three hours. Because when you've used up the protein you have in your body, you need to refill your reserves, and you've just got to eat, again and again. And that's extra tough while you're on steroids, because you know the time to grow is "now."

Martin is clearly also under the influence of gym lore and science when it comes to the body's absorption and metabolizing of protein and building muscles (see endnote 3). Yet regardless of the variations in specific user approaches, most of my informants agreed that sticking to your diet is crucial. As Adam explained, steroids alone just won't do the trick:

> Lots of people think this medicine is a wonder drug, but it's not, you know. It's the icing on the cake. Because if you don't get good sleep and do good workouts, and eat good food, then you can basically pump anything you want into your body and nothing will happen.

Strictly speaking, this is not correct. Take Jonas, a clear-cut YOLO type who talked about how he and his friends didn't worry much about the food they ate, just focused on training and steroids and continuously increased their muscle mass significantly. Anabolic steroids are actually so potent that a person on steroids will achieve more muscle growth and greater strength *without* workouts than they would working out with no steroids (Bhasin et al., 1996). Adam's point is still valid, though: With poor nutrition, users do not benefit nearly as much as they would otherwise.

Oskar also knows that to justify using steroids, they must be taken in conjunction with a highly disciplined dietary and training regime: "*Sure I know that if I just take a bunch of steroids and then eat hamburgers and pizza, I'm not gonna get that much out of it.*" Even though he described himself as serious, his story also shows that at times he has also lived a YOLO-type life. Based on this experience, he knows that combining steroids with bad food and a reckless lifestyle not only yields less benefit. It is also more risky, due to the greater strain on the user's health:

> If you party every single weekend and fill yourself with alcohol and do lines [cocaine], it's going to be at least three, four, maybe five days before your body's up to par, and of course that's really a nuisance, because then you won't get maximum benefit out of your workouts. Plus, you put an even bigger burden on your body than you have to. Because of course it's not healthy to dope yourself, but if at the same time you're getting drunk Friday, Saturday and Sunday, and going to parties with lines and that kind of stuff, things are bound to go off track.

For those who have left the YOLO lifestyle behind, much as Kasper described when talking about nutrition and calories, steroid cycles are planned in accordance with the season and the user's goals. A certain diet with a caloric surplus is often planned for the winter season, when the aim is to put on weight. Likewise, users plan their intake of steroids with various characteristics and effects according to their goals for a given season, as Jesper explained:

> Actually, you also plan your pharmaceuticals according to that, so the ones that cause a little bit of bloating [water retention], you take those in the winter, just like the really anabolic ones, you take those in winter too, and get your weight gain there. Because that's when it all has to happen. The winter battle is about gaining as much weight as you possibly can. The summer battle is about losing as much fat as possible, without losing muscle volume. These are the two "seasons," and it's precisely the same thing professional athletes do. They just do it in relation to competitions instead of seasons of the year.

Paradoxically, Rasmus — the most serious and active athlete in the group I interviewed — seemed a bit more relaxed about his diet. Unlike Anton, Martin and several other of my more junior informants, he did not attempt to justify his behavior with (pseudo-) scientific explanations about macronutrients and metabolic rates. When I asked him what he ate, he replied:

Rolled oats, fish oil, protein powder, and a supplement for breakfast. And then during the day I mainly eat rolled oats and egg whites because it's easy, and it's cheap. I whip up some pancake batter with egg whites, rolled oats, cinnamon and sweetener, then fry the pancakes in a little extra-virgin olive oil. And I eat that with three meals, and besides that we eat normal food that my girlfriend makes for supper. It's always some kind of chicken or beef or something, along with potatoes and rice and some vegetables and avocados and whatever. So, things that are pretty healthy. And I also take protein powder on the side.

Rasmus did know how much he was eating, however, and he had his total caloric intake under control, also adjusting it according to his cycles:

I'm in the range of 3,500–3,600 kilocalories per day, depending a little bit on the size and type of supper we have. It's not way up there, but then again I'm not doing steroids right now, only growth hormone. That's all. I've been doing this for a while now. But yeah, the steroids are going to come back at some point.

Outsiders may regard diets like these as excessive or exaggerated, or even as a manifestation of obsessive-compulsive behavior. Various researchers have observed such behavior with consternation and concern, which is why several studies have investigated whether such an atypical lifestyle is actually the expression of some sort of eating disorder or other mental illness. One Austrian study compared a group of 28 bodybuilders with two other groups: 30 college students with an actual eating-disorder diagnosis, and a control group of 30 healthy college students (Mangweth et al., 2001). Not surprisingly, the bodybuilders exhibited a level of preoccupation with food, body image and exercise that in many respects resembled observations of the group diagnosed with eating disorders, but which were not found in the control group. For instance, 74% of the bodybuilders stated that their meals were structured according to a preordained plan or schedule and not by hunger, as my informant Kasper also remarked.

But keeping a tight rein on calories and meal planning is not, in itself, a sign of illness. Nor is it necessarily aberrant for more than 80% of the bodybuilders in the study to have a bad conscience (like Martin and others described to me) when their meal plan went down the drain, causing them to avoid social situations, holidays or business trips where they would be unable to prepare their own food and so control their food intake. However, the researchers did not find any cases of obsessive-compulsive disorder (OCD), other mental illnesses or conditions that would clinically justify categorizing those in the bodybuilder group as having an eating disorder. All in all, the study was unable to demonstrate that bodybuilders exhibit a higher prevalence of mental illness than men in general. Admittedly, several of them had behavioral features that resembled features in people with eating disorders, such as weeks or months of deliberately going hungry or overeating. Meanwhile, this occurred primarily before and after competitions, which is understandable given the very specific requirements in competitive bodybuilding. Corresponding eating patterns can also be seen in elite athletes who do, for instance, lightweight rowing, horse racing, wrestling and gymnastics (Werner et al., 2013).

Self-perceived mood swings were also more frequent in the bodybuilder group compared to the control group, but not nearly as frequent compared to the eating-disorder group. What is more, the bodybuilders only experienced mood swings when coming off a steroid cycle. As mentioned earlier, a reaction can be anticipated in men who shift to lower testosterone levels in the blood, and it is therefore hardly reasonable to interpret this as expressing a predisposition for mental illness. This naturally does not mean mental illness does *not* occur among anabolic steroid users. Other studies that have focused not on food behavior but on the use of steroids and other drugs have found a relatively higher prevalence of various mental illnesses in steroid users compared with the respective control groups (Bjork, Skarberg, & Engstrom, 2013; Kanayama, Hudson, & Pope, 2009; Pope et al., 2014).

The point here is that although — based on the preceding descriptions of food and diets, and based on a number of corresponding findings in other studies — it seems fair to understand weight-training and disciplined dietary regimes as expressing behaviors reminiscent of OCD or eating disorders, these behaviors cannot scientifically be categorized as such (Fussell, 1991; Mangweth et al., 2001; Monaghan, 2001). Having said that, it is obvious that these patterns influence people's daily lives, for instance when users feel challenged in combining their dedication, strict diets and self-discipline, and other lifestyle factors with a social life among people who do not share their passion.

Girlfriends and parents

I asked Anton how his demanding dietary regime fitted in with having a girlfriend, which means you cannot always think of yourself and your own needs:

> They're not a very good match. Not unless it's a very, very understanding and really sweet girl. Because if you're living with a girl and leading the life I do, she can sometimes feel like she kind of gets ignored. But the girlfriends I've had have come to terms with it. Of course they think you eat a lot, and that it's expensive, but they accept it, because they know what they signed up for.

Organizing the practicalities of daily life can also be a challenge, as Kasper explained:

> So, let's take my girlfriend as an example. She's known me from before the time I started working out and up till now, when I'm past 90 kilos.

She gets annoyed when we're out shopping, because when I've been walking around for a couple of hours I've got to have something to eat. And if we go somewhere for eight hours, then we eat maybe two or three times. So in that sense people look at us as freaks. Because our eating is extreme. We eat constantly, and people notice that.

Kasper's parents were concerned about his workouts and dietary schedule, associating his larger body and his general lifestyle with the use of IPEDs:

Right at the start, stuff happens. You get stronger, and you also get more well-defined pretty fast. But since my parents saw me hang out with the big guys, they also started suspecting I was taking stuff, too. They were worried. Take protein powder: It was banned in their house. They associated it with doping. They believed it made your muscles bigger and enlarged your heart, so it must be dangerous. The same with creatine. But I'd just buy it on the sly. Later, they did accept that's just the way it was.

Anton also told me that although his girlfriends had accepted the situation, his parents were quite anxious about his lifestyle:

My parents think it's too much. They think I spend too much time on it. Last year, I really spent lots of time on it. At that point I was just shy of 100 kilos. But my mom thinks it's too extreme, too ugly, and too much.

Anton's altered physique shaped his parents' overall view of his lifestyle, and disagreements were quickly interpreted in light of this view. When he would visit them and they would disagree on some issue, his parents would automatically react by saying he probably had that opinion because he was on steroids. He also got stereotypical reactions to his size, style and clothing choices elsewhere: "*There are constantly these prejudices. If you're the size I am, people also like to be snide and say it's only because you're cheating; that sort of thing.*" He also had run-ins with his parents, who were not happy about his life choices:

This one time my parents found out I'd taken steroids, and they've been giving me grief about it ever since. As soon as my training's started to go well, even when I haven't been on steroids, if I've gotten bigger and I'm wearing a tight shirt, they always ask: "Are you *sure* you're not taking that stuff anymore?" They're constantly telling me that it's too much, that I shouldn't grow anymore, that I should go easy on all the working out.

Rasmus, who is ten years older, also knows what it is like when friends and family members worry. While his parents find it hard to come to terms with his choices, his friends have accepted his lifestyle:

> My parents don't think it's cool that I've taken steroids, but they've accepted it. I haven't actually told my dad, but he does know. I came right out and told my mom and it made her kind of sad, but when I'd talk to her about it she could hear I knew about these things, and that calmed her down a little bit.

During my interview with Rasmus in his apartment, his girlfriend came in. They had met each other at a physique competition, and she was into elite fitness training herself, so she knew the community from the inside. I asked her how she felt about her boyfriend using so much medicine in order to live as a competitive bodybuilder:

> Before I met him I was seriously against it. I'm really against putting things into your body that aren't supposed to be there, like alcohol, drugs and steroids. But it's like, after I met him, then … You see, I met him like this. He was taking these things. You know, it was part of the package. I don't know, I guess I just accepted it. And I also feel like I want to get bigger myself. I actually think that if I had the courage to do it, I probably would've been taking something too.

Others have drawn a very sharp line, as we saw Michael do, explaining how he and his girlfriend had a deal: If they were going to be together, she had to agree not to complain when she found one of the vegetable drawers in the fridge full of medicine. Jesper chose another approach and "sat down and dug deep," discussing steroid use with his girlfriend so she knew about the effects and side effects of the drugs. The same was true for Adam, the Well-being type, who did not believe any girlfriend could change the lifestyle he had chosen. Steroids were part of his life. When I asked him how he would react if he got a girlfriend who did not want him to take steroids, he immediately replied:

> I wouldn't accept that. Then she wouldn't be my girlfriend any more. It's such an integrated part of me as a person, and I would be another person without those things. On the other hand, I'd never fall in love with a girl who wasn't tolerant enough to say "That's okay."

Because of the obvious stigmatization from their surroundings, particularly as related by Kasper, Martin and Anton, it is worth asking: What makes people choose a lifestyle that is the object of so much scorn? Some might claim, in keeping with the American anthropologist Alan Klein, that what drives people to dedicate themselves to weightlifting and bodybuilding are "large doses of insecurity," and that therefore it is not something they "choose" (see Chapter 5, and Klein, 1993). The Welsh sociologist Lee Monaghan does not buy into this proposition. He underscores that being a bodybuilder is not a person's destiny but an expression of an active, reflected choice. Which brings us back to the question: Why choose this life, if your surroundings will stigmatize you as a big, stupid, muscle-bound brute?

Us and them

Among my informants, Kenneth was the one who most plainly expressed in words how, for him, lifting weights and being strong was part of his identity work, which also had to do with a fundamental sense of psychological insecurity. Clearly he had reflected on what his physical training had meant to his identity and his faith in himself:

> Ever since I was 18 years old and up till now, at 24, working out and the fact that other people could see it has meant a lot to me. Maybe I had a kind of talent for lifting weights, considering the discipline you've got to have. And I was able to lift quite a lot, and then you get some feedback on that, and you take that in, and then more and more it becomes a part of your identity. Maybe it's a substitute for something else if you don't ... Well, if you don't have enough faith in yourself, then that hole can be filled by weightlifting, and that creates an identity. For me, it probably has a lot to do with that.

Kenneth's account of what physical training means to his identity not only links to Klein's description of lacking self-confidence. It also ties in with the idea that identity is something you have to work on, and fight for, because it is linked to the recognition you get for the effort you make. But in addition to this unavoidable element in acquiring that identity — having to perform somehow to gain recognition from the others, as also seen in other sub-cultures — there is also a uniform and a style one must adopt. As Kasper explained, buzz-cut hair is one element:

> It's just like the punk rockers with their stand-up Mohawks: It's a style. It's an image. But it's also a style that has a practical side to it, because we're afraid of bacteria. In this sport, if you're sick for a week you drop two kilos. We don't want to do that, so we do everything we can *not* to get sick, and it's easier to stay clean if you have no hair on your head.

But even a buzz cut, the right clothes, and a membership card to the gym will not do the trick, in and of themselves. As we have heard, what is decisive for whether the new identity is experienced as strong and sustainable is that the person acts, achieves results, and by virtue of this gains recognition for their actions from people perceived as important. As also discussed earlier, the prospect of developing sex appeal and having sexual encounters is a key part of building an attractive body, and it can be a strong incentive for many a gym neophyte. Gradually, however, as a person's physique develops their focus will move beyond seeking attention and compliments from the opposite sex. Jesper described this shift:

> In the beginning, when I started working out, I wanted the girls to start looking. When I moved on and my weight rose over and above what most girls actually think is attractive, it was to make the guys start looking. Because when you get to the point where the *guys* start looking, man, you know they're impressed.

Kasper was in line with this view, stressing that although sex appeal is important, that doesn't mean compliments from women are more important than compliments from men:

> I prefer to get compliments from a guy who works out himself, and who knows what he's talking about. Let's say I'm at a club and some girl walks over and lays her hand on my chest. That doesn't mean anything, because she hasn't thought about how much work it represents. Sure, it's nice and all. But that's not what makes me tick. But if somebody walks over, maybe even a pro, who says things are looking good. I mean, if the alpha male gives you a pat on the back, you're doin' pretty good.

Among my informants, this view on compliments from women was a recurring feature. Everyone liked getting them, but they were not the most important thing. Rasmus didn't mince words: *"I'd much rather have a guy come up to me and tell me I look good. I don't give a shit about what the girls think."* He laughs, then elaborates:

> It really doesn't mean a thing to me. But I think it's totally cool when a guy who works out too walks over and gives me a compliment. Then you know you've been doing something right. Because if it's a girl, it might as well just be some stupid line to come on to you, and that doesn't count.

This last comment emphasizes how identity is not a role you can copy. You have to do something that is recognized by the right people. By way of example, you cannot simply walk into a bar in mountaineering shoes with a bag of talcum, ropes and snap hooks and expect everyone to see you as a mountain climber. You may fool a few non-climbers in the bar, but genuine, experienced mountain climbers will know you're not the real deal. Climbers don't walk into bars with their equipment. They use it on the mountain. The point is that young athletes who want to change their self-image have a tendency to over-identify with the external, visible codes of their sport before they really get to know the sport from within the community (Donnelly & Young, 1999). And that is why recognition does not really count until it comes from people who know what they are talking about. Female fawning and fussing may feel good, and it may even lead to a fun night on and off the dance floor, but as in all other walks of life the most important brand of recognition comes from people with status in the community.

Meanwhile, the odd eating and workout habits must be justifiable. One way to legitimize one's behavior — how you eat, work out, dress and cut your hair; the values to which you adhere — is to distance oneself from the things one is *not*, or with which one does *not* identify. Several of my informants noted the distinguishing contrasts in their own lifestyle and approach to physical training, as opposed to people with whom they would rather not be compared. Anton explained why he and his friend left the gym where they had originally started training:

> We'd go down there, and there'd be, like, four girls standing there looking in the mirror, plus some guys wearing a bunch of necklaces and stuff with their hair all waxed, posturing and preening. And they'd stand there and spend more time styling their hair and looking at each other than using the equipment. They spent more time trying to look good than they did lifting weights.

Rasmus, the bodybuilder, was also acutely aware of the types he did not identify with when I mentioned, during his interview, that some people work out because they want to look good when they go out. "*Yeah, the disco-pump guys,*" Rasmus explained:

> The kind of guys who work out to get the girls to look at them. Eye candy. They train some pecs and biceps but no legs at all. They have no calves, since all they ever think about is whether they look good in a T-shirt. It's not a lifestyle. I was never part of that crowd.

Rasmus was not implying there was only room for one type of person at his current gym. On the contrary:

> We've got old people, young people. And sure, you can see the difference, but that doesn't bother me. Not one bit. But I do know the disco-pump guys tend to work out at places like "Fitness DK" — which also has a nice, tidy feel to it when you walk in. People wear nice clothes, and there's a nice, mainstream pop channel playing on the radio. That's not so important down at our gym.

Michael's wording was even more blunt as he explained why he looked to bodybuilding rather than the more popular "fitness training" when he started seriously lifting weights: *"What I wanted was plainly something very different than fitness. And that became clear after just a month."* He quickly turned his back on exercise that would just be healthy and bring mainstream buffness:

> Totally. You know, I just thought what all those little fitness fairies were doing, it looked ridiculous. Prancing around in the big gym room, jumping over tires and doing stupid exercises that didn't take any real physical effort ... Christ, with a little practice anybody can do that. But the other stuff, sculpting a physique like a bodybuilder, that's really hard work.

Michael draws a very sharp line between "us" and "them"; between those who do things *"for real"* and those who don't. As he put it himself, the reason for his uncompromising position is probably his *"fire-and-ice"* personality. Either you do something 100% or not at all. You have to be dedicated to the things you get involved in, as he said, whether it's your job, your family or your sport. That is why he does not like people who say *"that's fine"* or are satisfied with mediocrity. Since earning his teaching degree he had been employed at a small private school with strong pedagogical values, and he described his work there:

> I'm insanely committed to my work. And this is where the arrogance comes in, because I'm really a great teacher. I'm the teacher who makes a difference for some of these kids, who might otherwise go through their entire school life and say: "Gee, going to school really sucked." But when they're sixty years old, I'm sure they're going to say: "Our teacher was a real buddy." A guy who wanted us to be team players, to give it our best shot, to shift our personal boundaries for what we think we can do. To move us away from "that's fine." Because it's not "fine." It's not even *good!* I hate it when parents say: "That's OK sweetie. You're doing fine."

It was this dedication which, in a few short years, brought about his metamorphosis from ambitious soccer player to highly respected competitive bodybuilder. But it was also, at least in part, the same attitude that drove him over the edge in his quest for a Danish championship title (as described in Chapter 6).

Not all my informants drew such solid lines. Adam, who was not as dedicated as Michael, sees no sharp distinction between people who want to cultivate bodybuilding and those with a more general goal of physical fitness:

> It doesn't seem to me there's any condemnation at the fitness center where I work out. We're very tolerant. People have different goals, and sometimes people's goals change. Maybe somebody from the fitness crowd moves into bodybuilding, or vice versa.

As long as people do something for their bodies and are committed to what they do, it's fine with Adam. But his tolerance hits a wall when he sees people who are overweight: *"I'm more judgmental now of people who don't do any kind of exercise at all. Especially if I see people who are really obese. Then I think: 'Oh, for cryin' out loud — get up and do something!'"* He explains that this attitude arose after he became more committed to his own physical training. *"It's something that's developed in me. I have to admit it's made me more judgmental. I'll think: 'Seriously, fellah — don't reach for that second helping of creamed potatoes.' It really isn't that hard."* I found this negative view of overweight people in several of my informants. Here, too, Michael offered the bluntest wording:

> Fat people, especially fat women — they really gross me out, man. I feel contempt, pure and simple. I see them as less worthy of my respect. The fact that they can't keep themselves under control. Why do they just stuff themselves with that crap? Why don't they go to the gym and exercise? Why don't they think about how they look? Why don't they think about what they shove into their face?

One might think a person who had lived with such high risks as Michael had, and taken so many unhealthy drugs, would be more accepting and less judgmental of others. However, Michael is not so much opposed to the unhealthy lifestyle but clearly associates obesity with a laxness and a lack of discipline and life commitment, which he finds very hard to accept.

Kasper had a slightly different approach. Perhaps because he has a number of friends who use steroids, and because he realizes his own training and dietary regimes do not fall within the conventional perception of "healthy," Kasper acknowledges that people are free to do with their bodies as they like, as long as they stand by their choices. He sees weight and obesity as a life choice:

> I don't mind people being overweight, but I'll be damned if I'm going to listen to them moaning and whining about it. People can do whatever they want to with their bodies. I don't start whining when I can't eat any more. But I just can't deal with those types on TV weight-loss programs who sit there complaining that they're oh-so-fat, and that their life is oh-so-tough. I'm like: There *is* actually a diet called "Stop pigging out!" It's not like you're going to get fat from eating nothing. You're doing something, and what you're doing is wrong. So no, I don't have a lot of respect for that. But it's a general thing, and no matter what the heck your problem is: I have no respect for people who don't have any discipline. Without it, you can't get a damned thing done. You know, we all have something we think is hard.

Even though the views of my informants may sound harsh and uncompromising, they differ little from the public view of overweight or obese people. In general, peoples' preconceptions declare obesity to be an outcome of one's personal responsibility, which is avertible by adopting the right lifestyle (Kim, Makowski, & von dem Knesebeck, 2019). A Danish opinion poll conducted by a well-reputed agency found that 82% of respondents indicated that people's responsibility for carrying excess weight lies, first and foremost, with themselves. Echoing Adam's sentiment, 32% answered that they think "Pull yourself together," when they see an overweight person holding a sugary soft drink or an ice-cream cone (Schmidt & Rasmussen, 2017). Interestingly, and contrary to the normalization hypothesis, it has been found that a comparatively high prevalence of obesity, like that seen in the United States, is associated with a higher level of obesity stigma compared to what has been found in a country such as Germany (Kim et al., 2019).

To people outside the gym community, a number of my informants seem to have chosen a dietary regime that is unnecessarily strict. They eat a lot, and often, affecting not only the protein synthesis in their muscles but also their personal finances and social lives, including their relations with families and partners. Many outsiders therefore believe these people have an obsessive-compulsive approach to food. Nevertheless, researchers have been unable to document any sort of psychological disorder among this group that would cause their unusual diets and eating habits.

Although my informant group was distinctive in their nutritional and dietary behavior, generally speaking they mirror a variety of commonplace sociological facts. We humans form groups with people who resemble us, and we create clear-cut distinctions and boundaries between ourselves and those with whom we wish to avoid comparison. Furthermore, we are able to rationalize our own odd behaviors — in this case relating to food and exercise — in the light of the goals we set for ourselves, whereas the behaviors and choices of other people seem less obviously "right" to us, and sometimes even repulsive.

One aspect shared by all my informants, but perhaps most clearly enunciated by Kasper, is that they expect people to be able to take care of themselves. Their statements are permeated by a fundamentally liberal approach to the effect that: (A) people can do whatever they want, as long as they don't prevent others from doing likewise; and (B) you can only achieve something in life if you make a personal effort.

As we saw above, Adam believed that his own view of overweight people and their level of self-discipline had changed after he began training himself. This suggests that workout regimes, and the physique people thereby achieve, also affect their views. We can hardly find any causal explanation, but since the statements from Adam and several other informants contained an element of contempt for weakness and poor self-discipline, this view seems to characterize the group. Further, this correlates with international research findings that show how physically stronger men tend to be more right-wing and less in favor of social and economic equality. One study showed a particularly strong correlation between the number of hours spent in the gym and having less egalitarian socio-economic beliefs (Price, Sheehy-Skeffington, Sidnaius, & Pound, 2017). We will return to this discussion in Chapter 10.

Although gym activities and gym culture are relatively new phenomena, the statements by the informants in my study — in this context and others — seem to confirm that weightlifting and bodybuilding have features from certain age-old circumstances where bodily strength impacted our perception of other people and our social interactions with others. Culture indisputably plays a crucial role to the norms and values that become dominant in various societies. But perhaps, in our discussions about values, gender, body images and the use of steroids we have forgotten that as human beings we have aspects of human nature and an evolutionary history that we carry within us, and that our bodies and appearance play a role in our values and attitudes towards other people. By gaining greater insight into these issues we can move towards a better understanding of the attraction of weightlifting, strength, muscles and anabolic-steroid use in our friendly neighborhood gyms and fitness centers.

Notes

1 Rolled oats is a typical Danish breakfast food (and has been so since the early twentieth century), containing relatively high levels of protein and slowly released carbohydrates.
2 Kasper's weight specifications for pasta and rice were dry weight, prior to cooking.
3 In 2017, the Journal of *The International Society of Sports Nutrition* published a position statement on this topic — a joint pronouncement from the professional community emphatically stating knowledge now considered as incontestably validated. Here the authors collected the existing body of knowledge they believe covers the correlation between protein intake, exercise and building muscle. The position statement said, firstly, that strength training combined with adequate protein intake, either before or after training, will stimulate protein synthesis in the muscle tissue (i.e. muscle growth). Therefore, to build up or retain muscle bulk, for most people "adequate protein intake" will amount to 1.4–2.0 grams of protein per kilo of body weight per day (g/kg/d). The general recommendation is 0.25 g of high-quality protein per kilo of body weight per meal, meaning a maximum of 20–40 grams per meal. However, recent research has demonstrated that +3 g/kg/d can be beneficial for people doing heavy resistance training. Ideally, protein intake should be distributed throughout the day on meals eaten at intervals of 3 to 4 hours. It is possible — even for dedicated gym-goers — to get sufficient protein by eating normal foodstuffs, but protein powders are a practical way to ingest the desired amounts of high-quality protein while limiting calories. Examples of food sources that provide 28 grams of protein include a 133-gram chicken filet (raw weight); a 126-gram pork chop (raw weight); 4 eggs (242 grams total weight); 1,400 grams of green beans; 560 grams of heavy, whole-grain rye bread; or 212 grams of rolled oats (Jäger et al., 2017).

References

Barland, B., Tangen, J. O., & Johannesen, C. A. (2010). Doping, muskler, mestring og mening. En kvalitativ studie av unge menns bruk av muskelbyggende medikamenter. Retrieved from Oslo: https://brage.bibsys.no/xmlui/handle/11250/175072.

Bhasin, S., Storer, T. W., Berman, N., Callegari, C., Clevenger, B., Phillips, J., ... Casaburi, R. (1996). The effects of supraphysiologic doses of testosterone on muscle size and strength in normal men. N Engl J Med, 335(1), 1–7. doi: doi:10.1056/NEJM199607043350101.

Bjork, T., Skarberg, K., & Engstrom, I. (2013). Eating disorders and anabolic androgenic steroids in males–similarities and differences in self-image and psychiatric symptoms. Subst Abuse Treat Prev Policy, 8, 30. doi: doi:10.1186/1747-597x-8-30.

Donnelly, P., & Young, K. (1999). Rock climbers and rugby players: identity construction and confirmation. In J. Coakley & P. Donnelly (Eds.), Inside Sports (pp. 67–76). London & New York: Routledge.

Fussell, S. W. (1991). Muscle: Confessions of an unlikely bodybuilder. New York: Avon Books.

Jäger, R., Kerksick, C. M., Campbell, B. I., Cribb, P. J., Wells, S. D., Skwiat, T. M., ... Antonio, J. (2017). International Society of Sports Nutrition Position Stand: Protein and exercise. Journal of the International Society of Sports Nutrition, 14(1), 20. doi: doi:10.1186/s12970-017-0177-8.

Kanayama, G., Hudson, J. I., & Pope, H. G. (2009). Features of men with anabolic-androgenic steroid dependence: A comparison with nondependent AAS users and with AAS nonusers. Drug Alcohol Depend, 102(1–3), 130–137. doi: doi:10.1016/j.drugalcdep.2009.02.008.

Kim, T. J., Makowski, A. C., & von dem Knesebeck, O. (2019). Obesity stigma in Germany and the United States: Results of population surveys. PLoS One, 14(8), e0221214. doi: doi:10.1371/journal.pone.0221214.

Klein, A. M. (1993). Little big men: Bodybuilding subculture and gender construction. Albany, NY: State University of New York Press.

Mangweth, B., Pope, H. G., Jr., Kemmler, G., Ebenbichler, C., Hausmann, A., De, C. C., ... Biebl, W. (2001). Body image and psychopathology in male bodybuilders. Psychotherapy and Psychosomatics, 70(1), 38–43. doi: doi:10.1159/000056223.

Monaghan, L. F. (2001). Bodybuilding, drugs, and risk. London: Routledge.

Pedersen, P. V., Ingholt, L., & Tjørnhøj-Thomsen, T. (2014). Disciplin og dedikation: Unges perspektiver på træning, kost og brug af muskelopbyggende og præstationsfremmende midler. Retrieved from Odense: http://si-folkesundhed.dk/upload/disciplin_og_dedikation.pdf.

Pope, H. G., Wood, R. I., Rogol, A., Nyberg, F., Bowers, L., & Bhasin, S. (2014). Adverse health consequences of performance-enhancing drugs: An Endocrine Society scientific statement. Endocr Rev, 35(3), 341–375. doi: doi:10.1210/er.2013-1058.

Price, M. E., Sheehy-Skeffington, J., Sidnaius, J., & Pound, N. (2017). Is sociopolitical egalitarianism related to bodily and facial formidability in men? Evolution and Human Behavior, 38(5), 626–634. doi: doi:10.1016/j.evolhumbehav.2017.04.001.

Schmidt, A. L., & Rasmussen, L. I. (2017, 5 April). Fede bærer selv ansvaret, mener stort flertal. Politiken, page 1, section 1.

Vinther, A. S., & Christiansen, A. V. (2019). Different users, different interventions. On the ideal typology of anabolic-androgenic steroid use and its implications for prevention and harm reduction. In K. van de Ven, K. Mulrooney, & J. McVeigh (Eds.), *Human Enhancement Drugs* (pp. 249–263). London: Routledge.

Werner, A., Thiel, A., Schneider, S., Mayer, J., Giel, K. E., & Zipfel, S. (2013). Weight-control behaviour and weight-concerns in young elite athletes: A systematic review. *Journal of Eating Disorders*, 1, 1–18. doi: doi:10.1186/2050-2974-1-18.

Zahnow, R., McVeigh, J., Bates, G., Hope, V., Kean, J., Campbell, J., & Smith, J. (2018). Identifying a typology of men who use anabolic androgenic steroids (AAS). *International Journal of Drug Policy*, 55, 105–112. doi: doi:10.1016/j.drugpo.2018.02.022.

Chapter 10

Manhood – powerful and precarious

Many devoted weight trainers and bodybuilders harbor what can fairly be called very traditional ideas of what being "really masculine" or "really feminine" means, as expressed in several studies (such as Andreasson & Johansson, 2014; Kanayama, Barry, Hudson, & Pope, 2006; Moberg & Hermansson, 2006). Alan Klein also stressed this point in his study of American bodybuilders on the West Coast, which led him to coin the evocative term "comic-book masculinity" to denote the stereotypical gender perception he observed among these groups (Klein, 1993). Generally, my interviewees, particularly some of my younger informants, also had fairly traditional perceptions of gender and muscles. This is evident in Anton's explanation of the kind of guy he believes girls typically fall for:

> Most girls like it when you look a little tough, with a touch of "bad boy." Most girls like that kind of guy. Maybe one out of twenty girls likes a guy who has that wussy kind of look, wears a scarf around his neck and stuff. But the rest want somebody who can take a hold of them and swing them around; who's rough and powerful and can really protect them, and at the same time be nice to them.

Boys have to be big, strong and protective. Girls have to be demure, sweet and sensitive. Clear-cut roles. That perception certainly does exist, but it hardly covers everyone, in fitness and gym cultures or elsewhere. Like most other subcultures these groups are also more diverse than they may seem at first glance. For instance, it is common knowledge that at least since the 1970s, gym culture at large has had a well-established homosexual component (Halkitis et al., 2008; Klein, 1993; Lanzieri & Hildebrandt, 2011; Luciano, 2007). Nevertheless, most advertisements for gyms and exercise magazines promote clear masculine and feminine ideals that are generally associated with heterosexuality. It was this schism which, at the time, motivated Klein to investigate the relationship between the imagined or *ideal* culture that bodybuilding communities used in their marketing, as opposed to the actual or *real* culture he observed. Using this conceptual pair as a lever, he was able to uncover a pervasive element of hypocrisy, since body-builders in fact talked about and idealized heterosexuality and autonomy, whereas their behavior and actions not infrequently hinted at or exhibited bisexual and homosexual conduct, as well as a dependency on people who held power in the organized world of bodybuilding sport (Klein, 1993).

Still, that observation does not change the clear links that exist between men, muscles and masculinity, which Anton rightly pointed to, and which Klein also noted. In fact, this link is not found merely among workout devotees. Rather, it is an essential cultural principle:

> Every man engages in some sort of dialogue with muscle; it does not matter whether he embraces or repudiates it — he holds an internal dialogue concerning muscle. It is an essential cultural principle and one that distinguishes men from women. Size matters when it comes to muscles.
>
> (Klein, 2007, p. 69)

Some readers may find this statement objectionable, but bear with me as I guide you through a small exercise, and you may find it less far-fetched than you thought at first. In a moment, I will ask you to close your eyes and think back to your school year in fifth grade. Try to recall your position in the physical hierarchy among your classmates. If you are a man, think back on the boys in your class: Who was stronger than you, and who was weaker? Likewise, if you are a woman: Which girls were stronger than you, and weaker? Now close your eyes and give it your best shot. Do you remember?

When I do this exercise in Denmark with my students at Aarhus University, virtually all the young men find it relevant and meaningful. They vividly recall the hierarchy and their place in it. Conversely, most of the young women see little point in doing the exercise. They have never dwelled on their own position in the physical hierarchy or felt its bodily consequences. The men have. In this way the exercise confirms Klein's claim that, generally speaking, muscles and physical strength are factors all boys and men think about, whereas girls and women do not.

In this chapter we will examine the role human biology and psyche play in our fascination with muscles, and in our perception of masculinity and femininity. In Chapter 2 we looked at some of the influential theories in the literature about the male fascination with muscles, and about why anabolic steroids have become so widely used. For obvious reasons, most of these theories take their cue from the cultural shifts the Western world has undergone over the past 50 years or so. They do this because there must be historical, cultural and sociological reasons why people today (as opposed to earlier generations) work hard to achieve their bodily ideals. Hence, the basis of these explanations has been the media's rise to prominence, the cultural exposure of attractive bodies, the crumbling of traditional gender roles, women's liberation, individualization, and the proliferation of surgical and medical interventions meant to bring people closer to their ideal. All these factors undoubtedly contribute, and precisely because they are pertinent we may tend to forget that human beings are not simply cultural beings. They are also animals, and as such they — *we* — have an evolutionary history that affects our psyche, behaviors, norms and aesthetic preferences, not least when it comes to sexually charged gendered interaction and our perceptions of "attractive bodies." If we fail to take these factors into consideration, we end up missing an important piece in the puzzle of why our culture, and the marketplace, have so successfully drawn people into fitness and gym culture, and why steroid use has grown to the proportions it has today. The hypothesis I investigate in this chapter is this: Is there a basic biological sounding board against which our marketplaces and cultures resonate?

Evolutionary psychology

In the context of evolutionary psychology, gender-based differences in norms and behaviors reflect adaptation to problems our distant male and female ancestors regularly had to face. The basic premise for studying gender differences in light of humankind's gradual development is that our brains have evolved in certain surroundings to cope with certain conditions that differ immensely from human surroundings and conditions today. What is more, the human brain has evolved under the influence of the same forces that shaped other biological phenomena. But although, on the one hand, the brain is the source of our behaviors, norms and values, on the other hand it has also evolved to think, learn and construct cultures. Humans are biological cultural beings. Therefore it would not be a fruitful approach to choose between explanatory models that emphasize *either* nature *or* culture; *either* cognition *or* learning. On the contrary, biology is a precondition for human culture, which makes it useful to know how it works on us, and within us. The American psychologist Douglas Kenrick and his colleagues have sought to show how the interplay between biological and social aspects are very clearly expressed precisely in the field of psychological differences between the male and female genders (Kenrick, Trost, & Sundie, 2004). They argue that in human biology we can trace back a number of universal, fundamental features concerning behaviors and norms, but that of course these are expressed in ways that are culturally specific.

One area where this becomes clear is in our efforts to find a mate or partner. Most people probably perceive the hunt for "a significant other" as a process controlled by flirting, romance and the search for someone with the right personality. Which it is. But under the surface, the subtle influences of human biology are at work. Despite legal equality in most areas, men and women are biologically different, and this affects our preferences and behaviors in ways that help us understand Anton's thoughts about what kind of guys most girls prefer.

In all mammalian species, males are more inclined than females to be aggressive and compete for dominance (Herbert, 2015). There are two evolutionary principles that explain this difference: the magnitude of their parental investment, and sexual selection. Generally, male and female mammals contribute very different amounts of effort to produce offspring. So too with humans. During a woman's life span she will release an average of 400 fertilizable ova, some ten of which may become offspring. This is not a large number, so she has to be careful about who gets to fertilize them. A man, on the other hand, can produce over 40 million sperm cells per ejaculation – which may occur every day from the time of sexual maturity until he is well over 60. Consequently, a man need not fret about the fate of his individual sperm cells, nor is there any biological quarantine or time lapse from the moment he contributes to one pregnancy until he can contribute to another. So whereas a man can increase his number of offspring many fold by having sex with many women, a woman cannot increase her progeny correspondingly by having sex with many men. This makes female reproductive capacity a limited resource, and so an object of male competition (Pinker, 2011). Since mistakes in the field of fertilization are far more costly for women than for men, women tend to be more selective than men are when choosing sex partners. What is more, a woman's absolute minimum investment in offspring is far greater than a man's absolute minimum investment. She must carry and nourish the child before and after birth, significantly draining her resources. The man's investment, on the other hand, does not have to demand any more than the energy it takes for him to have sex just the once. Nevertheless, it is clear that the child's chances of survival improve if the man invests more effort than that. But although, in humans, the male therefore most often makes much larger investment in parenting than most other species of mammal, his contribution is still considerably smaller than the female's, and the resources he brings to the venture are fundamentally different.

Because the two biological genders contribute different resources and invest unequally in parenting, men and women also look for different things — besides romantic love — when searching for a partner. In other words, their sexual-selection criteria differ. Women directly invest their physical, bodily resources in having children. Men invest indirect resources such as food, money and protection. That is why men search for fertile women of an appropriate age to conceive and bear children, whereas women search for men with resources that can help ensure a child's rearing and survival. Female fertility in humans peaks in the mid-twenties, then decreases and ends at menopause, which is why men of all ages instinctively turn their heads after women in their twenties. Given that male human reproductive capability is much less age-dependent, women have a stronger tendency to seek the things that can ensure their potential offspring a safe and comfortable upbringing. That is why they often turn their heads after men with resources — and "resources" may come in many shapes and sizes and are not necessarily age-dependent. Like other resources, the above-mentioned examples of food, money and security are often linked to social status. Even today, long after nature dictated these preferences by necessity, one can observe that women who achieve high social status generally do not shift towards preferring younger men, but continue to prefer men with resources (Kenrick et al., 2004).

Against this backdrop, from the perspective of evolutionary psychology one would expect to find universal behavioral traits in both genders. However, if one studies a particular culture, there are often more similarities than differences between women and men. What is more, the behavioral differences one can observe will be greater within a gender group than the behavioral differences between genders. Even so, this does not shoot down the hypothesis of universal behavioral differences. The fact is that these behavioral differences are not binary, like the gender-defined physiological differences between men and women. Rather, the behavioral differences are distributed on bell curves ranging from "less pronounced" to "more pronounced" in the same way height, strength and so on are distributed. That is, even though *a few* women will be physically stronger than most men, that does not change the curve indicating that men are *generally* stronger than women are. So too with behavioral differences. Although some women are more competitive than most men, that does not change reported findings that men are generally more competitive and dominance-oriented than women are (Kenrick et al., 2004).

A few examples will illustrate this point. One study that compared homicide rates in different societies found that men more frequently were murderers than women, and that the murder victim was most often a man.[1] Another study, on the division of labor in a variety of cultures, found that while the production of leather goods was evenly distributed between genders (some cultures mainly had male leather-goods workers; other cultures mainly female leather-goods workers; and yet others had both genders in almost equal measure), in 121 of the 122 cultures examined, the manufacturing of weapons was a job performed exclusively by males (with one culture where women participated in this activity). The third study showed that across 16 different categories for risk behavior, men were overrepresented in all except one: smoking. It further showed that the most significant gender differences were found where risk behavior involved testing physical prowess with a high probability of resulting physical and mental damage (all examples taken from Kenrick et al., 2004). Based on these observations it is easy to infer that men are more likely to become involved in risky, dangerous activities that can potentially increase their social status. The payoff in this would be that social status is highly valued by women seeking partners. So when young men on Pentecost Island, in the South Pacific nation of Vanuatu, jump off spindly wooden towers with vines tied around their ankles, it certainly displays the coming-of-age ritual in this particular culture. However, the behavior itself is linked to a universal male propensity to compete, show dominance and win status through publicly verifiable actions.

So here we have evolutionary psychology pointing to two circumstances that can help us understand why men use steroids in gym environments. One has to do with a certain type of bodily appearance that signals strength, resources and the ability to protect. The other has to do with how the male preference for competition and risk-taking behavior affects our perception of what a "real man" is. Let us look at these separately and see if they can help us understand Anton's statements about the kind of guys girls like best.

Universally attractive bodies

Reading the work of the American feminist writer Naomi Wolf, one might think there were no universal standards for physical beauty.[2] In her 1991 bestseller *The Beauty Myth*, she argues that beauty as an objective, universal trait does not exist. Putting an ironic slant on the biological perspective of beauty, she states that

> Women must want to embody it [beauty] and men must want to possess women who embody it. This embodiment is an imperative for women and not for men, which situation is necessary and natural because it is biological, sexual and evolutionary: Strong men battle for beautiful women, and beautiful women are more reproductively successful. Women's beauty must correlate to their fertility, and since this system is based on sexual selection, it is inevitable and changeless.
>
> (Wolf, 1991, p. 12)

However, she then asserts that "None of this is true," arguing instead that "'Beauty' is a currency system like the gold standard. Like any economy, it is determined by politics, and in the modern age in the West it is the last best belief system that keeps male dominance intact" (Wolf, 1991, p. 12). According to this interpretation, beauty is a cultural and political construction controlled by men, and aimed at repressing women. This echoes the perception that our quest to achieve a beautiful body expresses an ambition or wish inside us to adapt to a cultural prescription of what bodies are supposed to look like. A prescription which — we are told — is dictated through a particular discourse about body and normality, which is socially constructed through dominant, white, Western, male, heterosexual, middle-class values. Many academics have adopted this view, using its premises to point out that, as Wolf argued, we ought to leave behind the idea of beauty as anything but a social construct and not allow it to play any role in our lives. With this foremost in our minds, we can draw a sigh of relief and move on.

The only problem with this is that outside the confines of academia and the broader intellectual debate, beauty remains enormously important. No one has stopped looking at beautiful people because academics define beauty as a social construct. No one has stopped enjoying beauty, and many people certainly make a huge effort to acquire bits of it for themselves (Høgh-Olesen, 2019). Even though Wolf refutes them as untrue, these circumstances make the thought spring readily to mind that perhaps this preoccupation with beauty is, after all, a part of our natural human makeup (Ryan, 2018). That is precisely the idea Nancy Etcoff, a Harvard psychologist, pursues in *Survival of the Prettiest*, a book whose title reveals that she, too, is investigating an evolutionary path. Her premise, contrary to Wolf's, is that we are biologically adapted to take an interest in beauty. Our extreme sensitivity to beautiful people is embedded deep in our brains, because beauty in a person indicates a good genetic makeup. "We love to look at smooth skin, thick shiny hair, curved waists, and symmetrical bodies because in the course of evolution the people who noticed these signals and desired their possessors had more reproductive success. We are their descendants" (Etcoff, 1999, p. 24). Although modern humans try to avoid pregnancy in the vast majorities of sexual encounters, our sexual preferences are still controlled by age-old precepts that make us more strongly attracted to bodies that signal the best reproductive characteristics. Western culture, particularly in the United States, is often accused of being overly focused on appearance. However, a comparative study found that in one third of non-Western, non-North American cultures, appearance weighed more heavily than it did for college students in the United States. Researchers found that the decisive factor for how strongly individuals in a given culture value physical beauty in a potential partner was not based on their exposure to supermodels. It was based on how often they were exposed to parasitic diseases. In cultures where such exposure was common, unblemished skin and a slim, muscular body were visual confirmation of good health (Etcoff, 1999, p. 59).

Compared to other animals, we humans have clearly taken a more active role in engineering our beauty. We have developed cars, perfumes, music, fashion, surgery and a whole pharmacopeia to be employed in the service of sexual attractiveness. But, as the American evolutionary biologist Michael Ryan puts it: "to enhance one's beauty, either through the painstakingly slow process of evolution or the more immediate gratification of beauty-engineering, one must have some notion of what is beautiful" (Ryan, 2018, p. 2). The features women now find attractive and beautiful in a man are the same ones which, in earlier societies, made him able firstly to protect a woman, and secondly to intimidate and defeat other men. Evidently, being tall and having broad shoulders, narrow hips, well-defined muscles and a strong jawline is an advantage in love *and* war. Accordingly, men and women alike find that a pear-shaped body with narrow shoulders and broad hips is the least desirable male figure. Although not all cultures place as much emphasis on muscle as we do in the West, inversely no cultures see weak men as the most attractive (Gray & Ginsberg, 2007; Høgh-Olesen, 2019; Maisey, Vale, Cornelissen, & Tovée, 1999). The backdrop is that for tens of thousands of years humans lived as hunter–gatherers, depending on raw muscle power in our struggle to survive. During that era, cohabiting groups typically consisted of a couple of hundred individuals. Here, empathy, understanding and the ability to protect one's own group members were important. But it was equally important to be able to use one's strength and aggressiveness to defend the group, and possibly to attack other groups (Diamond, 1997).[3] Male brawn was not just an advantage when hunting and killing prey to obtain the proteins needed to supplement the fruit-and-nut diet gathered by the group. Physical strength also enabled the group to protect its women against predatory animals and other men, which in turn enabled the women to concentrate on protecting the children. The difference in strength between men and women is larger in the upper body than in the lower body. Stones, clubs and other weapons were thrown and wielded by hands and arms, making the men's greater upper-body strength an even greater advantage (Etcoff, 1999, p. 77). The musculature of the upper body is particularly sensitive to a surplus of testosterone in the blood, and usually these very muscles (in the arms, shoulders and chest) are the ones most vigorously trained by adolescent boys who join a gym. In other words, these young men are interested in increasing and reinforcing a gender difference that already exists. Darwin, in his day, already observed that human beings not only admire the characteristics nature has given them. Often, we also try to augment and exaggerate them (Etcoff, 1999, p. 168). As most readers will know, in bodybuilding competitions two of the key criteria for success are symmetry and size.

Women, like men, are attracted to symmetrical bodies and faces – even though symmetrical men tend to cheat on their partners more often than asymmetrical men do, and invest less in their relationships. This is probably because they are deemed attractive and so get more offers from other women. Symmetrical women also have more partners than their less symmetrical sisters. But not only do humans find symmetry attractive. As if by some built-in, prescient quirk of nature, this effect is reinforced at the most critical moment. A study of 30 women found that the asymmetrical features between the right and left sides of their body decreased by 30% when measured 24 hours before they ovulated (Etcoff, 1999, pp. 186–187; Scutt & Manning, 1996).[4]

In this light, it is little surprise that cross-cultural comparisons of the perceived "ideal body" are relatively uniform. In male bodies, an athletic figure is generally preferred. Deviations to this preference appear in societies where food is lacking, shifting ideals towards a stockier or fatter body. In conditions of scarcity, this ideal body type radiates access to the resources required to survive and foster children (and ensure their survival as well). When scarcity ends, the image of the ideal body shifts back towards an athletic figure, so cultural variations in the image of the ideal body are not first and foremost a question of cross-cultural coincidences. They seem to be largely explainable in terms of evolutionary psychology as an expression of resource accessibility (Dixson, Halliwell, East, Wignarajah, & Anderson, 2003; Swami et al., 2010; Swami & Furnham, 2007).

Across all cultures, beautiful people enjoy greater respect from their surroundings than their less fetching peers. They have higher incomes and more sexual partners, and other people treat them better. We are more inclined to confide in beautiful people, and we also let them have more personal space and generally try harder to please them (Etcoff, 1999; Høgh-Olesen, 2019; Ryan, 2018).

Some of my informants also have experiences that reflect this. One is Anton, who spoke in Chapter 5 about how reactions in his surroundings gradually changed as he became bigger and more muscular. He had never been bullied, but as his physique gradually grew, so did his self-confidence. He became more assertive, sensing that the people he knew changed the way they spoke to him and gave him more space and respect, thereby increasing his self-confidence (see page 81). Similarly, Anton described in Chapter 8 how his dealings with "girls" changed after he became more muscular. Earlier, he had found it hard to establish first contact, but after his transition he was constantly being approached by women who wanted his body (see page 138).

These experiences confirm the research findings. Human reactions to beautiful people contribute to reinforcing beauty as a sort of status, somewhat akin to being born into the aristocracy in earlier eras. In this sense beauty is profoundly unfair. Basically, it is a trait not attributed by merit, but those who possess it enjoy great advantages. Seen in this light, Wolf's point that we should not let ourselves be seduced by (the notion of) beauty is understandable — albeit the real villain here is neither the male gender nor capitalism, but Mother Nature. Nevertheless, Anton and many others have adopted the view that if you work hard, for instance at the gym, a piece of the beauty-pie can be yours. You are not simply predestined to make do with the body and the looks you have. As Anton explained about what initially got him to start working out: "My girlfriend was so pretty, I felt like I owed it to her to get a body that was handsome and fit." Then he started lifting weights. This is the very essence of what makes gyms and fitness clubs profitable enterprises: With hard work, we too can get closer to the beauty ideal and partake of the privileges that go with it.

As mentioned, women looking for a long-term male partner show a preference for resources and status. In our day, however, the factors that give men status and success are social background, education and intelligence rather than muscles and strength. If that were the backdrop for initiating an educational campaign against using anabolic steroids, it would be tempting to say that all young people have to do is pursue the culturally acknowledged paths to modern masculinity by getting themselves an Armani suit, an expensive car and a prestigious address. But realistically, not only is this path to masculinity inaccessible to most 21-year-olds, whereas a muscular, well-toned body is accessible and expresses strength and desirable traits in an easily decoded one-to-one ratio. There is also the biologically embedded human preference for a well-proportioned body, which still plays a decisive role when we look for partners, as clearly illustrated through Anton's experience. Beyond this, the teen years are the period when we find out how potential partners react to us. "It is not surprising," writes Etcoff, that "the preoccupation with bodies at this age cannot be overstated, and that adolescents are notoriously hypercritical and extremely attentive to their beauty" (Etcoff, 1999, p. 58). From this perspective it is understandable that adolescent boys are often attracted to weightlifting and bodybuilding. Still, a nice body and attractive appearance are not enough: Action is also needed. Just as humans have universal preferences for appearance, similar preferences evidently apply to our perception of what it means to be "a real man."

Be a man!

In their book *Thinking Sociologically*, British sociologists Zygmunt Bauman and Tim May establish that "Our 'sexual assignment', like anything else concerning our bodies, is not a quality that has been determined at birth" (Bauman & May, 2001, p. 105). Ponder this for a moment. It is quite a radical postulation. A lot of things relating to the body *are* actually determined at birth. However, with their interpretation of gender being a predominantly social construction, Bauman and May join ranks with many other influential sociologists and philosophers who, since the mid-twentieth century, have claimed that it is fruitless to perceive gender as an essential human trait. Their statement that gender determination is not established from birth is, however, far from straightforward. It seems to disregard the basic fact that the question of the child's gender is always the first question new parents get, and that they (almost) always answer the question as a matter of course. But this is not Bauman and May's point. Drawing on the notion of "plastic sex" in the modern age, introduced by Anthony Giddens, they continue: "'Being a male' or 'being a female' is a question of art which needs to be learned, practised and constantly perfected" (Bauman & May, 2001, p. 105). This observation is quite right, insofar as different cultures have different guidelines for demonstrating masculinity, and femininity. No young Greenlandic men are expected to kill a lion with the spear, and no young men from Botswana are expected to kill a seal while hunting from a kayak. Even so, this observation is superficial, as it overlooks the fact that both cultures expect young men, and not young women, to prove their gender status — their manhood — through decidedly physical, high-risk activities. Very few cultures have ceremonial methods involving similar physical ordeals where young women are called upon to prove their womanhood.

That is why, at the very least, it will take some qualification if we are to accept Bauman and May's further statements on manhood and womanhood:

> Moreover, none of the two conditions is self-evident, binding us throughout our lives and neither offers a clearly defined pattern of behaviour. [...] Humans were always born with either male or female genital organs and male or female secondary bodily features, but at all times the culturally patterned, taught and learned habits and customs defined the meaning of being 'male' or 'female.'
>
> (Bauman & May, 2001, pp. 105–106)

While it is correct that gender is not an essential feature that deterministically decides how our lives will unfold, their statements do not make us any wiser to what role gender does play for our psychology and behavior. In seeking to understand this role, it is not enough to ascertain that today a man can choose a profession like nursing, which would traditionally be termed a female profession, or that today a woman can choose a career as, say, a police officer, which was traditionally termed a male profession. Here, too, there are expectations to gender behavior, which demonstrate that "the culturally patterned, taught and learned habits and customs" rest upon a universal structure that is significant in determining "the meaning of being 'male' or 'female'."

Precarious manhood

This meaning and this structure are discussed by the two American psychologists Joseph Vandello and Jennifer Bosson in their review article entitled *Hard Won and Easily Lost: A Review and Synthesis of Theory and Research on Precarious Manhood* (Vandello & Bosson, 2013). Here they investigate the potential support for the hypothesis that manhood is a particularly insecure type of social status. On the face of it, this hypothesis may sound strange, given that above we saw how evolution has made men competitive and inclined to take risks. This, however, is precisely the point. Men who do not readily live up to the unspoken standards of masculinity, which are based on the expectation that men are minded for risk, action and competition, can feel a threat to their status as a man. The hypothesis of precarious manhood says that: (a) manhood is an elusive status that must be earned; (b) manhood is precarious and easily lost; and (c) manhood requires action and must be proved, preferably in public so it can be confirmed by others. Compared to womanhood, which is typically seen as a status resulting from natural biological development, manhood is something a person must deserve to achieve, then maintain through actions that can be seen and verified by others — preferably other men. What we have here is a cocktail of cultural and psychological consequences of men being more competitive and tending to take more risks than women. Vandello and Bosson review a large number of studies with different designs, comparing them with historical and anthropological descriptions to test how robust the hypothesis of precarious manhood is.

One of the first obvious signs that the idea has some legitimacy is based in language. Many languages, including Danish, have a variety of expressions about men becoming "soft"; being "a real man"; having to "be a man" in the face of adversity; or being asked whether they are "man enough" to handle a tough situation, which may leave the "last man standing." Conversely, you rarely hear anyone ask whether a woman is "a real woman," or "woman enough" to handle a given situation. Women can certainly be hassled and frowned upon for their actions, but their status as women is rarely called into question. On the other hand, men can temporarily lose their status if they fail as a man, or act too feminine in the eyes of others. In this way language reflects how manhood status is linked to actions, and also shows that there is a real risk of losing it in a way that does not equally apply to womanhood. That said, the mere fact that many of our languages point in this direction is no guarantee that the hypothesis is universally applicable.

Nevertheless, the expectation that men must practice a certain pattern resurfaces in a number of anthropological studies, which find, as suggested above, that manhood is achieved by the force of coming-of-age rites that often involve bodily risk and danger, where boys must prove they are men (Gilmore, 1990). As noted, comparably risky initiation rites are not found for girls, for whom the attribution of womanhood is most often linked to natural biological changes which, once assigned, are difficult to lose.

If the hypothesis is tenable, for one thing we will see that men experience more anxiety related to their gender status, and for another we will be able to observe that men will seek to reinforce their manhood if it has been threatened. If, however, the two genders show similar variations in situations that threaten their gender status, the hypothesis is not tenable. Meanwhile, most findings show that it is.

The following example provides evidence that levels of the stress hormone cortisol rise significantly in men placed in situations where their manhood status is threatened; and that these levels rise noticeably more than in women placed in similar situations. In addition, studies show that men who have a high level of testosterone — which can be used as a biological marker for status and dominance — show less rise in cortisol levels when their manhood is threatened. We also know that men (and other male primates) who rank higher in their hierarchy, or who win in competitive situations, have higher testosterone levels than men who lose competitions or rank lower in their hierarchy (Herbert, 2015; Mazur, 2005). Furthermore, the willingness to run risks to reinforce manhood rises in men when their male status is threatened. In a study that was described to participants as "a study of physical coordination," men were asked to braid the hair on a wigged female mannequin, then finish the braid with pink bows. A control group did a mechanically identical (but gender-neutral) braiding activity framed as a rope-strengthening task. The participants were then asked to choose between two follow-up activities: a gender-neutral puzzle task, or a masculine punching-type task. More than twice as many men in the mannequin-hair-braiding group chose the punching task, and they also hit harder than men in the rope-strengthening group who chose the punching task as follow-up. And their choices worked. When measuring cortisol levels in their subjects, the researchers found that in subjects who had the opportunity to punch, cortisol dropped more quickly than in men placed in a control-group situation where that option had been removed after braiding the mannequin's hair. In another study presented as "a marketing study", men were asked either to test a fruit-scented hand lotion or a power drill. After this, they were asked to participate in a gambling-type game where they could win real money. The men who had tested the lotion subsequently placed much riskier bets than those who had tested the drill. So it seems that men have a need to reestablish their masculinity after it has been threatened, and that public activities that are aggressive or risk-based help them do just that (all examples are from Vandello & Bosson, 2013).

Overall, the evidence supporting the hypothesis of precarious manhood is fairly solid. Beyond that, it even seems to apply across historical eras and cultures and thus is not linked to modern Western cultures. Naturally, as Bauman and May explain, there are specific cultural and historical markers of masculinity and manhood. Nevertheless, the general structure — which seems to be universal — is that manhood is perceived as something that requires action; something one must earn through action(s) that have to be confirmed (preferably by other men); and something that can be lost (Vandello & Bosson, 2013).

Muscles, masculinity and strong views

Ironically, the very absence of formalized coming-of-age rituals in modern secular societies can be part of what makes men more insecure about their gender status. While they know they must perform, there is no formalized ritual through which they can do so, which can cause anxiety as to whether their actions are good enough. In this situation, the gym offers a solution. Most other sports do too, but the gym offers multiple opportunities: showing you can do (or lift) certain things, developing expertise that commands peer recognition, and building an attractive body that universally signals health, strength and an ability to protect.

Martin gave this explanation of why the girls in his social circle are fascinated by guys who work out:

This thing about protecting them, I think, is really important. Making them feel safe. So that's why they like their boyfriends to be masculine. Being masculine isn't just being able to take care of yourself, it's being able to take care of them, too. Masculinity does mean a lot in our culture. In some cultures it's good to be fat, because it signals affluence. For us, here, masculinity is important. You know, it's a package deal, because you get more than one thing. I know it sounds kind of primitive, but it's the reptile brain that kicks in and says: Here's a good mate, because he's an alpha male.

Basic evolutionary psychology is not unknown territory for 22-year-old Martin. Bearing out the above, in the company of friends he had experienced how the strength they emanated after having become bigger and stronger could be perceived as something other men could test and challenge. Martin explained that in the various settings where their lives unfolded — in the city's night life, and at the vocational college they both attended — if another young man could confront or rile up a big guy, he would win "street cred," somewhat like counting coup in certain Native American tribes. That is why men with his sort of conspicuous physique must sometimes tolerate provocations from others, not least in clubs and bars:

But there's also a negative side to getting bigger, because some people feel like they want to test you. We've had that happen when we go out for a beer. My friend hardly ever gets a chance to just chill out. There's always some drunk dude who starts pushing him around. Then my friend has to shout at him to make him go away: "Listen man, I don't want to get thrown out of here for fighting with you!" So people have to test themselves against the big guy to see if they can knock him over.

This expresses, in very practical terms, the Darwinistic alpha-male competitive mentality often seen in night-life settings. To earn credibility, to make your mark and move up in the social hierarchy as a young man, the reward is always greatest if you dare to challenge high-ranking individuals in that hierarchy. This mirrors other social and professional contexts. A person does not win the same respect by besting those who rank lower. Among young people out on the town, a muscular physique can be an eye-catching marker of a social position some people feel called upon to challenge.

The hypothesis of precarious manhood, along with the need to have one's status confirmed by other men, also explains why most of my informants would rather reap praise and recognition for their body and skills from other men at the gym rather than from girls, as we saw in Chapter 9. Praise from other men reassures them of their status, and it positions them within a male hierarchy in a way praise from women cannot.

Further to this, one can imagine that the male members of a workout community — especially those who take steroids to build muscles, identity and masculinity — hold more conventional or conservative views of a man's role. As noted, Alan Klein described the general outlook of bodybuilders as part of his "comic-book masculinity" concept, but others have sought to determine whether they could actually measure a higher degree of classical or stereotypically masculine virtues in practitioners of strength training or weightlifting who either use or do *not* use anabolic steroids.

One such group is Gen Kanayama and some of his colleagues at Harvard Medical School. They examined 89 heterosexual men who did strength training, to study their views on the male role. Of these informants, 48 had experience with anabolic steroids, while 41 did not. Their views were measured using a questionnaire tool called the Male Role Attitude Scale. The higher the scores, the more the respondent agreed with traditional, conservative views on manhood. The questionnaire included statements such as: "A guy will lose respect if he talks about his problems." "It bothers me when a guy acts like a girl." "Men are always ready for sex." As it turned out, the researchers found no real difference in the scores of the two groups. There was a slight tendency for steroid users to score marginally higher than non-users, but being statistically insignificant, these discrepancies could be coincidental (Kanayama et al., 2006). This means that even though building muscles and perhaps achieving a hypermasculine appearance through steroid use could be a way to confirm one's manhood, there was no measurably more conservative masculine ideology among steroid users than among non-users.

Nevertheless, this does not justify discarding Klein's notion of comic-book masculinity, since it represents a type of ideal image that cannot necessarily be measurably operationalized in a male-role scale. In other words, there could well be a link between well-defined muscles and clearly defined views.

The thing is, Klein's point that muscles and strength play a key role for men seems to influence the quality or nature of their views, rather than influencing their propensity to harbor certain types of conservative views. At least that is what one Danish–American study suggests (Petersen, Sznycer, Sell, Cosmides, & Tooby, 2013). Here, researchers investigated the link between physical strength, compared to how clearly and strongly subjects expressed their views. Unlike Kanayama's study, which measured a certain type of conservative, masculine ideology, this study examined the link between men's upper-body strength and how clear and strong their views were on economic redistribution in society. The research team collected information from 1,502 respondents (757 women; 745 men) about their socio-economic status and their views on social-benefit programs and economic redistribution policies. The team also measured the size of each respondent's flexed upper arm. To reduce statistical noise from very diverse cultural and historical backgrounds, the study included 486 American, 223

Argentinian and 793 Danish respondents. Most of the factors that explain people's views on economic redistribution are based on history, culture and social models (primarily according to rational-choice theory), but the findings of this study point in a new direction. They showed that men with high socio-economic status and greater upper-body strength were the respondent segment most clearly against economic redistribution, whereas those with high socio-economic status but less upper-body strength were less staunchly averse to it. A corresponding but inverted pattern occurred in men with low socio-economic status, as stronger respondents in this group were more in favor of redistribution, whereas their weaker peers had more moderate demands to redistribution. Among women respondents, those with high socio-economic status were against redistribution, while those with low socio-economic status were in favor, but their views did not vary in line with their physical strength (Petersen et al., 2013). The research group has explained these findings as follows: Although we live in a society where it is no longer rationally meaningful for men to base their views about resource redistribution on physical strength, during the history of humankind this parameter has been crucial in conflict situations. Hence, as a parameter, it is still a part of our psychological apparatus today.

So it is that the theory of evolutionary psychology can also explain why men have different attitudes to the question of economic redistribution, even though they belong to the same socio-economic group. The Danish–American study actually took its cue from a well-known evolutionary theory of how animals act in conflicts that involve resources. This theory basically says that if you are in conflict with a person to whom you are physically superior, you should escalate the conflict and attempt to gain control of the resource in dispute; if you are physically inferior, you should withdraw (Petersen et al., 2013). Transplanted into our modern political reality, this means that the more upper-body strength a man has, the more probable he is to have a political view that will increase his share of society's resources, so physical strength influences the extent to which men dare to pursue or promote their own interests. Taking this further, the theory can also explain why men with low socio-economic status and less upper-body strength were also more moderate in their redistribution demands than strong men with low socio-economic status. But although the study shows that a correlation exists, it says nothing about any underlying causality. Consequently we cannot say whether men will change their view of, say, economic redistribution if they train rigorously and become stronger, or if they stop training and become weaker.[5]

Affluence and body dissatisfaction

These insights from evolutionary psychology bring us closer to a new understanding of the widespread body dissatisfaction discussed earlier, in Chapters 2 and 5. The cultural studies I reviewed in Chapter 2 could seem to suggest that many people's dissatisfaction with their own body, and their quest to achieve a body image that differs from their own body, is solely a product of the media's manipulation of our perception of the ideal body. On the face of it, this perception is supported by observations of how, in some cultures and some historic eras, obesity has been elevated as an ideal. This is part of the backdrop against which some have claimed that bodily ideals among men and women must be understood as pure social construc-tions (Bordo, 2000; Wolf, 1991). As we have seen, this is hardly the case. Instead, what we can consistently observe is a clear link between body-weight ideals and the (in)security of access to resources, with heavier bodies preferred in cultures and eras where the access to resources (affluence in general, and food in particular) is poor or unpredictable. This indicates that one of the primary functions of fatty tissue is to store calories, which in turn shows that the amount of body fat carried by a given individual is a reliable way of predicting their access to food. In eras or cultures with insecure access to resources, people will therefore idealize heavier bodies, because overweight is associated with resource access.

This idea is supported by recent research findings that demonstrate a nega-tive link between socio-economic status and ideal body weight. One study, conducted across ten regions around the globe, showed that the lower the socio-economic status among a population, the greater the value it placed on heavier women (Swami et al., 2010). In keeping with these findings, a cross-cul-tural study of women and men from the United Kingdom and Malaysia showed that, in *both* countries, women and men with high socio-economic status had the same ideal for the opposite sex, whereas women and men from poorer parts of Malaysia preferred heavier members of the opposite sex (Swami & Tovée, 2005, 2007). A corresponding pattern has been identified for men's and women's assessments of the most attractive figure for females in South Africa. In urban areas (Cape Town), both sexes have a slimmer female body ideal than people in poorer rural areas (KwaZulu-Natal). Around the world there are minor differences in the type of female figure found most attractive by men *and* women, with a grouping of, respectively, North America and Southeast Asia on the one hand, and Western Europe and Scandinavia on the other. North Americans and Southeast Asians have a female ideal that is slightly slimmer than Western Europeans and Scandinavians. However, the largest differences are observed internally in these various regions — between affluent urban areas and disadvantaged rural areas. Seemingly, when it comes to explaining body dissatisfaction, socio-economic status is a better indicator than culture. Or put differently, when seen in isolation the local socio-economic conditions give a better basis for explaining body ideals than regional culture does (Swami et al., 2010). Naturally this does *not* mean that other factors, including exposure to Western media and the media's promotion of a certain beauty ideal, are unimportant. As the informants cited in Chapter 5 explained, their image of the ideal body was also shaped by media influences.

Even though our human biology has been a constant, unchanging factor (at least in historical times), this factor is not beyond the influence of culture. But rather than "a constant," biology ought to be seen as the foundation on which culture stands. This allows us to see how very diverse cultures and eras have either accentuated or disregarded this foundation. For almost a millennium, the Greeks and Romans took an intense interest in the muscular male body, as even a cursory look at much statuary from Antiquity will confirm. Consider ancient sculptures of Hercules, the Laocoon group, pankration fighters, Myron's discus thrower or Michelangelo's *David*. Such sculptures make it hard to ignore the well-muscled athletic body's significance as an aesthetic ideal. Conversely, the body's physical appearance was paid little heed during the heyday of Christian culture, from around 1000 until the late 1800s, when sport and open-air movements arose (Bonde, 1996; Mangan, 2013). Nevertheless, judging from Leonardo da Vinci's famous drawing of *The Vitruvian Man* from around 1490, his model could just as well have been a modern-day Olympic decathlete. Incidentally, this drawing, done to show the ideal proportions of the human body, shows that even in a historic period when the body was not in the cultural spotlight, the actual body ideal was the same as the one we know today as the athletic, muscular body.

Human nature

People are fascinated by beautiful, symmetrical, strong bodies. It is "deeply embedded in human nature to value physical strength and power," as the Danish philosopher David Favrholt writes. "It lies deep within us that we experience strength and power as something appealing, something beautiful, and that the will-power underlying the manifestation of strength and power fascinates us in a positive way" (Favrholt, 2002, p. 80, my translation). Despite being a philosopher, Favrholt is clearly drawing on evolutionary biology when pointing out a link here between sport and aesthetics.[6]

One reason I have gone to such lengths to explain this topic from the perspective of evolutionary psychology is that I believe it can help us understand the success of gyms and workout facilities, as well as the use of anabolic steroids. Another reason is that this perspective has been all but absent in most other analyses of this phenomenon. So why has the biological element — including the emphasis on a universal aesthetic preference for strong, muscular, symmetrical bodies — been left unexplored in most of the literature on fitness, bodybuilding and the male (and female) fascination with the muscular body? Perhaps for fear of attracting accusations of social Darwinism or, worse still, accusations of fascism (Tännsjö, 2000). However, as Favrholt asserts, it is impossible to deny that as human beings we are fascinated by symmetrical, strong bodies, and that we find them beautiful and attractive. As we have seen, this is also in step with the personal experiences of a number of my informants. Obviously, this does not mean we can explain everything about young men's appetite for muscles from the perspective of evolutionary psychology. Meanwhile, the market and the media would not be able to force any values on a culture if the people in that culture were unreceptive to those values. To paraphrase the biologist Michael Ryan, as cited above: we must have some notion of what *is* beautiful before we can pursue an ambition to *be* beautiful (Ryan, 2018). Being strong and muscular was once a biological, evolutionary advantage. That biological advantage became an aesthetic preference. Personal tastes, historical periods and particular cultures have, of course, shaped these preferences, but they did not create them any more than the Coca-Cola Company or McDonald's created our craving for sugary drinks or salty, greasy food. In this way the perspective of evolutionary psychology helps us understand various basic circumstances regarding muscles and steroids and allows us to see how these circumstances create the foundation that markets, media and the manufacturers of multifarious products can exploit and reinforce.

On the other hand it is indisputable that because these circumstances of biology and evolutionary psychology are universal, they are only able to explain our attraction to and fascination with muscular bodies at a very general level. They cannot explain how these things are expressed in a particular culture, or why, say, only a small percentage of the male populations in most Western countries have personal experience in increasing their muscle mass using steroids. To understand these questions, we can seek aid in the theory of precarious manhood, dealt with above.

If we are not aware of our biologically founded, psychological preferences, we cannot know which things our cultures and marketplaces are reinforcing, affecting and exploiting. Nor does it avail us to claim that we are under the influence of various cultural conventions, if we are incapable of explaining what gave shape to these conventions. As the Swedish biologist Per Christian Jersild once observed, knowledge about human nature, and the nature of humans, is decisive if we wish to change the world we inhabit:

> Humankind will hardly undergo changes in the nature of its biology. Making the world a better place calls, instead, upon political and cultural changes. Still, if we learn more about the biological nature of humankind, we can come to better understand the warning signs in situations where the cultural veneer is threatening to crack.
>
> (Jersild, 1998, p. 10, my translation)

Notes

1 This hardly reflects a historical coincidence. According to Steven Pinker's book *The Better Angels of our Nature: A history of violence and humanity*, "The one great universal in the study of violence is that most of it is committed by fifteen-to-thirty-year-old men. Not only are males the more competitive sex in most mammalian species, but with Homo sapiens a man's position in the pecking order is secured by reputation, an investment with a lifelong payout that must be started

early in adulthood" (Pinker, 2011, p. 125). In line with this, the American anthropologist Donald Brown's long list of "human universals," across cultures, cites the following: "males more aggressive, males more prone to lethal violence." This list is printed in (Pinker, 2002, p. 135 ff).

2 My introduction to this section is inspired by (Etcoff, 1999).

3 This is why it is erroneous to phrase the question of whether humankind is "fundamentally good or evil." Human beings evolved in an environment where, in order to survive, they had to have both aggressive and empathic traits.

4 It has been verified that the symmetry of body parts such as breasts and fingers changes during the menstrual cycle. This scientific study measured the differences (the asymmetry) at four different body sites: between the right and left ears, middle finger, ring finger, and little finger. Findings showed that, beginning on the day before ovulation (measured using ultrasonographic techniques), body asymmetry was reduced by an average 30% (Scutt & Manning, 1996).

5 Also, these findings do not necessarily contradict the findings by Price and colleagues mentioned in the concluding section of Chapter 9 (Price, Sheehy-Skeffington, Sidnaius, & Pound, 2017). Both the experimental design and the measurement tools were quite different in the two studies.

6 However, the fundamental thinking behind his claims is not necessarily as recent as evolutionary biology. In Praise of Athletic Beauty, a book by the German–American philosopher Hans Ulrich Gumbrecht, finds support in Immanuel Kant's theory of aesthetics when explaining the elements in sport that fascinate us at the most visceral level (Gumbrecht, 2006). In this context, one of Kant's key concepts is "subjective universalism," the paradoxical circumstance that although we know our judgments of what is beautiful are our own, and are subjective, we implicitly expect others to agree with them, and expect that they are universally applicable. Kant's arguments for this view build on a complex analysis of the judgment of taste, but the conclusion is remarkably concordant with findings from evolutionary psychology — which indicate that there is a universal standard for what humans generally find beautiful, healthy and viable.

References

Andreasson, J., & Johansson, T. (2014). The global gym: Gender, health and pedagogies. Houndmills, Basingstoke, UK & New York: Palgrave Macmillan.

Bauman, Z., & May, T. (2001). Thinking sociologically (2nd ed.). Oxford: Blackwell Publishers.

Bonde, H. (1996). Masculine movements: Sport and masculinity in Denmark at the turn of the century. Scandinavian Journal of History, 21(2), 63–89. doi: doi:10.1080/03468759608579317.

Bordo, S. (2000). The male body: A new look at men in public and in private. London: Macmillan.

Diamond, J. M. (1997). Guns, germs, and steel: The fates of human societies. New York: W.W. Norton.

Dixson, A. F., Halliwell, G., East, R., Wignarajah, P., & Anderson, M. J. (2003). Masculine somatotype and hirsuteness as determinants of sexual attractiveness to women. Archives of Sexual Behavior, 32(1), 29–39. doi: doi:10.1023/A:1021889228469.

Etcoff, N. (1999). Survival of the prettiest: The science of beauty. London: Little, Brown.

Favrholdt, D. (2002). Æstetik, fascination, spænding – parametre til vurdering af sporten. In V. Møller & J. Povlsen (Eds.), *Sportens forførende skønhed: En antologi om sport og æstetik* (pp. 74–95). Odense, Denmark: Syddansk Universitetsforlag.

Gilmore, D. D. (1990). *Manhood in the making: Cultural concepts of masculinity*. New Haven, CT: Yale University Press.

Gray, J., & Ginsberg, R. (2007). Muscle dissatisfaction: An overview of psychological and cultural research and theory. In K. J. Thompson & G. Cafri (Eds.), *The muscular ideal: Psychological, social, and medical perspectives* (pp. 15–39). Washington, DC: American Psychological Association.

Gumbrecht, H. U. (2006). *In praise of athletic beauty*. Cambridge, MA.: Belknap Press of Harvard University Press.

Halkitis, P. N., Moeller, R. W., & DeRaleau, L. B.. (2008). Steroid use in gay, bisexual, and nonidentified men-who-have-sex-with-men: Relations to masculinity, physical, and mental health. *Psychology of Men & Masculinities*, 9(2), 106–115. doi: doi:2048/10.1037/1524-9220.9.2.106.

Herbert, J. (2015). *Testosterone: Sex, power, and the will to win*. Oxford: Oxford University Press.

Høgh-Olesen, H. (2019). *The aesthetic animal*. New York: Oxford University Press.

Jersild, P. C. (1998). *Darwins ufuldendte: Om menneskets biologiske natur*. København, Denmark: Samleren.

Kanayama, G., Barry, S., Hudson, J. I., & Pope, H. G. (2006). Body image and attitudes toward male roles in anabolic-androgenic steroid users. *Am.J.Psychiatry*, 163 (4), 697–703. doi: doi:10.1176/appi.ajp.163.4.697.

Kenrick, D. T., Trost, M. R., & Sundie, J. M. (2004). Sex roles as adaptations. An evolutionary perspective on gender differences and similarities. In A. H. Eagly, A. E. Beall, & R. J. Sternberg (Eds.), *The psychology of gender* (2nd ed., pp. 65–91). New York: Guilford Press.

Klein, A. M. (1993). *Little big men: Bodybuilding subculture and gender construction*. Albany, NY: State University of New York Press.

Klein, A. M. (2007). Size matters: Connecting subculture to culture in bodybuilding. In J. K. Thompson & G. Cafri (Eds.), *The muscular ideal: Psychological, social, and medical perspectives* (pp. 67–83). Washington, DC: American Psychological Association.

Lanzieri, N., & Hildebrandt, T. (2011). Using hegemonic masculinity to explain gay male attraction to muscular and athletic men. *Journal of Homosexuality*, 58(2), 275–293. doi: doi:10.1080/00918369.2011.540184.

Luciano, L. (2007). Muscularity and masculinity in the United States: A historical overview. In J. K. Thompson & G. Cafri (Eds.), *The muscular ideal: Psychological, social, and medical perspectives* (1 ed., pp. 41–65). Washington, DC: American Psychological Association. (Reprinted from: Not in File).

Maisey, D., Vale, E., Cornelissen, P., & Tovée, M. (1999). Characteristics of male attractiveness for women. *The Lancet*, 353(9163), 1500.

Mangan, J. A. (2013). *Making European masculinities: Sport, Europe, gender* (J. A. Mangan Ed.). Abingdon, Oxon, UK: Routledge.

Mazur, A. (2005). *Biosociology of dominance and deference*. Lanham, MD: Rowman & Littlefield Pub.

Moberg, T., & Hermansson, G. (2006). *Mandom, mod och morske män: Anabola androgena steroider – medicinskt, rättsligt och socialt* (Manhood, courage, and contentious men). Göteborg, Sweden: Mediahuset.

Petersen, M. B., Sznycer, D., Sell, A., Cosmides, L., & Tooby, J. (2013). The ancestral logic of politics. *Psychological Science*, 24(7), 1098–1103. doi: doi:10.1177/0956797612466415.

Pinker, S. (2002). *The blank slate: The modern denial of human nature*. New York: Penguin Books.

Pinker, S. (2011). *The Better angels of our nature: A history of violence and humanity*. London: Penguin Books.

Price, M. E., Sheehy-Skeffington, J., Sidnaius, J., & Pound, N. (2017). Is sociopolitical egalitarianism related to bodily and facial formidability in men? *Evolution and Human Behavior*, 38(5), 626–634. doi: doi:10.1016/j.evolhumbehav.2017.04.001.

Ryan, M. (2018). *A Taste for the beautiful: The evolution of attraction*. Princeton, NJ: Princeton University Press.

Scutt, D., & Manning, J. T. (1996). Ovary and ovulation: Symmetry and ovulation in women. *Human Reproduction*, 11(11), 2477–2480. doi: doi:10.1093/oxfordjournals.humrep.a019142.

Swami, V., Frederick, D. A., Aavik, T., Alcalay, L., Allik, J., Anderson, D., ... Zivcic-Becirevic, I. (2010). The attractive female body weight and female body dissatisfaction in 26 countries across 10 world regions: Results of the International Body Project I. *Personality and Social Psychology Bulletin*, 36(3), 309–325. doi: doi:10.1177/0146167209359702.

Swami, V., & Furnham, A. (2007). *The body beautiful: Evolutionary and sociocultural perspectives*. Houndmills, Basingstoke, UK & New York: Palgrave Macmillan.

Swami, V., & Tovée, M. J. (2005). Male physical attractiveness in Britain and Malaysia: A cross-cultural study. *Body Image*, 2(4), 383–393.

Swami, V., & Tovée, M. J. (2007). The relative contribution of profile body shape and weight to judgements of women's physical attractiveness in Britain and Malaysia. *Body Image*, 4(4), 391–396.

Tännsjö, T. (2000). Is it fascistoid to admire sports heroes? In T. Tännsjö & C. M. Tamburrini (Eds.), *Values in sport: Elitism, nationalism, gender equality, and the scientific manufacture of winners* (pp. 9–23). London: E & FN Spon.

Vandello, J. A., & Bosson, J. K. (2013). Hard won and easily lost: A review and synthesis of theory and research on precarious manhood. *Psychology of Men and Masculinity*, 14(2), 101–113.

Wolf, N. (1991). *The beauty myth. How images of beauty are used against women*. London: Virago.

Chapter 11

IPED policy and regulation – the Danish experience

The Danish authorities have addressed the use of anabolic androgenic steroids with a number of political and legislative measures. As mentioned in the introduction, I will use Denmark as a case, not only because that is where my research originates, but also because, with two decades of experience in this area, the Danish authorities have had to face many of the challenges arising when trying to intervene in IPED use in gyms. Doping and IPED use in gyms and fitness centers began attracting the attention of the governing bodies in Danish sports in the early 1990s, and it entered the national political agenda ten years later. The Danish NADO's changing perceptions of, and approaches to, the issue since the turn of the century can therefore serve as an illustrative case, showing the challenges facing any larger bodies aiming to intervene: How best to distinguish doping in gyms and fitness centers from doping in elite sport? What are the aims of regulating and intervening? How far can authorities go, and how do they legitimize their preventive efforts? In Chapter 13, I will compare the Danish approach to alternative strategies – most notably the British harm-reduction strategy. However, to understand why the Danish anti-doping policy has taken the shape it has, we must briefly go back 20 years in time.

Paradoxically, attention was drawn to IPED use or "doping" among Danish fitness and weightlifting practitioners through a very different sport — road cycling — whose athletes had other and very different ambitions than building muscle. The doping scandal in the 1998 Tour de France sent shockwaves through the international sports world, and many were forced to ask themselves whether sport as such was actually infected by doping, as this was certainly the impression anyone would get from the media coverage. To assess the scope of this problem in Denmark, in February 1999 the country's then minister of culture, Ms. Elsebeth Gerner Nielsen, set up a committee tasked with preparing a fact-finding report on doping in Denmark. The aim of this report was to "create a total overview of the background, scope and consequences of doping-substance abuse" (Danish Ministry of Culture, 1999). Considering the large number of disciplines, leagues, practitioners and athletes in the Danish sports world, it is not surprising that this ambitious aim was not reached. However, if the report's analyses were to be trusted, Danish politicians had little cause for concern. Back in the days when caffeine was still on the doping-substance list, it turned out that "extremely few" (0.6%) respondents stated having any doping experience. The committee's investigation showed that doping was not an epidemic phenomenon in Denmark but was isolated in certain top-level athletic circles, cycling in particular — where the use of caffeine was and still is widespread — and to athletic disciplines that required strength. But there was one area that spiked in the numbers: 7.8% of the male respondents who used gyms and fitness centers reported having experience with doping substances, and 5% had experience with anabolic steroids (Danish Ministry of Culture, 1999; Pedersen & Benjaminsen, 2002). Informed by the conclusions of the fact-finding report, and following the growing international momentum in anti-doping awareness, in spring 2000 the Danish government made a collaborative agreement with the country's sports organizations to establish a body called Anti Doping Danmark. Following a five-year test period, this body was made permanent as a non-profit organization established by law, whose aim was to prevent doping in sports, notably through "control and information measures" (Steele, Bang, Brandt, & Kirkegaard, 2010, p. 22).

Building on the report's mandate, from its inception one of Anti Doping Danmark's main tasks was to develop anti-doping efforts at Denmark's gyms and fitness centers. From 2003, the Danish facilities willing to pay to join a national program would be able to have doping controls done on site by Anti Doping Danmark staff. This arrangement was truly unique, since no other country in the world was doing anything similar. Though it may seem strange that based on the Tour de France doping scandal Denmark was testing recreational, non-competitive gym-goers, at the same time this was a logical consequence of the fact-finding committee's work. Their report had just shown that problematic IPED use was extremely rare in Denmark, except in elite athletic circles (and even here the data volume was fairly sparse) and in Danish fitness centers. So given that Denmark, having found no pervasive doping problem, still chose to set up Anti Doping Danmark, it would have been odd indeed if the one area reasonably representing some level of problem behavior did not fall under the scope of the new body's work.

However, getting commercial fitness centers to back actual anti-doping efforts proved to be quite a challenge. The Danish legislation that makes it possible to doping-test recreational, non-competitive users is based on the anti-doping work done in elite sports, which rests on two key arguments: ensuring fair play (the moral argument), and safeguarding athlete health (the health argument). These two arguments are deemed to be weighty enough to justify doping control in top-level sports (Evald, 2011; Houlihan, 2002). On the other hand, the situation in the Danish fitness centers is altogether different, and IPED use is primarily a health issue since very few IPED users participate in competitions — as the fact-finding report also demonstrated. Doping control in fitness centers was therefore mainly legitimized with the health argument — ensuring members' health — partly through the deterrence assumed to result from the testing regime, and partly by getting rid of negative role models younger members might look up to (Steele et al., 2010). The minimum precondition for a control regime is therefore a solid argument that such a regime can and will improve health — or that health would be worse off without it. This argument is necessary for several reasons, not least to justify the interference in people's private life that controlling entails. Compellingly proving this argument is not easy, so generally speaking the basis for the control regime is weak. Other dangerous shoals also lurk beneath the surface of the legally muddy waters Anti Doping Danmark must navigate as they work to reach the country's gym and fitness communities.

Control or dialogue?

Early in the new millennium, doping stopped being an internal affair in the world of sports. It is true that the Canadian lawyer Dick Pound, the first director general of the World Anti-Doping Agency (WADA), argued that the use of doping substances ought to be regarded as breach of a sports rule — on a par with using your feet in European handball, or taking a short-cut in a marathon race (Teetzel, 2007). If Pound's argument was sound, it was meaningless to involve national authorities in the fight against doping, which is, however, precisely what is happening as governments around the globe ratify the UNESCO anti-doping convention, thereby undertaking to adhere to the World Anti-Doping Code (WADC) (Houlihan, 2014; UNESCO, 2005; WADA, 2015).

The involvement of national governments in anti-doping efforts indicates support for the view that doping is not merely some infringement of arbitrary sporting rules, but that doping is also a broader health-related and ethical problem for society as a whole. An article written by UNESCO program specialist Paul Marriott-Lloyd explains the rationale behind the convention:

> Doping poses one of the biggest threats to sport today. It harms athletes, destroys fair play and equitable competition and does irreparable damage to the credibility of sport. However, the impact of doping goes far beyond the athletes concerned or sport itself. It is a problem that affects all of society by undermining the intrinsic value of sport.
>
> (Marriott-Lloyd, 2010)

This line of argument seems obscure. It is understandable that doping can be problematic because it adversely affects sports and athletes. It is harder to see how it ostensibly affects society by "undermining the intrinsic value of sport" — mainly because Marriott-Lloyd says nothing about what he considers "the intrinsic value of sport" to be. What he can hardly be thinking of in this context, a key feature of elite sports, is the dedicated athlete's uncompromising will to win, which is precisely one of the things that can tempt athletes to dope themselves. He is more likely referring to the widespread albeit somewhat vague ideas of the educational and character-forming value of sport, and of its capacity for spreading happiness, health and a sense of common purpose; the sort of ideas politicians are inclined to praise in public speeches and toast at dinner parties. But he could also be referring to something completely different. In either instance, the fact that the text is open to interpretation means that nations can use its assessment of doping's socially detrimental effects as a way to also become involved in preventing doping outside the confines of elite sport.

This is no simple undertaking, however, since for practical reasons the WADA definition of doping cannot be used outside elite sport.[1] So on the one hand we hear that "doping" is not just an issue for top-level sports to deal with, while on the other hand the word carries a different meaning when we talk about recreational or non-competitive sport. This lack of clarity does, however, tie in well with the slightly vague ideas in the UNESCO wording about what sport is, it's "intrinsic value" in and to society. Understood in a Danish context, it means that what we are fighting in Denmark's non-competitive communities is not "doping," but rather the use of specific IPEDS that improve the user's physical performance and appearance. This clouds the message and has caused confusion on several counts, also within Anti Doping Danmark, which for many years interpreted the call to "address problems in the fitness community" primarily as a mandate to conduct doping tests and run information campaigns.

As a parallel to introducing doping tests in Danish fitness centers and gyms in 2003, Anti Doping Danmark launched a campaign under the slogan "It's open season in fitness centers across the country." One campaign element was a series of postcards and posters of bodybuilders in various silly poses hiding behind pillars, potted plants and waste baskets. Presumably the humorous message behind the campaign — to expose bodybuilders as ridiculous muscle fetishists who, like little kids, thought they could hide behind the furniture — and the actual messages were uniformly stigmatizing: Dopers cannot hide from us; they're a bunch of vain simpletons; and we will find them and root them out.[2]

Anti Doping Danmark's efforts in fitness and gym communities has changed considerably since 2013. The head of the Danish NADO's non-competitive sports efforts, Senior Consultant Malene Radmer Johannisson, concedes that previously, especially in 2008–2010, the organization was highly focused on doping controls as its decisive tool against steroid use among fitness and weightlifting enthusiasts. At the same time, however, she finds it regrettable that doping control and testing measures still dominate public and private conversations (Danish and transnational) about Anti Doping Danmark's work with fitness centers and gyms; regrettable in the sense that the NADO has so many other preventive initiatives that are far more important than testing. As one of the keynote speakers at the *International Conference on Doping and Public Health*, held in June 2017, Johannisson began by explaining that in its early years the Danish system was not well suited to its purpose, despite massive efforts and high ambitions. Anti Doping Danmark disseminated comprehensive information about side effects and also launched a national campaign entitled "Steroids are stronger than you." The signature illustration showed a male figure going through three stages: As his appearance gradually grew larger, stronger and more aggressive, inside he became progressively smaller and more twisted (see Figure 11.1). The humorous approach had been replaced by a sense of sinister urgency, but like the 2003 campaign this was also perceived as scare tactics, and the gym community felt similarly stigmatized by its portrayal of steroid users as mental wrecks. This led to a situation where users and non-users alike did what they could to discredit and speak out against Anti Doping Danmark on various Internet forums. Meanwhile, the country's fitness centers reacted to the lack of campaign efficiency by requesting even more testing. It all seemed very ineffectual, and in hindsight Johannisson characterized the efforts of those years as being "too random, too inflexible and ineffective."

The whole state of affairs generated widespread opposition to Anti Doping Danmark among dedicated weightlifters and gym-goers, and as a result the NADO had difficulty reaching its target group at all. Summing up the results of its efforts, Johannisson concluded that "The members were frustrated, the gyms were frustrated, and we were frustrated."[3] This was, in fact, a remarkable statement. It was the first time, at any international conference, that I had heard a representative of any NADO or international anti-doping organization so frankly concede to making a mistake and approaching the problem from the wrong angle. After several years this experience led Anti Doping Danmark to rethink and revamp its entire strategy. Presumably, Anti Doping Danmark would prefer for everyone to forget its past focus on doping controls and testing, concentrating instead on the present dialogue-based approach. Nonetheless, the reality is that doping tests at fitness centers were, and still are, the crucial issue, not only for Anti Doping Danmark but also for law-makers, fitness centers and gyms, members and steroid users.

Danish legislation

The two most important laws that regulate the work of Anti Doping Danmark among recreational and non-competitive practitioners is the 1999 *Act on Prohibition of Certain Doping Substances* and the 2004 *Act on Promotion of Doping-Free Sport*, the latter of which was renamed in 2015 as the *Law on Promoting Integrity in Sport* (Retsinformation, 1999, 2004, 2015).[4]

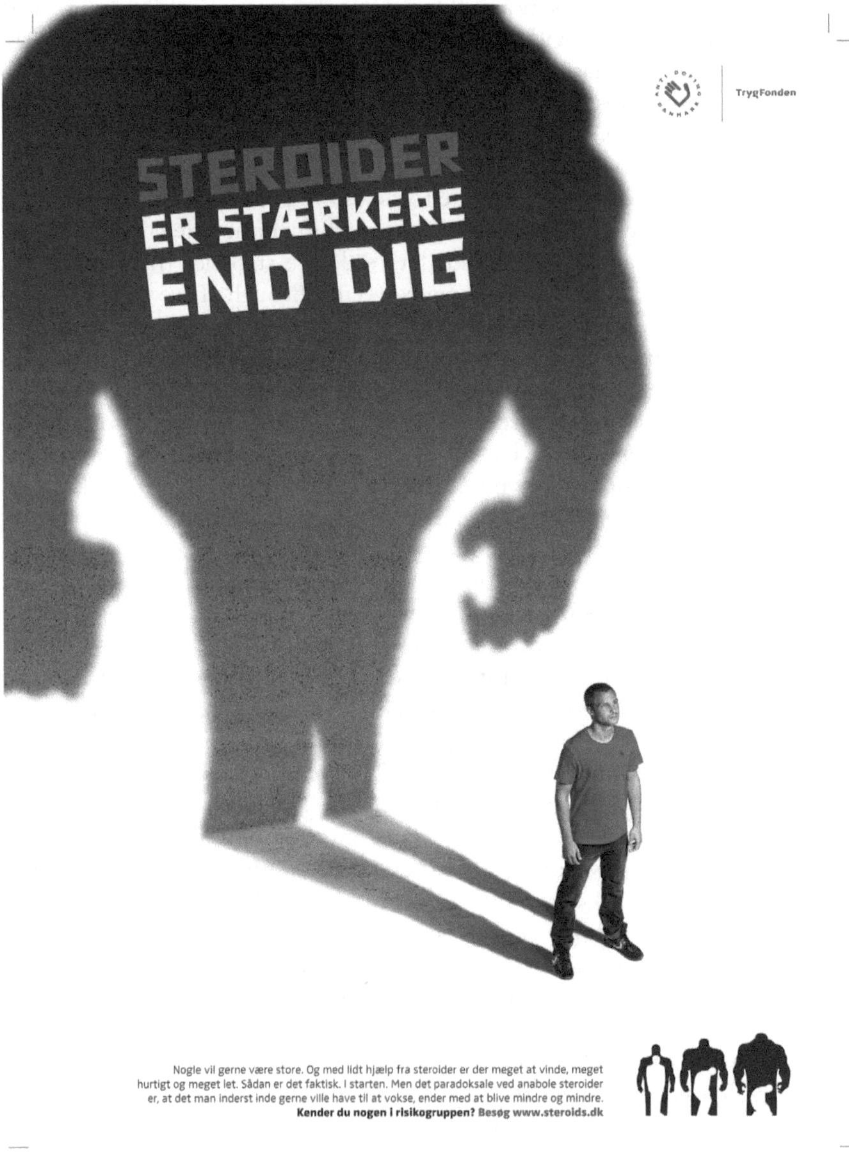

Figure 11.1 Wording on poster: "Some people want to be big. With a little help from steroids, you can make real progress, real fast and real easy. That is actually what happens. At first. But the irony of anabolic steroids is that deep down inside, what you really wanted to grow ends up getting smaller and smaller. Do you know someone in the at-risk group?" © Anti Doping Danmark

The renamed 2015 act stipulated that Anti Doping Danmark was to "seek collaborative agreements" with commercial fitness centers "to combat doping." According to this act, however, information and educational work is not enough. At centers and gyms that have an agreement with Anti Doping Danmark the organization must also ensure that "doping tests and sanctions [are implemented] in a manner that complies with the guidelines applicable to the sport organizations" (Retsinformation, 2015). This means: (A) that doping control must be performed; and (B) that the procedures and potential sanctions for infringements must follow those that apply to elite sports. This framework also complies with the UNESCO convention. Consequently, even if someone were to get the idea that steroid use ought to be regarded as a kind of substance-abuse or public-health problem, then legally speaking, doping control as a tool to counteract steroid use in fitness centers is still seen as a sports-based countermeasure. Despite all this, the health argument is the strongest pillar in the fight against recreational and non-competitive doping, as mentioned earlier.[5]

Against this backdrop it is understandable that Anti Doping Danmark has, at times, found it hard to make its practices live up to the letter of the law.[6] In the first decade of its life the NADO was actually obliged to test recreational fitness-center members for precisely the same range of substances as elite athletes competing under the WADC were tested for. This was because Danish legislation used precisely the same definition of "doping" as WADA did (see endnote 1). Hence, at least in principle, regular people exercising at fitness centers also had to be tested for asthma medication, cough medicine, EPO, blood-doping and the roughly 300 other substances on the list. By the same token, in principle, older men receiving testosterone replacement therapy and kidney patients receiving EPO were supposed to apply for a Therapeutic Use Exemption (TUE) before applying for membership at a fitness center that had signed a collaboration agreement with Anti Doping Danmark. Most people could see the absurdity in this, given that the campaign did not target kidney patients on EPO but young men on anabolic steroids. Therefore, after a decade in force the wording was changed in 2013 to enable Anti Doping Danmark to stop acting against the letter of the law, which it had done up to that point, at least to a degree. After this change the commercial fitness centers and gyms were able to only test for the substances stipulated in the *Act on Prohibition of Certain Doping Substances*.[7] These are androgenic anabolic steroids, testosterone, human growth hormone, EPO and masking agents for anabolic steroids (Retsinformation, 2013). So even though EPO remains on the list, the TUE issue remains problematic and the NADO's difficulty in complying with the law remains unresolved, at least now the Danish legislation is more in accordance with what has been the NADO's actual practice from its inception: that testing at Danish fitness centers and gyms is aimed at curbing the use of anabolic steroids among recreational and non-competitive workout enthusiasts.

Ephedrine and other stimulants

The paradoxes do not end here. Another oddity is that the focus on steroids is skewed in terms of gender. Given that the Danish legal basis for testing is primarily rooted in the health-promotion argument, one might expect the law to aim at ensuring the health of both men and women. As previously mentioned, very few women use androgenic anabolic steroids, and the female-to-male user ratio has been estimated to be as low as 1:50 (Pope et al., 2014). In this context it is often forgotten that the drug clenbuterol, which is classified as an androgenic anabolic steroid, is probably one of the substances female dopers avail themselves of because it can facilitate weight loss. Female users generally take substances that can reduce appetite and increase fat-burning. Indeed, in the Danish fact-finding report discussed above, 88% of female respondents reported exercising to achieve a smaller body, as opposed to 24% of males reporting this, and twice as many women as men reported having personal experience with slimming products – figures that are mirrored in other studies (Andreasson & Johansson, 2019; Barland & Tangen, 2009; Danish Ministry of Culture, 1999). Besides clenbuterol, users take drugs like ephedrine, which stimulates the central nervous system (CNS), and sometimes also amphetamine or cocaine, substances that can be as harmful as anabolic steroids. The reason ephedrine is used as a slimming drug is that it reduces appetite and increases fat-burning. Although importing ephedrine into Denmark is illegal the substance is sold over the counter in many other countries, including the United States and Canada. Among the various side effects of ephedrine-based dietary supplements the US Food and Drug Administration lists high blood pressure, heart palpitations, nerve damage, muscle damage, nausea, psychoses and amnesia. Ephedrine has even been reported to cause heart attacks, strokes and death (Miller & Waite, 2003), and the effects from amphetamine and cocaine are even graver (WHO, 2004).

All three of these substances are on the WADA doping list, so they would be obvious candidates for drug testing in Danish fitness centers. This is not being done, however, even though in 2010 more than one in four fitness centers felt it would be appropriate (Steele et al., 2010). This is quite understandable in light of the many situations and users where ephedrine could be more harmful than anabolic steroids.[8] Again bearing in mind that the Danish doping-test legislation relies on the health argument, and that ephedrine has an immediate, short-term stimulating and performance-enhancing effect, ephedrine testing in elite sport is only done in-competition and not out-of-competition. The same goes for the other listed CNS stimulants. Since a test at a fitness center, health club or gym by definition is an out-of-competition test, the reasoning goes that authorities would subject recreational athletes to a more rigid control regime than elite athletes if they decided to test for stimulants in gym settings. This is not permitted when the testing and legislation rest on UNESCO's anti-doping convention and, by extension, on the WADC. Legally, this argument is logical, yet it goes against the intention of Danish legislation: to ensure the health of athletes and exercise practitioners. Put differently, apart from the fact that some women also use clenbuterol,[9] in practice the Danish legislation with its focus on steroids is solely aimed at ensuring the health of men in the gym and fitness communities.

The Danish "smiley" program

Anti Doping Danmark adjusted its testing patterns and its focus after testing began in 2003 and up until the mid-2010s, as described above. Between 2003 and 2008, doping tests were virtually the only intervention the Danish NADO conducted in the country's fitness centers and gyms. Early on, less than 250 tests were done annually, but in 2008 Anti Doping Danmark entered into formalized anti-doping agreement with the industry's umbrella, the Danish Fitness & Health Organization (DFHO) and at the same time intensified testing in commercial exercise facilities. These were the years when resistance to Anti Doping Danmark in the workout community grew strong. The participating facilities would expect two control visits each year, with two tests per visit. One result of this was that the number of tests more than tripled — from 232 in 2007 to 751 in 2009 (Storm, Toft, & Bang, 2015). Interestingly, increasing the number of tests did not change the proportion of positives, which remained at 20–25%, just as the smaller number of tests in the early years had showed (see Table 11.1). This was one factor that made facilities propose even more testing.

In 2009 the Danish "smiley program" for fitness centers and gyms was introduced, obliging those that had made a collaboration agreement with Anti Doping Danmark to visually indicate this with a sticker showing a

Table 11.1 Doping and test statistics for commercial fitness centers and gyms in Denmark, 2005–2011

Year	Number of tests	Number of positive cases	Number of positive cases as % of tests
2005	106	24	23
2006	216	46	21
2007	232	51	22
2008	463	111	24
2009	751	151	20
2010	669	139	21
2011	510	118	23

Source: (Anti Doping Danmark, 2019; Storm, Toft, & Bang, 2015).

"happy smiley" and featuring the text "☺ We work with Anti Doping Danmark on doping controls." Conversely, facilities who did not collaborate and were not part of the smiley program were obliged to visually indicate this with a "sad smiley" and the text "☹ We do NOT work with Anti Doping Danmark on doping controls." A 2010 evaluation showed that especially the larger fitness centers with more than 2,000 members quickly joined the program, whereas small centers with less than 500 members more often opted out. In total, about half of all commercial exercise facilities in Denmark joined the smiley program, but because this half included most of the large gyms and chains, roughly 80% of Danish fitness-center and gym customers were working out at a facility that was in the program.

Most centers in the program expressed general satisfaction with Anti Doping Danmark's work, although many said the program was too inflexible and the tests too few and far between. The facility representatives believed testing was the right thing to do, and that the fight against recreational and non-competitive doping was important, but they looked differently at participation. For one thing, the majority responded that responsibility for the fight against doping lay mainly with the fitness industry and gyms themselves. At the same time, however, 60% of gyms said that besides signing up for the smiley program they had implemented no other measures to counteract doping, thus placing responsibility for solving the problem with Anti Doping Danmark and their individual members. Most customers and members were also satisfied with having a control and testing program. More than 70% found it important that their fitness center or gym had an agreement with Anti Doping Danmark.

The facilities that were not part of the smiley program were generally less satisfied, and many did not publicly display the sad-smiley sticker. A series of random site checks showed that only 5 of 30 facilities who were not in the testing program had posted their signage correctly. Most facilities outside the program stated, as their reason, that it was too expensive; that doping was not a problem at their facility; or that the facility handled doping issues internally. However, a small minority of 7% responded that they would lose customers or members if they joined the testing program (Steele et al., 2010). Some gyms even featured statements in their PR material indicating that gym-goers could *not* be tested while working out there. One was Angergym, which explicitly wrote in its Danish material that they had "no collaboration with Anti Doping Danmark," followed by the English text: "We accept all hard-working athletes."

Such ironic comments to the smiley program were not a prominent feature in the general picture, but they do point to an unintentional consequence of the smiley program for gyms: The obligation to have signage indicating non-collaboration could also be exploited in advertising to target IPED users.

More dialogue, less control

The pent-up frustration among dedicated fitness and workout practitioners and the opposition against Anti Doping Danmark — combined with the organization's own realization that focusing solely on control, monitoring and side-effect information was problematic — led the NADO to change course from 2012 onwards. Their work at recreational fitness centers was separated from their elite sports and competitive efforts, and they set up a separate program where centers and members could play a much more active role (Storm et al., 2015). A key element in this new direction was more focus at Anti Doping Danmark on dialogue, mutual cooperation and user involvement. Instead of having Doping Control Officials (DCOs) come knocking at the door of each facility, the NADO employed a number of fitness consultants who visit the facilities and make themselves "available for dialogue and counseling for everyone at the center," and who also conduct the doping controls that are still a central part of the program (Anti Doping Danmark, 2018).[10] The irony is that most of the new fitness consultants are in fact trained police officers who have taken this on as a second job. So, even if the ideal of the consultants' dialogue work is to promote positive values among non-users, the reality is that they mostly focus on removing so-called "negative role models" from the fitness centers.[11] Even so, in Anti Doping Danmark's assessment, today the fitness centers and their members have a better testing experience, knowing that fitness consultants (rather than elite-sport DCOs) conduct the tests on site.[12] The new consultants come more often, are to some extent acquainted with the staff, and perhaps even know some members, so they no longer have the same tough no-nonsense attitude they may have deemed necessary under the earlier strategy (see note 8). What is more, most visits involve no testing, and the number of tests has been more than halved since 2009. At the same time, the previous two visits per year with two tests have been abandoned in favor of more targeted selection of gyms and individuals for testing. Additionally, and unlike the earlier strategy, today centers can ask to have certain members or clients tested. The numbers from recent years illustrate this development (see Table 11.2).

In 2015, Anti Doping Danmark carried out 728 visits among Denmark's commercial fitness centers and gyms. Of these, 515 focused mainly on dialogue work and no testing was done. During the remaining 213 visits dialogue work was supplemented by control work, and a total of 278 people were called in for testing. In 133 cases either the test was positive (64) or the person refused to submit to testing (69), which carries the same sanctions as testing positive. In Denmark the sanction is typically a two-year ban from all fitness centers and

Table 11.2 Visits by Anti Doping Danmark (ADD) at commercial fitness centers and gyms in Denmark, 2012–2018. Data for dialogue-only visits only available for 2015–2018

Year	NADO/ADD visits to commercial facilities (total)	Dialogue-only visit	Visit with doping test	Persons selected for testing	Persons tested positive	Test-taking refused	Total cases	Total cases as % of tests
2012	410	141		339	38	66	104	31
2013	668	439		272[13]			101	37
2014	753	504		343			147	43
2015	728	515	213	278	64	69	133	48
2016	1,029	736	293	356	87	100	187	53
2017[14]	926	697	229	271	71	69	140	52
2018	937	727	210	248	51	63	114	46

Source: (Anti Doping Danmark, 2019; Storm et al., 2015).

gyms in the program, plus a four-year ban from all organized sports in the country.[15]

Since then the Danish NADO has intensified its efforts. Their consultants pay approximately one thousand visits to commercial fitness centers per year while downscaling testing to 250–350 individuals. Still, around half of these either test positive or refuse to submit to testing (Anti Doping Danmark, 2019).

Compared with the early 2000s, when about one in five tests was positive, in recent years Anti Doping Danmark has evidently become much better at targeted testing and at selecting people who have used illegal substances. The higher hit rate is also a result of the facilities' new option to contact Anti Doping Danmark directly and ask for testing of individuals they perceive as dubious in terms of substance use. Still, this percentual rise in the number of cases tells us nothing about how many steroid users there are in Denmark, nor does it indicate a rise in use.

The NADO's new focus, abandoning the previous "police-like" approach (Storm et al., 2015, p. 33) (by engaging police officers as consultants), has been well received at Danish fitness centers and gyms. A 2015 study showed that about half of all commercial facilities were part of the program, covering approximately 80% of all members. While these statistics mirror the situation in 2010, in the meantime the absolute number of facilities and their membership figures have increased. As initially mentioned, an estimated 1 million of the country's roughly 5.8 million Danes hold membership at a fitness center, health club or gym. According to the 2015 survey, 95% of the facilities in the program stated they had joined because they wanted to take responsibility for combating doping in non-competitive fitness and workout communities. Most facilities were also pleased with their cooperation with the new fitness consultants, though almost half of facilities would have liked to see Anti Doping Danmark have even greater visibility and local presence. At the same time, however, they still found controls to be an important part of the preventive strategy. Most were thus satisfied with Anti Doping Danmark's new quick-response practice, arriving quickly to do a test if the facility suspected specific individuals of using doping substances, and 83% of centers that were in the program found testing of members to be "important" or "very important" for optimal anti-doping prevention (Storm et al., 2015, p. 62).

In 2015, the main reasons given by fitness centers and gyms opting out of the program were largely the same as in the 2010 survey.[16] Generally speaking, facilities in the program were clearly more satisfied with Anti Doping Danmark's work than those that had opted out, and two out of three in the latter group were still not displaying their sad smiley (Storm et al., 2015). As one owner of an opt-out facility explained, justifying his decision not to post his sad smiley as prescribed:

It's totally idiotic to force gyms to post a sign saying people can train without any drug testing. This attracts a lot of undesirables, which means that we personally have to screen every single new sign-up to make sure our local community doesn't get the idea that the fitness center is a place where people can dope themselves without any risk. We go to great lengths to make it clear that doping is *not* acceptable at this gym. And the sad smiley undermines that.

(Storm et al., 2015, p. 86, my translation)

Unlike Angergym, which actively used the sad smiley in their marketing, there were opt-out facilities that were frustrated at the risk of attracting doping-substance users because they were forced to publicly display that they were not cooperating with Anti Doping Danmark. In 2016 information requirements to the facilities were changed, and the happy smiley was replaced by a check mark, and the mandatory no-cooperation sticker simply reads: "We have no cooperation agreement with Anti Doping Danmark."

Another new initiative arose from Anti Doping Danmark's recognition that it was not enough to use mass communication to educate people about side effects and similar issues. The NADO realized the need, firstly, for user involvement and, secondly, for locally rooted, cross-disciplinary efforts focusing on prevention and early identification. The first point meant that communication-wise the NADO moved its focus away from the small minority with undesirable behavior (doping-substance use) to the majority showing positive behavior by training without drugs. The inspiration for this shift came from behavioral psychology and other disciplines, building on the idea that behavioral changes do not stem from *information* but from *motivation*. Working with three athletes (a power-lifter, a crossfit athlete and a fitness athlete) to serve as role models, Anti Doping Danmark created a social-media presence with Danish hashtag campaigns whose titles translate as "#PureTraining" and "#PureStrength," the aim being for young people rather than Anti Doping Danmark to create the content (see Figure 11.2). The campaign has gained a certain following among younger fitness enthusiasts, who use the two hashtags when posting pictures and stories on Instagram and Facebook (Anti Doping Danmark, 2016).[17]

A new direction

Based on the above, it is safe to say that Anti Doping Danmark's work in and with the fitness and workout community has changed considerably in recent years. The NADO's early focus, which was mainly on scare campaigns, control, testing and information about side effects, has now come to include dialogues with workout facilities, members and other outreach initiatives, a shift that began in 2012 and noticeably gained momentum in and after 2015. In 2018 Senior Consultant Johannisson illustrated the NADO's new trajectory by saying that if we consistently "vocalize the use of doping substances as risk behavior, we overlook that doping can be a

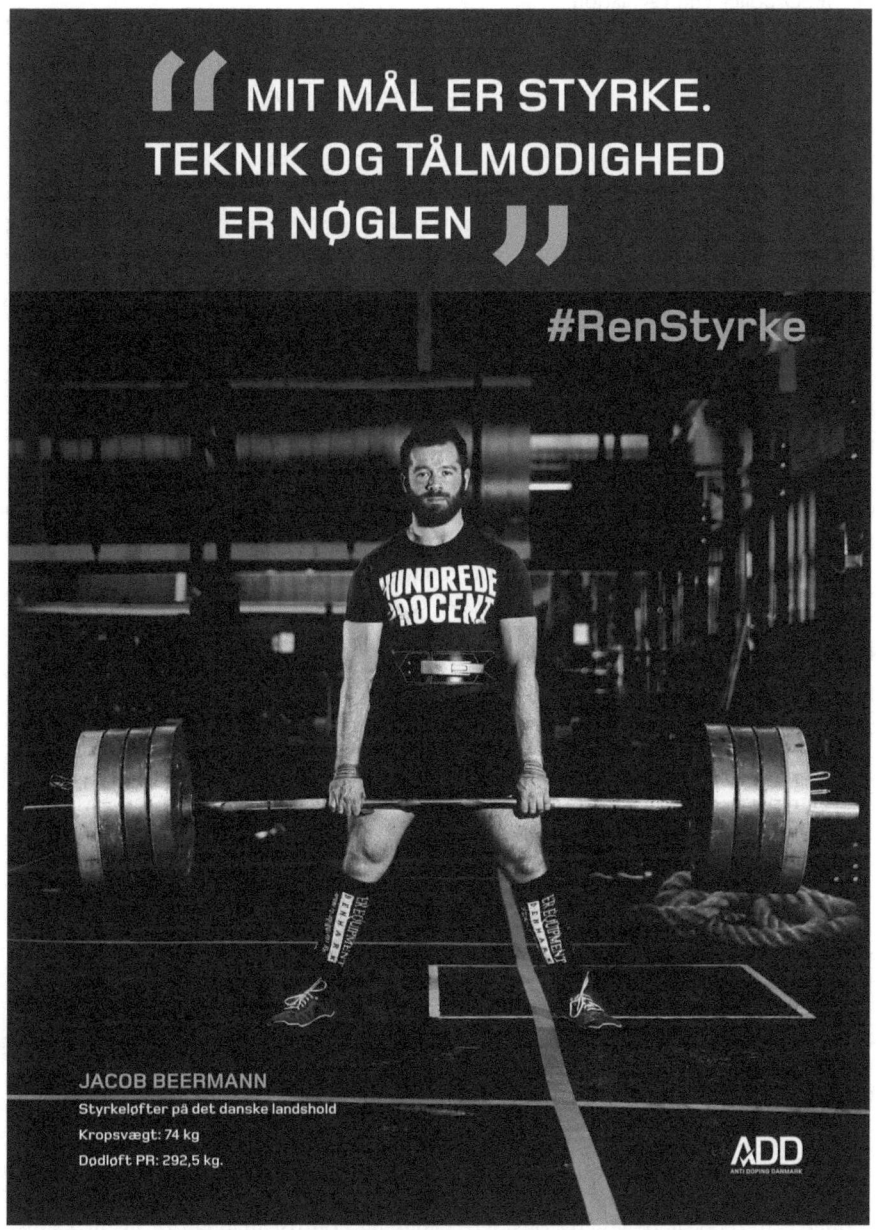

"MIT MÅL ER STYRKE. TEKNIK OG TÅLMODIGHED ER NØGLEN"

#RenStyrke

JACOB BEERMANN
Styrkeløfter på det danske landshold
Kropsvægt: 74 kg
Dødløft PR: 292,5 kg.

ADD
ANTI DOPING DANMARK

Figure 11.2 Anti Doping Danmark's campaign in 2016 plainly showed the altered strategy. Instead of communicating about side effects and targeting "wrongdoers," the campaign built on user involvement and focused on people who were doing something positive. The "clean" theme of the hashtag campaign, expressed as #RenStyrke and #RenTræning (roughly: "pure strength" and "pure training"), aimed to get young people to create content themselves by sharing pictures and social-media stories. Focus shifted from information to motivation. © Anti Doping Danmark

solution, a coping strategy, for young people who feel under pressure to constantly perform in all areas of life." For Anti Doping Danmark this is a whole new way of talking about doping in non-competitive fitness and weight-lifting communities. So instead of doping simply being an immoral, unhealthy form of cheating, as the Danish NADO previously tended to say, it can also be understood as a way for young people to handle their feeling of being under greater pressure to perform. Visibility, dialogue and understanding have become guiding ideals. The control element is still present, but it has been toned down. Also, campaigns have shifted their focus from information to motivation, thereby moving to a more positive and less stigmatizing message. The chairman of the Anti Doping Danmark board, Mette Hartlev, has highlighted the strategic shift in the organization's work with the fitness and workout community by stating that the NADO no longer see eradicating IPEDs as its goal, but rather described their work as an effort to help "ensure that young people have a right to an open future."[18] This message has two key points: the dialogue with young people, combined with a policy that also aims to reduce the harm IPED use can cause.

Notes

1   WADA does not have a lexical definition of the term "doping." Rather, it has the following ostensive, or indicative, definition: "Doping is defined as the occurrence of one or more of the anti-doping rule violations set forth in Article 2.1 through Article 2.10 of the Code." However, Articles 2.1–2.10 pertain not merely to use of the 300 or so substances on the list. They also pertain to the possession of such substances; to attempts at aiding and abetting in doping-rule violations; and to associating with others who have had doping-related sanctions imposed. A definition this broad is impossible to enforce in Danish fitness centers and gyms (WADA, 2015).
2   The postcards and posters are reproduced in (Mogensen, 2011).
3   This and the above quote is from senior consultant with Anti Doping Danmark, Malene Radmer Johannisson's talk at the International Conference on Doping and Public Health held in Oslo, Norway, on June 9, 2017.
4   "Retsinformation" literally translates as "legal information" and is a database of all Danish laws and acts and the associated documents.
5   Denmark has long had a government-run "smiley program" covering a wide range of publicly accessible locations or facilities, which includes mandatory checks and subsequent display of the official "smiley" given to that location to reflect its level of quality, cleanliness, and/or compliance. Ironically, the explanatory notes to the law establishing the Danish "anti-doping smiley program" — which was introduced in 2008, and which considered making control mandatory at all Danish fitness facilities — stated that the "abuse of doping substances among recreational sports practitioners is a health problem, and solely a health problem. This is not something we can control our way out of. What is needed is an increased educational effort and a voluntary testing program" (Retsinformation, 2008, item 4).
6   The level of enthusiasm observable in Anti Doping Danmark's lobbying to amend Danish legislation is a whole different question. Between 2000 and 2010 the late Finn Mikkelsen was the director of Anti Doping Danmark, and he

generally expressed satisfaction with the legal framework and with Anti Doping Danmark's work in recreational and non-competitive workout communities. Seen from a distance, he did not seem to be actively working to change the impracticable and unsuitable aspects of testing procedures or of Danish law. The new course in this field was set after 2011, when Lone Hansen took the helm at Anti Doping Danmark. She remained in the director's seat until 2014, after which Michael Ask took over in 2015.

7 In Denmark, fitness centers and gyms registered as membership organizations under the two umbrella organizations, the Sports Confederation of Denmark (DIF) and Danish Gymnastics and Sports Federations (DGI), are still subject to the unabridged WADA list.

8 Several informants also found it odd that Anti Doping Danmark only tested for steroids, not for stimulants. Kasper, who had never used steroids, expressed his surprise at the lack of ephedrine testing as follows: "They test for all the anabolic steroids, but what about ephedrine? Why don't they test for that? Say there's this girl who weighs 45 kilos and she just ate four Thermapower tablets [an ephedrine-based slimming product]. That puts her just as much at risk of keeling over as the 120-kilo guy who just took a shot of insulin. Actually, he's probably got a better chance of making it through safe and sound than the girl has." Kasper knows that ADD does not test for insulin either. The reasons for this are largely technical rather than legal or health-related. However, his point is a different one: If health risks were the decisive argument, then in certain situations using ephedrine is almost sure to be even more risky than experimenting with something as dangerous as insulin.

9 In 2018, Anti Doping Danmark initiated 248 tests in Danish commercial gyms. Of these, 19 were done on women, and 9 were positive (Anti Doping Danmark, 2019).

10 Experiences with former DCOs suggest this was a good idea. Kenneth, who had never been tested himself but had seen them at work at the fitness center, said: "*In my experience, I've never seen them being aggressive or anything. It's all pretty low-key, nice and easy, you know. They don't look at you like they're challenging you or anything.*" Kasper, who had been tested himself, had experienced things differently: "*These people who come out and do the testing, it's like they think they're cops or something. No wonder they get into trouble sometimes. When I was tested, this little guy walked over to me — and I was annoyed that it was this little guy who was going to test me. It seemed totally wrong. But they act like they're police officers, and their style was very direct. It's an approach I really don't care for. The big people don't talk to them like that. And I was frisked before I went in to give my sample, and you're not allowed to do that. But he did. And he frisked me all the way down, so he was sure that I didn't have a bag full of fake urine I could press on. They've been cheated before, see.*" His story was quite intense. Still, I've only heard about such extensive frisking in this one instance, and I therefore have no reason to assume it was part of their general practice. Nevertheless, Kasper was not the only one who experienced a heavy-handed approach from the DCOs. After saying goodbye to his former YOLO lifestyle, Jonas, who took a very positive view of Anti Doping Danmark's work, had undergone a test that also involved stern, no-nonsense DCOs: "*I said 'yes, sure you can test me' and then they told me to go with them out to the back. They were kind of callous, a little negative, the kind of attitude like 'Boy, are you in for it now.' That was their attitude, but I was trying very consciously all the time to be nice and polite to them, because, you know, they're just doing their job, and it also benefits me, them coming up there. They kept up this really tough face. And they took their test, and then it took a month, maybe five weeks before I got the results. But they were very strict and very direct. And I thought about it afterwards, quite a lot, and I think maybe that style must be a result of their being used to getting negative vibes from people. And probably it's not really that much*

fun, having to walk over to a bodybuilder who weighs 320 pounds and looks like someone who could eat your mother for breakfast."

11 Personal communication with Danish scholar Anders Schmidt Vinther, who has interviewed the fitness consultants as part of his research on how to design effective interventions to prevent steroid use in gym cultures.

12 Quote from Malene Radmer Johannisson, a senior consultant with Anti Doping Danmark, at the International Conference on Doping and Public Health held in Oslo, Norway, on June 9, 2017.

13 The smaller number of tests stated for 2013 stems from a laboratory error. A total of 352 tests were taken in Danish commercial fitness centers and gyms in 2013, and 121 cases were opened. Due to errors in the analytical work done at the Danish Technological Institute, 20 sanctions were repealed, 2 cases were dropped during processing (of tests found positive), and 58 samples were declared "inconclusive" and therefore canceled (11 of which, when re-analyzed elsewhere, were found positive). This calculation, 352 – (20 + 2 + 58), brings the number of non-canceled samples to 272 (Anti Doping Danmark, 2014).

14 As for the 2017 numbers, in total, that year saw fewer visits in Danish commercial fitness centers and gyms with collaboration agreements. This was because, as part of the agreement between Anti Doping Danmark (ADD) and the Ministry of Culture, ADD was tasked with following up on whether commercial facilities with no agreement were correctly displaying the new signage (introduced in autumn 2016). As part of the follow-up efforts ADD visited all (identified) gym and fitness facilities and took the opportunity to inform them about potential collaboration with ADD, and about the content and costs of an agreement. In 2017, ADD conducted 426 such visits to non-collaborating commercial facilities — in addition to its planned visits to facilities with agreements.

15 "All organized sports" means all sport activities organized under the auspices of the three umbrella organizations: the Sports Confederation of Denmark (DIF), the Danish Gymnastics and Sports Federations (DGI), and the Danish Workers' Sports Association (DAI).

16 According to the 2010 evaluation, the cost at the time — 12,000 Danish kroner (roughly 2,000 US dollars) — was a decisive factor for many of the facilities that chose not to join the program. The cost has since been reduced more than once, most recently in 2017, to DKK 4,000 kroner for facilities that are members of the Danish fitness-industry umbrella DHFO, and to DKK 6,000 for independent collaboration agreements (Anti Doping Danmark, 2017).

17 As role models, the Danish athletes face tough competition from prominent figures outside Denmark. Recalling the examples in Chapter 2, as of September 2019 the crossfit athletes Sara Sigmundsdóttir (Iceland) and Richard Froning (USA) both had more than 1.3 million followers. By comparison, as of October 9, 2019, the most popular of the campaign's three Danish role models — powerlifter Jacob Beermann — had just over 14,000 Instagram followers. The other two — body-fitness athlete Stine Spuur Hansen and crossfit athlete Pelle Rune Jensen — had 7,663 and 886 followers, respectively.

18 Quoted from Anti Doping Danmark's conference on cooperation with Danish municipalities 15 March 2018.

References

Andreasson, J., & Johansson, T. (2019). *Fitness doping: Trajectories, gender, bodies and health.* Cham, Switzerland: Palgrave Macmillan.

Anti Doping Danmark. (2014). Årsberetning 2013. Retrieved from Brøndby: www.antidoping.dk/sitetools/downloadcenter/aarsberetninger.

Anti Doping Danmark. (2016). # ren-kampagne. Brøndby: Anti Doping Danmark.

Anti Doping Danmark. (2017). Kommercielle motions- og fitnesscentre får ny samarbejdsaftale [Press release]. Retrieved from: www.antidoping.dk/om-add/a ktuelt/2017/01/kommercielle%20motions-%20og%20fitnesscentre%20f%C3%A5r %20ny%20samarbejdsaftale.

Anti Doping Danmark. (2018). Samarbejde med motions- og fitnesscentre. Retrieved from: www.antidoping.dk/dopingkontrol_i_danmark/samarbejde-med-fitnesscentre.

Anti Doping Danmark. (2019). Statistik 2018. Retrieved from: www.antidoping.dk/om-anti-doping-danmark/statistik/statistik-2018.

Barland, B., & Tangen, J. O. (2009). Kroppspresentasjon og andre prestasjoner: En omfangsundersøkelse om bruk av Doping (2009:3). Retrieved from Oslo: https://a ntidoping.no/sitefiles/1/dokumenter/pdf/omfangsundersokelsen.pdf.

Danish Ministry of Culture. (1999). Doping i Danmark: En hvidbog. Retrieved from København: https://kum.dk/publikationer/1999/doping-i-danmark-en-hvidbog. English summary: https://kum.dk/uploads/tx_templavoila/Doping_in_denmark_a_white_ book.pdf.

Evald, J. (2011). Sports law in Denmark: Doping and sport. In R. Blanpain (Ed.), International Encyclopaedia of Laws (1 ed., pp. 61–69). Alphen aan den Rijn, Netherlands: Kluwer Law International.

Houlihan, B. (2002). Dying to win: Doping in sport and the development of anti-doping policy (2nd fully revised ed.). Strasbourgh, France: Council of Europe Publishing.

Houlihan, B. (2014). Achieving compliance in international anti-doping policy: An analysis of the 2009 World Anti-Doping Code. Sport Management Review, 17(3), 265–276. doi: doi:10.1016/j.smr.2013.10.002.

Marriott-Lloyd, P. (2010). International Convention against Doping in Sport. UNESCO, 9. Retrieved from UNESCO website: http://unesdoc.unesco.org/ima ges/0018/001884/188405e.pdf.

Miller, S. C., & Waite, C. (2003). Ephedrine-type alkaloid-containing dietary supplements and substance dependence. Psychosomatics, 44(6), 508–511.

Mogensen, K. (2011). Body punk: En afhandling om mandlige kropbyggere og kroppens betydninger i lyset af anti-doping kampagner. Roskilde, Denmark: Forskerskolen for Livslang Læring, Institut for Psykologi og Uddannelsesforskning, Roskilde Universitet.

Pedersen, I. K., & Benjaminsen, L. (2002). Doping og anvendelse af andre præstationsfremmende midler blandt brugere af danske motions- og fitnesscentre: En statistisk analyse. Sociologisk rapportserie, 9(2002).

Pope, H. G., Kanayama, G., Athey, A., Ryan, E., Hudson, J. I., & Baggish, A. (2014). The lifetime prevalence of anabolic-androgenic steroid use and dependence in Americans: Current best estimates. Am J Addict, 23(4), 371–377. doi: doi:10.1111/ j.1521-0391.2013.12118.x.

Retsinformation. (1999). Lov om forbud mod visse dopingmidler. Retrieved from: www.retsinformation.dk/Forms/R0710.aspx?id=21128.

Retsinformation. (2004). Lov om fremme af dopingfri idræt (Act on Promotion of Doping-free Sport). Retrieved from: https://english.kum.dk/uploads/tx_templa voila/Act%20on%20Promotion%20of%20Doping-free%20Sport.pdf.

Retsinformation. (2008), Lov om ændring af lov om fremme af dopingfri idræt. Retrieved from: www.retsinformation.dk/eli/ft/200722L00089.

Retsinformation. (2013), Bekendtgørelse af lov om fremme af dopingfri idræt. Retrieved from: www.retsinformation.dk/Forms/R0710.aspx?id=160267. English version: https://english.kum.dk/uploads/tx_templavoila/Act%20on%20Promotion%20of%20Doping-free%20Sport.pdf.

Retsinformation. (2015). Bekendtgørelse af lov om fremme af integritet i idrætten. Retrieved from: www.retsinformation.dk/Forms/r0710.aspx?id=174633.

Steele, R., Bang, S., Brandt, H. H., & Kirkegaard, K. L. (2010). Indsatsen mod motions-doping i kommercielle motions- og fitnesscentre: En evaluering af mærkningsordnin-gen (The fight against doping in commercial fitness centres: An evaluation of the labelling scheme). Retrieved from København: www.idan.dk/vidensbank/for skningoganalyser/stamkort.aspx?publikationID=bbd99a70-1a98-4232-a6e9-9e3000e57 a68&/Vidensbank/Forskningoganalyser.aspx?currentstart=0&ResultPrPage=5&Kort visning=False&emneID=873805be-6673-4d78-b326-25899e74736f.

Storm, R. K., Toft, D., & Bang, S. (2015). Motionsdoping i Danmark. Evaluering af indsatsen mod motionsdoping i kommercielle motions- og fitnesscentre (Use of IPEDs in Denmark. An evaluation of the intervention in commercial gyms in Denmark). Retrieved from København: www.idan.dk/vidensbank/downloads/m otionsdoping-i-danmark/382b209b-fd84-4c04-9a6a-a50f0113101b.

Teetzel, S. (2007). Respecting privacy in detecting illegitimate enhancements in ath-letes. Sports, Ethics and Philosophy, 1(2), 159–170.

UNESCO. (2005). International convention against doping in sport 2005, ED.2005/CON-VENTION ANTI-DOPING Rev C.F.R. Retrieved from: http://portal.unesco.org/en/ev. php-URL_ID=31037&URL_DO=DO_TOPIC&URL_SECTION=201.html.

WADA. (2015). World Anti Doping Code 2015. Retrieved from: www.wada-ama. org/sites/default/files/resources/files/wada-2015-world-anti-doping-code.pdf.

WHO. (2004). Neuroscience of psychoactive substance use and dependence. Retrieved from Geneva: www.who.int/substance_abuse/publications/en/Neuroscience.pdf.

Chapter 12

Anti-doping efforts as perceived by IPED users

As explained earlier, most of the interviews were conducted in 2009, so obviously none of my informants could speak of the work done by Anti Doping Danmark (the Danish NADO) after its policy shift in 2012.[1] Interestingly, however, at the time of the interviews user frustration with Anti Doping Danmark was at its peak. This may be reflected in the criticisms some informants voice in this chapter, whereas others acknowledge the NADO's work and find doping tests and controls a necessary measure.

Jesper, who was critical of Anti Doping Danmark's work, accepted what they were doing, even though he knew it might have consequences for his peers or himself:

> When I joined the gym I also signed a form allowing them to test me. And I don't have a problem, either, if they test me, and if I test positive and I'm kicked out. No problem at all. That's just the way it is. That's the way the rules are, and I can't do anything about it.

At the time of the interviews Anti Doping Danmark had recommended that gyms and training centers remove all dumbbells weighing more than 30 kilos, as a preventive measure (Anti Doping Danmark, 2009). Oskar, who had extensive experience with virtually every available muscle-bulking substance, did not believe this would help, but he did have another recommendation:

> People are just going to take steroids anyway. The guys who take steroids are still going to be big even if you remove the dumbbells, so that's not going to work anyway. So control and testing, that's the best way. That's my opinion. No doubt about it.

To test his views on this point, I took on the role of the Devil's advocate, offering an alternative scenario. I asked why he didn't just say that because he wasn't entering any competitions, just working out and taking the steroids he had decided on — in a controlled manner, and making sure his liver values were checked — the authorities ought to just keep their nose out of his affairs. In short: Was there any reason to have strangers from the NADO watch him pee in a cup to check on what he was doing in his spare time? Oskar did not rise to the bait:

> Well, the situation is that I've chosen to work out at a gym where this is mandatory, or where you have to submit to testing if they ask you to. That's the way the rules are, you know, so you just have to accept that. Society has these rules, see? And they've done a good bit of thinking about various things, so you've got to respect that.

When I asked about his views on the effectiveness of doping control, Oskar — having used steroids himself — replied that they had a preventive effect that was analogous to speed checks on the roads: *"It's just like doing 130 [km/t] and there's a sign that says 90, and you know the traffic cops are around. Then you've got to be pretty stupid if you keep going 130!"* Even while maintaining that he found doping control to be a good idea, Oskar was very pragmatic about the risk of being tested. While he had been "speeding" himself, he moved his workout activities to a gym that had opted out of the Anti Doping Danmark program:

> Yeah, well, I left my fitness center while I had some of the stuff in my body that was traceable for a long time. Then I stayed at that place for about three years, until I was sure there was nothing left.

In other words, when Oskar says the rules must be respected, it does not mean "respected by not using steroids"; it means you should not complain about work being done to ensure a doping-free environment in the gym you use. He has no sympathy for people who gripe about the work Anti Doping Danmark does, or holler and cuss if they get picked for testing. People know the score, and if they still want to use IPEDs they have to take the trouble to find a workout location with no testing.

Kenneth, who had felt tempted to use steroids several times but ultimately decided against it, believed testing might deter people who were contemplating steroids as an option, as he once had:

> I think for people who are considering taking something, it's a strong argument that they risk getting caught, and risk public humiliation. You see them getting tested, then suddenly they're not working out at your gym anymore. That must be a deterrent. Without control or testing there's nothing to hold them back.

This view about the weight of potential public humiliation fits in with the rest of Kenneth's story. As we heard in Chapter 5, a powerful motivation for his training was personal insecurity, and he spent quite a lot of time thinking about other people's opinion of him and about how he might become part of the circles or cliques with *"the in crowd, the cool kids."* At the time of his interview, Kenneth finally felt he had reached that point: *"It's the first time in my life I'm in a circle with the in crowd."*

A researcher must be careful not to search for psychological factors when analyzing motivation. Still, these and other statements from Oskar and Kenneth make it easier to understand the difference in their views on the effectiveness of doping control. Oskar, who was older and presented as a stable, self-confident person, was able to think pragmatically about the risk of being tested, whereas Kenneth, a slightly insecure medical student who was very preoccupied with what other people thought of him, perceived the potential "public humiliation" of testing positive as an effective deterrent. Ironically, Kenneth's self-preoccupation meant that to showcase his disciplined training and the results he achieved *without* drugs, he would actually have liked to be selected for testing. This would have been a strong and useful signal to his surroundings — but it had never happened:

No, I've never been tested. At one stage I almost felt kind of insulted that they didn't pick me, because I wanted them to think I was doping. But I've never been tested, even though I've walked past them lots of times when they were at the gym. But I've never used anything, so you could say I've never had anything to fear.

Kasper, who didn't use doping substances either, but had work-out buddies who did, accepted the testing. Unlike Kenneth, however, he did not believe it was effective:

You know, Anti Doping Danmark are okay. And it's fine that there's some control going on. And it's fine that they're trying to fight doping. But they spend loads of money on testing, and it hasn't gotten them anywhere.

Kasper had been tested himself, and it had also boosted his vanity. Yet the experience was not entirely positive, since he also had his work to think of, as a trainer and role model for children and young people:

I really have mixed feelings about it. One is pride. It's cool to be suspected of being on 'roids without being on them, I have to say that. You know, it's a big pat on the back; a real thump. But at the same time it's really irritating. You're being treated on a par with somebody who commits illegal acts. That's not very nice. And here I am, working with young people, even in my spare time and all. Of course it's not cool to have parents think that this guy coaching their boys is probably on something. Yeah, that's a problem. So I have mixed feelings about it. Do you want my opinion as the beast I am at the gym, or do you want my opinion as the coach? As the beast, it's pretty awesome; as the coach, it's not cool at all.

Whereas Oskar and Kenneth were warmly in favor and Kasper and Jonas accepted Anti Doping Danmark's work with a shrug, other of my informants were against it. Adam, who spoke of steroids as *"such an integrated part of me, and I would be another person without those things,"* emphasized steroid use as a personal lifestyle choice. He took the drugs because they made him feel better about himself, and he could not comprehend why any public authority should have the right to interfere with that:

> I'm against doping in competitive sports. I think it's wrong there, because it gives a clear advantage to the people who dope themselves. But why test people like me, who do it out of vanity? I fail to see how this is any different than having a breast augmentation, or pumping neurotoxins like Botox into your face to get rid of wrinkles. And, you know, it's completely acceptable for people to do that sort of thing. In my view, that's just an incredible example of double standards. I don't think they should interfere with that sort of thing, at all.

Here Adam hits a pain point in the debate about recreational and/or non-competitive doping at fitness centers and the legislation that governs it: How can you justify giving a guy from a local fitness center, who uses IPEDs to feed his vanity, the same punishment — typically a two-year ban from all fitness centers — that you would give a professional top athlete who uses drugs to win an Olympic medal, international fame and lucrative contracts? As Adam rightly points out, Danish law does not punish people who embark on other risky bodily interventions motivated by vanity. If the good-health argument is to undergird the fight against "vanity doping," it is understandable that some people wonder why the authorities do not also interfere with other, similar practices that can harm a person's health. Here, Adam is on the same page as the Danish doping scholar Verner Møller, who has likewise stated that "a consistent policy would demand corresponding interventions against the 'vanity doping' that takes place at beauty clinics." Møller, like Adam, also points out the lack of clarity as to

> why vain bodybuilders are prohibited from using hormones in the quest to achieve the perfect body, while vain men and women are allowed to remove wrinkles, for example, using the poisonous nerve substance Botox, which can also have serious side effects. In a similar vein, it would also be reasonable to demand the closure of [tanning parlors], where for the sake of vanity people allow themselves to be artificially tanned and as a consequence increase the risk of contracting skin cancer.

Penis enlargements, piercings, silicone implants, and hair dyes are other examples, for which consideration for the nation's health could give cause for prohibition, monitoring and other control strategies.

(Møller, 2009, p. 22)

Møller's analogy seems somewhat overstretched. For instance, the authorities could choose to prohibit smoking without simultaneously prohibiting inactivity, even though both factors increase the risk of premature death. And imagine prohibiting tanning beds, which would also imply an official ban on sunbathing at large if such a measure were to be consistent. It would also be a gross infringement of personal freedom.

As previously explained, in Denmark we are fighting steroids (and not tanning beds) because we signed the UNESCO anti-doping convention. Thus, a consistent line of argumentation defending the use of doping tests and control in gym environments means that we cannot legally accept Adam's motive for using steroids — vanity, or image — as his only reason. The fact that steroids have a performance-enhancing effect, thereby increasing his chances of winning competitions he is *not* taking part in, must necessarily be included as a parallel motive. Otherwise it is not possible to justify testing.

Objections to testing as a matter of principle

For Rasmus, the Athlete type, the performance-enhancing effect of steroids is decisive to why he takes them. He is a competitive bodybuilder and has consciously chosen to work out at fitness centers and gyms that do not cooperate with Anti Doping Danmark. When stating the reasons for this choice, however, he does not emphasize the risk of testing positive, but lists three other issues that are matters of principle more than anything else: (1) the individual's right to decide over their own body; (2) the central-database registration of people who test positive; and (3) the test situation's violation of a person's right to privacy. Echoing Adam's sentiments, Rasmus was the first informant to point out the fundamental absurdity he saw in the authorities' testing of recreational or non-competitive gym-goers:

It's just working out, you know. Just let people do what they want. They come in to socialize, and to have fun, and to work out. Some people are serious and dedicated; some aren't serious. And everybody's using something. Or no, they're not using, but some'll be smoking cannabis, others will be on narcotics, or using steroids, and I just think it's wrong to kick people out based on that. But yes, if they'd been causing trouble or acting inappropriately or something, I'd understand it. But it's not like they're hurting anybody just because they're on steroids.

The way Rasmus sees it, the important thing is for people to be judged by their behavior and their actions, not by what drugs they are taking. Further to this, the two evaluations of the testing program conducted by the Danish Ministry of Culture point out that some fitness centers think their agreement with Anti Doping Danmark can be used as an excuse for not laying down anti-doping rules or enforcing their own house rules or code of conduct (Steele, Bang, Brandt, & Kirkegaard, 2010; Storm, Toft, & Bang, 2015).[2] Seen in that light, we can take the point Rasmus made to mean that if a member of the fitness center acts in an unpleasant or inappropriate way or breaks the house rules, the management ought to ask that person to act appropriately or, if that has no effect, to revoke their membership. If, instead, the management contacts Anti Doping Danmark to have the person tested, in order to be able to kick him out (based on the idea that his bad behavior is probably due to his steroid use), the management will be in a weak position if he tests negative and is not generally banned from membership.

It was clear from the quote, and indeed throughout the entire interview, that Rasmus has a fundamentally liberal mindset, and he believes people ought to be allowed to do whatever they want, as long as they do not hassle or harm others or stand in the way of other people's freedom to think and act as they like. That is also why the surveillance and monitoring built into the control system rubs him the wrong way. Everyone who tests positive is recorded in a central database (Retsinformation, 2013), which Rasmus does not like:

> See, it's just *more* surveillance. And then they just have to get even more data on you. I think that sucks, big-time. I'm not comfortable at all with having that data floating around out there. It's like a kind of abuse. I don't think there's any call for that; monitoring people like that.

That also explains why he has chosen to train at a gym that does not cooperate with Anti Doping Danmark, which is why he has never been tested, as he explains, elaborating:

> And I wouldn't like it either, if I had to be tested. To me that's like a violation of my privacy, having somebody stand there watching you piss in a cup. I mean seriously, how many people walk around with a fake urine test in their pocket? Nobody does that. And they test it [the sample] right after you've peed, to see whether it's okay [if it has been tampered with]. And I guess I just think it's pretty weird. At least they could let people piss in private. I think it's gross, and it sure oversteps my personal boundaries. They could at least give people their freakin' thirty seconds of privacy.

Technically, when a person is selected for doping control they are asked to partially undress in front of the doping-control officer, pulling their undergarments down to their knees and lifting their T-shirt above their navel, leaving their private parts clearly visible. The person is then asked to urinate while the official watches, viewing the process from the front or side. As the international WADA standard stipulates, "The DCO/Chaperone shall ensure an unobstructed view of the Sample leaving the Athlete's body" (WADA, 2016, p. D.4.9). Unlike Rasmus, Kasper had actually been in that situation. He found it very uncomfortable, and because of the awkwardness of being under observation he had difficulty passing his urine then and there:

> It's unpleasant. We can all do it down at the bar, but it's not easy with somebody watching. And it's not easy at all when you're under suspicion all the while, because then you're nervous too. And there you are with this stupid little cup you have to make it go into, and you can really make a mess of it, and I thought that was really unpleasant. This guy was standing right up behind me, with his chin over my shoulder, looking down at my dick while I was peeing. He had to, to visually check that I didn't have some rubber tube or something else tricky hanging out. I don't even know if they're allowed to do that? Isn't that invading your privacy, or indecent exposure or something? And at the same time the other DCO, who's a lady, is sitting in the changing room next door. She can't see anything, but there aren't any doors between the rooms, so she can hear everything that's going on.[3]

There is no doubt that this type of doping control oversteps the boundaries of the private, personal sphere. In this sense a test is a state-sanctioned violation of people's privacy, as also conceded by leading Danish doping lawyers and by David Howman, former director general of WADA (Evald, 2009).[4] Naturally, this argument can be shrugged off by contending that people who choose to work out at a gym that is part of the program voluntarily accept this potential violation. In short: If they don't like it, they can leave it — and find another gym, like Oskar did. One could likewise argue that privately owned commercial facilities have the right to decide which partners they want to cooperate with, and as long as joining the program is voluntary for facilities and as long as the members are informed about the cooperation when they join, they can hardly object to potentially being selected for a test. On the other hand, it is reasonable to question whether such privacy violations, despite being voluntarily accepted, are defensible. Firstly, there are reasons based on principle. Secondly, 80% of people holding fitness-center memberships in Denmark fall under program, and a number of small towns across the country have no alternative fitness centers for people who, as a matter of principle, would not wish to be tested.[5]

In an article about the legal boundaries for doping, the Danish law professor and arbitrator at the Court of Arbitration for Sport (CAS), Jens Evald, who is also a former chairman of Anti Doping Danmark, has observed that the World Anti-Doping Code has no rules limiting doping control to respect privacy. But both Article 71 of the Danish Constitution and Article 8 of the European Convention on Human Rights (ECHR) have provisions concerning the individual's right to privacy, and the laws and conventions currently in force in Denmark also cover the world of sport. Based on this, the Danish law professor has argued:

> given that respect for the right to privacy, and the protection of citizens' personal integrity, can be deduced from the provisions in the [Danish] Constitution, in laws, and in international conventions, then in a democratic nation governed by the rule of law, norms regarding these topics must be attributed a weight that is not insignificant — also in connection with formulating the rules for doping control, and with administrating these rules.
>
> (Evald, 2009, p. 72, my translation)

The ECHR states in Article 8, section 1, that "Everyone has the right to respect for his private and family life [...]," and further, in section 2, that "There shall be no interference by a public authority with the exercise of this right except such as is in accordance with the law and is necessary [...] for the protection of health [...]" (Council of Europe, 1950, Article 8). The national government indisputably plays an important role in doping control in Denmark, given that: the Danish state has ratified UNESCO's anti-doping convention; the national treasury funds a considerable part of the NADO's (Anti Doping Danmark's) budget; and the Danish minister of culture appoints the chairman of the NADO's board. Hence, the national government is responsible for ensuring that doping-control work is conducted in accordance with Article 8 of the ECHR. Professor Evald has explained what this means:

> Pursuant to Article 8, section 2, the state may only intervene in the private life of citizens when there are substantial reasons to do so. At the same time there must be proportionality between the nature of the intervention and the purpose it seeks to achieve. The proportionality requirement means the state must choose between a less invasive, rather than a more invasive, type of restriction, and that the measure must be reasonable when compared with the purpose described.
>
> (Evald, 2009, p. 82, my translation)

So the question is whether there are "substantial reasons" to test as the authorities do, and whether the interference in the individual's right to privacy (during doping controls in Danish fitness centers) is thereby justifiable. Evald concludes that such interference is defensible in elite sports, partly because this helps to protect athlete health and partly because it is necessary to maintain the fair-play ideal in sport. However, although the fairness and health arguments are both valid in elite sports, all things considered, it is only the health-protection argument that holds any relevance in fitness and workout communities. Consequently, if one is to defend the way doping control interferes with the citizens' right to privacy, one must argue that it is necessary in the interest of protecting health. But this is difficult. Not because of lacking evidence that steroids harm health, but because it is impossible to obtain evidence that doping control can reduce steroid use in fitness and gym environments — either because fewer people start using or because people who are caught using stop doing so and change to a healthier lifestyle. This may well be happening, but no evidence has been found to prove it is happening. It therefore seems that doping controls in gyms and fitness centers do not live up to the proportionality requirement, which calls for authorities to choose an intervention that is less comprehensive or restrictive.

Seen in this light, Anti Doping Danmark's shift in recent years from control to dialogue makes good sense, dialogue being a considerably smaller "intervention" and, based on the available knowledge and evidence, one that is probably equally efficient in promoting health. However, as long as the Danish parliament maintains the legislation currently in force, Anti Doping Danmark will still be obliged to control and test gym-goers at the facilities that have joined its program — and the problem of government-sanctioned violations of citizens' privacy will continue to exist.

As we have seen, health promotion is the undergirding argument for efforts that target recreational and non-competitive doping, and this points us towards a final challenge facing anti-doping efforts in Denmark. This final question is: When the aim is to ensure the health of non-competitive sport practitioners, is the target group only the people who do what the authorities want, or does the target group also include those with health problems caused by steroid use?

Help for abusers

The potentially grave side effects of using androgenic anabolic steroids have already been described. Some users end up in abuse or dependency they may find hard to escape. While in recent years politicians have discussed options for treatment, in Denmark there is no specific program for the group that ends up with health problems. Considering the intense focus on doping control in Denmark back in 2009, Jesper expressed his criticism of Danish doping efforts with unveiled sarcasm:

> They test some people, then they go and find out: "Gotcha! You're doping, so out you go!" But when do they get a hold of people? When

do they go in and say: "Do you have an actual problem? Are you moving into abuse? Are you doing any harm to yourself, or other people?" Nobody's doing stuff like that.

Typically, the penalty for testing positive for IPEDs at a fitness center is a two-year ban from all gyms and centers in the program, plus a four-year ban from participating in any other organized sport in Denmark. Anti Doping Danmark does subsequently contact people who test positive, but for all intents and purposes these people are left to their own devices, just like everyone else who ends up having an "actual problem" with steroids. The series of articles from 2012 in the Danish daily *Politiken*, dealt with in Chapter 1, described the situation at that time:

> When the dream of the perfect body ends in steroid dependency and psychological collapse, the pumped-up doping addicts must find their own way out of their nightmare. Because although doctors, psychiatrists and organizations see how muscle-fixated Danish men become slaves of doping substances, and in some cases develop the eating disorder megarexia, there are no targeted public treatment options for them in Denmark. The catch is, the Danish Health Authority does not have anabolic steroids on its list of addictive substances, in addition to which it does not have megarexia — roughly, an aberrant urge to attain a larger body — on its list of diagnoses.[6] And without that sort or recognition, the public health system cannot offer treatment.
>
> (Heide-Jørgensen & Brock, 2012)

As of 2019 the situation has not changed significantly. There seems to be a wicked irony in this, reading the comments to the 2008 legislation, which introduced the smiley program, which stated: "The abuse of doping substances among recreational sports practitioners is a health problem, and solely a health problem" (Retsinformation, 2008, item 4). Even with such unconditional recognition of the problem, it is currently being met primarily with prevention efforts in the form of control, information, education and dialogue — not with treatment for those who have, in fact, contracted health problems.

As the article excerpt shows, part of the explanation for this is that, unlike alcoholism or cannabis and drug abuse, there are no clear-cut diagnoses in this field. Although there are a few recent studies suggesting that both mental and physical dependency on anabolic steroids can occur, the results are not conclusive. As discussed in previous chapters, it is beyond doubt that a person can become dependent on the feelings, experiences and social benefits associated with steroids: "the pump," quickly gaining muscle bulk, getting a motivational boost during workouts, and gaining recognition from friends and acquaintances. After a cycle, when testosterone levels decline, so does the user's mood, muscle-mass gain and motivation, which makes it tempting to start another cycle. This can result in a vicious circle, as Michael described in Chapter 6.

Another plausible explanation for the lack of treatment options has to do with the stigmatization of steroid users. While drug addicts and alcoholics are, to a certain extent, seen as victims who need help, the side effects of steroid use are perceived as self-induced. They occur in strong people as a consequence of a conscious choice, not in vulnerable people who in their darkest hours fall prey to drugs or alcohol. A recent study has confirmed that the health system may also have a stigmatizing bias towards steroid users. The American clinical psychologist Jessica Yu and her colleagues have demonstrated that health professionals react more negatively to a vignette describing a steroid user than to corresponding stories describing, respectively, a non-user and a cocaine user (Yu, Hildebrandt, & Lanzieri, 2015). When the center-left politician Ulla Astman, who chairs the health committee of the association Danish Regions was asked in 2012 to comment on the fact that steroid users were contacting the public health system for help to have undesired mammary tissue removed, she stated to the newspaper journalist from *Politiken*: "That's misuse of the resources in the public health system. It's not reasonable that we should spend money on medical testing and operations when these people have brought this damage on themselves with eyes wide open" (Brock & Heide-Jørgensen, 2012, my translation). If this is meant to express that the public health system cannot expend resources on people who have "brought [...] damage on themselves with eyes wide open," then Astman would also have to turn away smokers with lung cancer, or obese citizens with diabetes and cardiovascular disease, at the doors of Danish hospitals. At any rate, lifestyle diseases people have contracted by legal use of their knives and forks, or an equally legal inactive lifestyle as couch potatoes, are perceived as less stigmatizing in the health system than diseases caused by the illegal use of performance-enhancing drugs in the gym.[7] In all events, whatever the explanation, this lack of specific treatment options means that most IPED users are treated for acute physical problems, either by their own physician or at the cardiology and endocrinology wards in hospitals, but find there is no treatment for IPED abuse or dependency.

Some other countries do have specific treatment options for people suffering mental and physical health problems after anabolic steroid use. Likewise, certain countries also assist, inform and educate IPED users in ways that radically differ from the Danish approach.

Notes

1 As mentioned in Chapter 1, as a thesis supervisor and external examiner I have read a number of interviews with Danish anabolic-steroid users done by students in 2012–2019. None of these interviews offered radically new insights into user experiences with anabolic steroids, nor did they call into question the fundamental variations my study revealed in user views on Anti Doping Danmark's work. Consequently, although these views do not directly address the shift of focus in

the Danish NADO's efforts after 2012, I have no reason to assume that the range of views voiced by my informants would differ significantly from what one would find in a corresponding survey or study done today.

2 In 2015 the head of one gym outside the anti-doping program stated the reasons for deciding not to join: "Giving over responsibility for doping abuse can easily lead to complacency, and you can avoid the highly unpleasant task of confronting people who are obviously doped. That means most of the people who dope can just go ahead and keep doing it. In my own experience, what happens is that when one person gets confronted and expelled from the gym the other abusers vanish, for fear of being next. Understood in the sense that if the 'doping police' is the gym itself, they feel like they're under surveillance all the time, as opposed to the risk of being selected when there's a visit from Anti Doping Danmark. Every time I've expelled someone who was clearly doped, a small group has always disappeared too, and it's funny how they always moved to a gym that's signed on with Anti Doping Danmark." Quoted from (Storm et al., 2015, p. 60, my translation).

3 Kasper is not alone with his experience of having difficulty urinating when others are watching. According to the German sport psychologist Anne-Marie Elbe this phenomenon also occurs among professional athletes, many of whom find it difficult to urinate while being observed. In the context of doping control this problem is not merely physiological (as when an athlete has just used the bathroom or is dehydrated after a training session or competition). There can also be psychological reasons such as difficulty urinating under surveillance or within hearing range of others. According to Elbe, concerns about not being able to pass water can cause athletes to develop paruresis (Elbe et al., 2016). Also known as "shy bladder syndrome", paruresis is a phobia that means a person cannot urinate while others are watching or are (assumed to be) nearby. See also https://en.wikipedia.org/wiki/Paruresis (accessed on October 10, 2019).

4 "It is a breach of privacy rights to have to pee in front of some stranger. But it is [a means that is] proportionate to the aim [to catch dopers in elite sport]." WADA Director General David Howman, speaking at the International Network of Doping Research (INDR) conference *Anti-doping: Rational Policy or Moral Panic*, held at Aarhus University on August 18–19, 2011.

5 The following propositions are based on (Christiansen, 2011).

6 As mentioned in Chapter 2, the term "megarexia" has been replaced by the technical term "muscle dysmorphia," which does not appear on the Danish Health Authority's diagnosis list either.

7 One could, of course, argue that the "fairness" in the public health-care system's principle of treating lung cancer, cardiovascular diseases and other lifestyle diseases (but not the long-term effects of steroid use) lies in the fact that smokers and overweight citizens have contributed large sums to the public coffers by purchasing cigarettes and soda, which carry a heavy product or sales tax. Unlike these groups, steroid users have illegally imported their health-harming substances, courting misfortune without contributing to society's common pool of funds.

References

Anti Doping Danmark. (2009). *Håndbog for fitnesscentre. Råd og vejledning om antidoping* (J. Berget & M. R. Johannisson, Eds.). København, Denmark: Anti Doping Danmark.

Brock, J. L., & Heide-Jørgensen, C. (2012, 23November). Muskelmænd udnytter lægehjælp (Muscle men exploits medical treatment). *Politiken*, section 1, page 1.

Christiansen, A. V. (2011). Bodily violations: Testing citizens training recreationally in gyms. In M. McNamee & V. Møller (Eds.), *Doping and anti-doping. Ethical, legal and social perspectives* (pp. 126–141). London: Routledge.

Council of Europe. (1950). *Convention for the Protection of Human Rights and Fundamental Freedoms (ECHR)*. Retrieved from: http://conventions.coe.int/Treaty/en/Treaties/Html/005.htm.

Elbe, A. M., Jensen, S. N., Elsborg, P., Wetzke, M., Woldemariam, G. A., Huppertz, B., … Butch, A. W. (2016). The urine marker test: An alternative approach to supervised urine collection for doping control. *Sports Med, 46*(1), 15–22. doi: doi:10.1007/s40279-015-0388-6.

Evald, J. (2009). Retlige grænser for dopingkontrol. In A. V. Christiansen (Ed.), *Kontrolsport: Big brother blandt atleter og tilskuere* (pp. 71–88). Odense, Denmark: Syddansk Universitetsforlag.

Heide-Jørgensen, C., & Brock, J. L. (2012, 25 November). Dopingvrag står uden hjælp (Doping wrecks receive no help). *Politiken*, section 1, page 25.

Møller, V. (2009). Conceptual confusion and the anti-doping campaign in Denmark. In V. Møller, M., McNamee, & P. Dimeo (Eds.), *Elite sport, doping and public health* (pp. 13–28). Odense, Denmark: University Press of Southern Denmark.

Retsinformation. (2008). Lov om ændring af lov om fremme af dopingfri idræt. Retrieved from: www.retsinformation.dk/eli/ft/200722L00089.

Retsinformation. (2013). Bekendtgørelse af lov om fremme af dopingfri idræt. Retrieved from: www.retsinformation.dk/Forms/R0710.aspx?id=160267. English version:https://english.kum.dk/uploads/tx_templavoila/Act%20on%20Promotion %20of%20Doping-free%20Sport.pdf.

Steele, R., Bang, S., Brandt, H. H., & Kirkegaard, K. L. (2010). *Indsatsen mod motionsdoping i kommercielle motions- og fitnesscentre: En evaluering af mærkningsordningen* (The fight against doping in commercial fitness centres: An evaluation of the labelling scheme). Retrieved from København: www.idan.dk/vidensbank/forskningoganalyser/ stamkort.aspx?publikationID=bbd99a70-1a98-4232-a6e9-9e3000e57a68&/Vidensba nk/Forskningoganalyser.aspx?currentstart=0&ResultPrPage=5&Kortvisning=False& emneID=873805be-6673-4d78-b326-25899e74736f.

Storm, R. K., Toft, D., & Bang, S. (2015). Motionsdoping i Danmark. Evaluering af indsatsen mod motionsdoping i kommercielle motions- og fitnesscentre (Use of IPEDs in Denmark: An evaluation of the intervention in commercial gyms in Denmark). Retrieved from København: www.idan.dk/vidensbank/downloads/m otionsdoping-i-danmark/382b209b-fd84-4c04-9a6a-a50f0113101b.

WADA. (2016). The World Anti-Doping Code International Standard for Testing and Investigations (ISTI) January 2017. Retrieved from: www.wada-ama.org/sites/ default/files/resources/files/2016-09-30_-_isti_final_january_2017.pdf.

Yu, J., Hildebrandt, T., & Lanzieri, N. (2015). Healthcare professionals' stigmatization of men with anabolic androgenic steroid use and eating disorders. *Body Image, 15*, 49–53. doi: doi:10.1016/j.bodyim.2015.06.001.

Chapter 13

Harm reduction as an alternative strategy

Looking at the national anti-doping organizations (NADOs) across Europe, some of the most well-developed educational and dialogue measures to reach groups in fitness centers and gyms are found in Denmark, Holland and Norway. Sweden and Finland have also done much in this respect, but their anti-doping efforts in gym circles are handled outside the country's NADOs, which leads to other approaches.[1] In the United Kingdom, most work in this area is not only detached from the NADO, it has also taken a completely different approach, focusing on harm reduction. In this chapter, I discuss measures that differ from Danish efforts, the aim being to compare alternatives and discuss pros and cons of the different approaches.

Unlike in Denmark, the health authorities in Holland, Norway and Sweden have all established clinics for steroid users seeking treatment and help to stop using, and there is clearly a need in this group for access to such treatment (Havnes, Jorstad, & Wisloff, 2019). These clinics are physically located in or near conjunction with hospitals and they are not directly related to the anti-doping effort in sports. In my estimation the most comprehensive treatment setup is found in Sweden, where the Örebro Län Region has had a facility called *Dopningsmottagningen* ("the doping reception unit") since 2012. This unit has a wide variety of expert professionals including psychiatrists, psychologists, endocrinologists and other doctors to help and treat steroid users who have ended up in abuse or dependency (Region Örebro Län, 2019). Norway has a health facility called *Hormonlaboratoriet* ("the hormone laboratory") under Oslo University Hospital with an affiliated clinic for outpatient treatment (Oslo Universitetssykehus, 2019). In Holland, the *Spaarne Gasthuis* (Spaarne Guest House) in Harlem has a similar outpatient clinic that offers treatment for steroid abusers (Smit & de Ronde, 2018; Spaarne Gasthuis, 2019). However, neither Holland, Norway, nor Sweden has actual health checks or counseling for anabolic steroid users on, for instance, correct injection techniques and similar topics.

Countries that do offer such services in multiple locations include Australia, Ireland and the United Kingdom, and the UK model with "Needle and Syringe Programs," "steroid clinics" and outreach initiatives has both attracted a fair amount of discussion in the UK-based literature and also been one element under consideration as an addition to the existing policies in Scandinavia (Bates, 2019; Bates, Tod, Leavey, & McVeigh, 2019; Christiansen & Bojsen-Møller, 2012; Evans-Brown & McVeigh, 2009; Kimergård & McVeigh, 2014a, 2014b). These programs originally emerged in the mid-1980s in Merseyside in the north of England, primarily in response to concerns about HIV and hepatitis B and C transmission among heroin users. The aim was to avoid epidemics among drug users by handing out sterile needles and syringes, as well as educating people about correct injection techniques. In other words, their basic aim was not to eradicate drug abuse, but to reduce the scope and severity of the harm users and abusers risked bringing upon themselves and those around them. In short, these were harm-reduction initiatives. In general, harm reduction initiatives encompass

> interventions, programmes and policies that seek to reduce the health, social and economic harms of drug use to individuals, communities and societies. A core principle of harm reduction is the development of pragmatic responses to dealing with drug use through a hierarchy of intervention goals that place primary emphasis on reducing the health-related harms of continued drug use.
>
> (Rhodes & Hedrich, 2010, p. 19)

There is solid evidence showing that these clinics had the desired effect on the original target group of infected drug users (Bates, 2019; Kimergård & McVeigh, 2014b). Things then developed gradually, and unintentionally, to the point where several of these clinics observed that more and more of those they served were steroid users rather than traditional drug users. Because it was a known fact that steroid users can also have risky injection practices, for instance sharing needles or using needles that are too thin, this group was also allowed to frequent the needle-exchange clinics. As a result, some clinics of this type in Northwest England have a clientele of over 80% steroid users (Kimergård & McVeigh, 2014b). Thus, healthcare targeting people who use IPEDs in the UK is mainly delivered through substance use services and pharmacy-based needle and syringe programs that provide a variety of interventions and support services for people who use a range of drugs. Some of these clinics focus specifically on steroids and have staff who are specifically educated to deal with steroid issues. Still, the services offered at the individual clinics that are part of the needle and syringe program vary greatly. In most clinics, users can come to get new, sterile needles and hand in old ones, and they may be offered interviews with healthcare staff and education about proper injection techniques. Some clinics also offer health checks to measure blood pressure and cholesterol, screen for blood-borne viruses and check liver values, all with the view of encouraging users to stop taking steroids if the results are negative. As part of the outreach program, some clinics are located in gyms, where there is also counseling about weight-training techniques and diets that can lead to the desired bodily improvements without steroids. A few clinics even give advice on dosing and combining various types of steroids in order to avoid overdosing and inappropriate "stacking" of drugs and "polypharmacy" (Kimergård & McVeigh, 2014b). While all clinics have the same basic ambition of harm reduction, the actual practices and services among the clinics as well as the users' reception of the clinics vary greatly (Bates, 2019).

It is worth noting that in the UK, steroids have a different legal status than they do in Denmark and many other countries, which is a key factor when considering this work. In the UK, anabolic steroids are controlled as a class-C drug under the 1971 *Misuse of Drugs Act*, which means that possession of anabolic steroids is not a criminal offense, provided they are for personal use. Conversely, it is illegal to manufacture, import or possess large amounts of steroids with a view to sale. The latter is an offense punishable by up to 14 years in prison, which is significantly higher than, say, the Danish maximum steroid-peddling sentence of 6 years (Bates, 2019; McVeigh & Begley, 2017).[2]

Besides the needle and syringe programs themselves, the UK has a wide variety of information material in the form of flyers, pamphlets and magazines that describe drugs, drug groups, brand names, effects and side effects, advantages and disadvantages of tablets and injections, and correct injection techniques. As an outsider embedded in the Scandinavian approach to IPED use, I was quite surprised the first time I saw this large body of material. Up until then, similar material I had seen had all focused on side effects, sometimes taking the form of scare-campaigns, but the graphics, style and aesthetics in the British material often emulated what is found in physical-fitness and bodybuilding magazines. Pictures of extremely fit, well-oiled bodies with tensed muscles next to fact boxes and exhaustive information about needle sizes, injection techniques and production locations, as well as drug names, brands, effects and side effects. As with the needle and syringe program, the whole purpose of providing detailed, frank and factual information to steroid users is to give them knowledge and information and thereby reduce the harm that can occur, rather than attempting to frighten people to keep them from starting on steroids.

The most obvious result of such direct use of harm-reduction strategies to reach steroid users is that the element of condemnation that has generally dominated the discussion of doping issues is absent.[3] Rather than holding onto the ideal of a doping-free future, which can only be achieved by rooting out the evil, a policy of harm reduction takes its cue from an imperfect reality; a reality where people do stupid and potentially dangerous things. So the basic premise is not: "We want to win the fight against doping." Instead, the premise is: "We know people do inappropriate and harmful things, so let's at least make sure they harm themselves as little as possible while they're at it." Framed in the language of ethics, one could say: "While much of conventional anti-doping policy takes its cue from deontological ethics and is concerned with the intention ("cheating" in elite sport; or "vanity" in recreational sport), a policy of harm reduction, is based on utilitarian ethics and therefore more concerned with the consequences of actions.

The question is whether a harm-reduction approach works. The simple answer is: We do not know. The reason is that, as yet, there has been no systematic, scientific evaluation with uniform measurements that has compared the effects of the various policies and approaches — neither on the number of users, on the harm they cause to themselves or on the total amount of pressure this puts on the public health services. However, the assessment of researchers in the field is that the effectiveness of the efforts varies considerably, depending on where their focus lies and how committed and knowledgeable the staff is (e.g. Bates, 2019; Kimergård & McVeigh, 2014b). Andreas Kimergård and Jim McVeigh, from Liverpool John Moores University, have observed and interviewed users and staff at the UK clinics, and they describe how in some places steroid users simply walk in to load up on needles and syringes for themselves and their friends, then leave without ever engaging in a conversation. At other clinics there is a good dialogue, frequent conversations and ongoing follow-up on the users who come in. As Kimergård and McVeigh conclude in their study of the clinic-based initiatives, this huge variation in initiatives stands in contrast to other areas of health-service provision in that there is no best practice when it comes to reducing harm for anabolic-steroid users. Even so, in light of the experience from similar interventions they assess that the harm-reducing effect is greatest when multiple initiatives are offered in combination, such as sterile equipment, health checkups and conversations with educated personnel (Kimergård & McVeigh, 2014b).

In many respects, drug researcher Geoff Bates, also from Liverpool John Moores University, echoes this assessment. He believes that harm-reduction initiatives are needed for health workers to remain in professional contact with IPED users who, seen as a group, are very sexually active, to prevent them from attracting and spreading diseases, not least the hepatitis C virus. However, when it comes to the clinic's effectiveness in their ambition to change behavior and reduce prevalence, Bates is less optimistic. As he concludes in his study on initiatives that support men who use anabolic steroids: "There remains, however, no evidence to date beyond anecdotal accounts to demonstrate that services (including pharmacy NSPs [needle and syringe programs], substance use services or AAS [anabolic androgenic steroids] clinics) are effective in influencing AAS choices or changing behaviours" (Bates, 2019, p. 171).

The information paradox

Imagine being a spin doctor for the minister of culture, who (at least in Denmark) is responsible for sport and therefore also responsible for doping, and being asked which strategy is best and most clearly communicable. The obvious choice would be an "anti-doping" message, based on the "zero tolerance" principle. The easiest route is unequivocal rejection: "IPEDs are harmful." "Doping is cheating." "Join the fight against doping." These are messages people understand and largely support, also in Danish gym and fitness communities (Storm, Toft, & Bang, 2015). Nevertheless, though total rejection is the easiest message to communicate, it is not necessarily the best message. Alternatively, one could recommend a multifaceted approach consisting of information, dialogue and aims of including treatment and potential harm reduction, after the fashion of the British approach. Jonas presaged this when he rhetorically asked why the system doesn't help the people who have a problem.

The reason why "anti-" and "zero"-type messages are easiest to communicate is mainly that the very nature of information and education is a paradox. You can give people knowledge and insight, but you have no way of knowing what they are going to do with it. I personally found myself confronted with this dilemma while attending a conference in June 2016, at Liverpool John Moores University. Besides researchers, health professionals and representatives from authorities I knew from previous conferences in the field, the participants included people who plainly had very personal, years-long experience with steroid use. Very large men in very snug T-shirts. It was odd to witness how, after the various presentations, they would unabashedly offer comments and ask about topics like police work, Internet trading, distribution chains, the quality of certain drugs and substance dependency. Never before had I seen such keen interest in research findings from the actual users. Our non-British research colleagues were particularly uncomfortable when asked about how the steroid dealers and traders operated, or which drugs were purest and safest. They could hardly come right out and say they did not wish to share what insights they had gained, but at the same time it was quite obvious that the conference's abundantly muscled participants took a different interest in these topics than the academics did.

This example — along with the difference between the English and Danish approaches — frames two fundamental conflicts inherent in education and information initiatives in this field. The first question is: If health authorities provide detailed information about risks and correct drug-handling and injection techniques, does your position as an authority contribute to legitimizing steroid use and giving an impression that steroids can be taken safely, without risking adverse effects? The second is: If you provide information about these things, is it possible to differentiate the information given to different groups, so that a 20-year-old who has not yet started using steroids does not receive the same information as the 30-year-old seasoned user? Some of the staff providing services in the British clinics felt caught in a dilemma when doing health checks on steroid users, fearing they might consequently have some understanding that their use was not risky since it was monitored by trained health staff (Kimergård & McVeigh, 2014b). Thus, it is possible to imagine that users experiencing safety and security, and possibly also fewer unpleasant side effects, may develop a longer-lasting and more risky use pattern, which in the long term will increase their risk of more severe health problems. Herein lie the main arguments against harm-reducing initiatives: There is a risk that the efforts of health consultants may cause some people to use steroids for longer; and the presence of trained health staff as advisors may tempt some people to try steroids who otherwise would not have done so. The counter-argument is: If we know there are people out there exhibiting risky or dangerous behavior, which can be prevented using relatively limited resources, then society has a moral obligation to try and steer them away from such behavior. Or inversely, if it is possible to do this by expending relatively limited resources, then it is morally unacceptable to refrain from taking action that may prevent people from harming themselves.

It is very clear that if harm-reduction initiatives for steroid users are to gain any significant measure of popular support outside the UK-based needle and syringe programs, and if the people who run them are to avoid accusations of having double standards, then these initiatives must be anchored in a location or a body that is distinct and separate from efforts against doping in elite sports. The mixed messages would simply be too confusing if the same institution was battling doping with one hand and educating doping users about correct injection techniques with the other. Therefore, if Denmark, or any other country where the NADO leads IPED prevention among gym and fitness enthusiasts, wished to introduce a system that also includes harm reduction and treatment, the country would have to anchor this effort outside the Ministry of Culture and the local NADO, for instance placing it instead, organizationally, under the Ministry of Health. That would also make it easier to communicate a more flexible and graduated message than "anti-" and "zero"-type messages are. In a scenario such as this, the NADO could continue to be responsible for dialogue and for the primary prevention efforts in fitness centers and gyms, as in the case of Anti Doping Denmark. But the NADO would not be responsible for secondary prevention efforts in the form of harm-reduction initiatives (as exemplified in the British clinics) or for tertiary prevention, which (like the Swedish, Norwegian and Dutch clinics) deals with detox and treatment programs (Vinther & Christiansen, 2019).

It is worth noting that one type of prevention does not rule out other types, since the three prevention levels have different aims and different target groups. The primary prevention level addresses behaviors that have not yet occurred; the secondary addresses current behaviors; and the tertiary addresses behaviors in the past. When it comes to prevention, one size definitely does not fit all.[4] Just as dialogues and consultations should be tailored to suit a YOLO type, an Expert and so on, as profiled in the ideal typology in Chapter 7, conversations must also be tailored to suit, say, 20-year-old Mike, who as yet is only tempted by steroids, or 30-year-old Peter, who has years of experience. The former conversation ought to focus on counseling for healthy eating and training, realistic goals and healthy body ideals, whereas the latter might focus on safety, harm reduction, downscaling and/or potentially quitting steroids. Recalling Chapter 11, an example of primary prevention would be Anti Doping Danmark's 2016 "pure"-themed hashtag campaign, because it focuses on people with positive behaviors (dedicated gym-goers who don't use steroids), while a conversion with an experienced user would be at the secondary and tertiary level, depending on the user's situation. At present, in 2020, Denmark has no secondary or tertiary prevention measures for steroid users. Sweden and Holland have primary and tertiary, but no secondary prevention. In the UK, primary prevention through information campaigns comes from the same sources who issue information about drugs generally, and which therefore have little to do with the organizations UK Anti Doping or UK Sport. The UK has secondary prevention through providing needles, education and user consultations at the steroid clinics, but it has no tertiary prevention dedicated to steroid users, who can, however, seek treatment through the same system as other substance abusers.

Moving back to Denmark as a hypothetical case study, if the national authorities chose to introduce prevention at all three levels it would be tantamount to recognizing that it is not possible to eradicate IPED use in the country's non-professional gym and fitness communities. Recognizing this is a reasonable step, firstly because the alternative sets the scene for ever-more-rigid interventions as long as the goal of eradication is not met, and secondly because it is solidly based in empirical evidence. I make the second observation not because there is solid scientific data demonstrating the effectiveness of various types of regulations on anabolic steroid use. As explained earlier, such data does not exist, which means that researchers have no way of quantitatively comparing the impacts of different types of political interventions (legislation, harm reduction, doping control and so forth (Bates et al., 2017)). However, there are other experience-based arguments that would justify recognizing that IPED use in recreational, fitness, weightlifting and similar exercise environments cannot be eradicated.

First and foremost, consider the general observation that no country has so far succeeded in doing this. That in itself is a strong indication that total eradication is not possible. Other arguments are even more compelling. In assessing the possibility of how far the authorities can get through various interventions, there seems to be a lower limit to the number of steroid users in any population. Looking back on the prevalence rates (the percentage of the population with personal experience of steroid use) dealt with near the end of Chapter 2, the lower limit seems to be 1–2% for men. Then add this general assumption: If there are high prevalence rates for a certain drug or substance, say alcohol or tobacco, educating the population and changing the law, especially to reduce accessibility, can lead to changes in prevalence. However, on an issue where prevalence is already low, it is difficult to see the effects of stricter *and* of softer legislation. This assumption is substantiated by a review study of the impacts of legislation on the use of cannabis in various European countries. Here, the researchers found no single type of impact on prevalence resulting from either more rigid or more lenient legislation on cannabis. In some countries stricter legislation led to higher prevalence; in other countries, to lower prevalence. The introduction of softer legislation led to a pattern that was equally unclear, as in some countries prevalence rose; in others, it fell (European Monitoring Centre for Drugs and Drug Addiction, 2017).

Various reservations must be taken, of course, when comparing legislation on cannabis and on anabolic steroids. First, cannabis is more easily accessible, being easier to manufacture. Secondly, many more people use cannabis than steroids. Thirdly, cannabis is used to obtain an effect here and now, whereas steroids are used to achieve a much longer-term goal that will affect the user's appearance and performance. Nevertheless, despite these reservations I believe that in Denmark, for instance, we would see correspondingly unclear patterns in the prevalence of steroid use, whether laws were made stricter or softer. This view reflects the prevalence data I presented in Chapter 2, where I explained that it was not possible to identify clearly derived effects when comparing different countries with similar cultures but different legislation on this area. But that view also reflects other analyses presented in this book, which have shown how a variety of psychological, social and cultural forces influence us as human beings, and how attractive, well-trained bodies hold a universal appeal, even in our modern day and age.

I therefore reason that we have a solid foundation on which to assume that it will never be possible to eradicate the use of IPEDs in fitness, gym and workout environments. Naturally, this does not mean I believe we should refrain from educating people about the harm steroid use can entail, nor do I believe we should tell police and customs officers not to interfere with the activities of distributor and dealer networks. I do, however, believe we ought to give up the ideal of a doping-free future, taking instead a more pragmatic approach to how this particular culture and the market forces, as well as our human biology and psychology, affect modern people's goals, ambitions and dreams of achieving an attractive body.

Doping problem or public-health problem?

Increased monitoring, more sanctions and tougher punishments for people who use IPEDs may feel right and just. Meanwhile, there are no empirical or experience-based studies that show these things improve health — at a personal level, or among the population as a whole.

The alternative is to take a pragmatic, utilitarian approach to handling steroid use in recreational and non-competitive settings. Such an approach will also regard IPED use more as a public-health problem than as a problematic issue related to cheating in professional sports, bearing in mind that it was originally addressed as the latter in Denmark, based on the fact-finding report investigation from 1999 described earlier. If we imagine that Denmark, or any other country where the task of preventing IPED use lies with the NADO, officially accepted that the number of users is sufficiently high to view non-competitive steroid use as a public-health problem, this would also mean that the interventions, campaigns and rules put in place ought to be guided by public-health ethics rather than sport and "fair play" ethics. Obviously the norms applied to public-health interventions are not based on sports-related rules and values but seek instead to clarify when it is reasonable to try to achieve general-health goals among the entire population (such as promoting health, and reducing illness, pain and suffering), even though the resulting intervention or interference might be in conflict with the population's civil liberties (such as the right to freedom, privacy and secrecy).

In light of such reasoning, in 2002 a group of researchers with academic backgrounds in medicine, law and public health proposed five conditions that must be fulfilled to justify any intervention that infringes upon the civil rights of individuals (Bernheim, Childress, Bonnie, & Melnick, 2015; Childress et al., 2002). These five conditions are: (1) effectiveness; (2) necessity; (3) least infringement; (4) proportionality; and (5) impartiality.

So firstly, one must ensure that the intervention is *effective* relative to the public-health goals it seeks to address. Although it may be effective, however, it may not be *necessary* in order to reach the goal. Perhaps voluntary measures might achieve results that were just as good. The burden of proof to demonstrate that the intervention is necessary lies with the authority that wants to implement it. If the first two conditions are met (and the intervention is arguably effective and necessary), the authority moves on to the third condition, and it must always seek to determine which intervention will cause the *least infringement* of general moral considerations (for instance autonomy, privacy or confidentiality). This ties in with the fourth condition, which requires the authority to ensure *proportionate balance* between the anticipated total benefits of the intervention (such as lower risk of illness) with the probable negative effects (such as interfering with citizens' private lives). Once these four criteria have been fulfilled, the authority must ensure compliance with the fifth and final condition, namely that the intervention is carried out impartially and independently so as not to discriminate against or stigmatize any specific groups.

Each particular initiative would naturally require a more thorough analysis, done in context. Having said that, doping control as practiced in Danish fitness centers and gyms would hardly make the grade itself, as the nature of the intervention seems to be problematic on all five conditions. In other words, the five ethical criteria for intervening in the public-health domain show that the way we think about and approach IPEDs changes dramatically when our perspective shifts from "cheating in sports" to "improving health" or "promoting public health."

Politically regulating non-competitive doping

A group of researchers, politicians and stakeholders published a report on behalf of the European Commission in December 2014 entitled *Study on Doping Prevention – A Map of Legal, Regulatory and Prevention Practice Provisions in EU 28*. This report made one thing clear: Although two thirds of the then 28 EU member states found it "important" or "very important" to fight doping outside elite sports, there was no common set of rules or guidelines on how to do so. There were good intentions across the board, but the operational initiatives were only good enough for three member states to say they were "satisfied" or "very satisfied" with the information available in their country on how to prevent IPED use in recreational and non-competitive sport environments (Backhouse et al., 2014).

At a structural level only one third of member states had a formal, structured collaboration between their NADO and customs, police and health authorities (Backhouse et al., 2014). As for involving commercial gyms and health clubs in anti-doping work, the picture was even more diverse. Some countries (like Denmark) have their own legislation governing fitness centers, whereas doping prevention in all forms is institutionally based in the sports-governing bodies. Other countries (like Sweden and the UK) organizationally have different institutions for handling doping prevention for gym-goers on the one hand, and issues in the wider world of recreational club-based sports on the other hand. Yet other countries have no legislation, beyond having signed the WADC, which formally covers club-based sports but in practical terms is only applied to top-levels sports and athletes and has no influence over commercial workout facilities. Consequently, based on the ambition of sketching out a best practice for this area, the 2014 report recommended launching work that could create a foundation for a common, coordinated European doping policy that could apply to wider club-based sports and recreational activities across all EU member states. However, such an overarching European framework seems to lie on a distant horizon, and if and when it is established it is unlikely that commercial gyms and fitness centers will fall under the joint-framework rules since — unlike most sports clubs and locally rooted sports activities — they are part of the private market.

Clearly, no single country has all the answers. Some are looking to Denmark for inspiration because of our long track record (the longest of any single country) for having information and educational campaigns, legislation, doping control and fitness-center regulations. This combination of measures has enabled Denmark to gather experience on what works and what does not work, as previously described. Still, it remains equally clear that the entire area is a hard one to regulate, and policy-makers everywhere must do their best to chart a safe course through difficult waters, beset on one side by moral condemnation, human striving and personal vanity, and on the other side by the protection of individual rights, the promotion of good health and the appetites of an insatiable marketplace.

Notes

1 PRODIS in Sweden (runs the program 100% Pure Hard Training) (https://www. renhardtraning.com/), and Dopinglinkki in Finland (https://dopinglinkki.fi/en).
2 In Denmark, up until 2013 this offense was punishable by just 2 years in prison. Only with the legislative amendment that year was the maximum sentence raised to 6 years in prison (Retsinformation, 2013). In other words, although for possession and personal use the UK has more lenient laws than Denmark, the UK is much tougher on sale and distribution.
3 The non-judgemental ideal may, however, sometimes be lacking. As Geoff Bates demonstrates in his work on the support of men who use steroids in the UK, in some instances service providers do take a moralizing tone or fail to enter into a genuine dialogue with users. One participant described it in this way: "If you have this moralizing approach you're not going to get anywhere. If you're coming across like 'steroids are bad, you shouldn't take them' it's going to get people's backs up straight away and you're losing them straight away. They're not going to listen to you, and they probably won't come back. Lots of them have experienced this and it kind of sums up what they think people in services are going be like" (Bates, 2019, p. 98).
4 A more recent model in this area splits prevention measures into three categories: "universal prevention," "selective prevention" and "indicated prevention." Universal prevention strategies can be aimed at the entire population or parts of it, going through channels such as elementary schools or workplaces. Selective prevention efforts are aimed at risk groups, going through channels such as commercial nightlife environments or vulnerable residential areas. The involved actors include public authorities, health professionals, social caseworkers and similar professionals. Indicated prevention, with preventive measures for at-risk individuals, differs from selective prevention in being aimed at single persons rather than groups in the general populace. Professionals seek to reach this target group using a "high-risk" strategy with a proactive approach of personal contacts, one-on-one conversations, and the like (Brotherhood & Sumnall, 2011).

References

Backhouse, S., Collins, C., Defoort, Y., McNamee, M., Parkinson, A., & Sauer, M. (2014). *Study on doping prevention. A map of legal, regulatory and prevention practice provisions in EU 28.* Retrieved from Luxembourg: https://ec.europa.eu/assets/eac/sport/news/2014/docs/doping-prevention-report_en.pdf.
Bates, G. (2019). *Supporting men who use anabolic steroids: A sequential multi-methods study.* (PhD Doctoral), Liverpool, UK: Liverpool John Moores University. Retrieved from http://researchonline.ljmu.ac.uk/id/eprint/11012/.

Bates, G., Begley, E., Tod, D., Jones, L., Leavey, C., & McVeigh, J. (2017). A systematic review investigating the behaviour change strategies in interventions to prevent misuse of anabolic steroids. *J Health Psychol.* doi: doi:10.1177/1359105317737607.

Bates, G., Tod, D., Leavey, C., & McVeigh, J. (2019). An evidence-based socioecological framework to understand men's use of anabolic androgenic steroids and inform interventions in this area. *Drugs: Education, Prevention and Policy, 26*(6), 484–492. doi: doi:10.1080/09687637.2018.1488947.

Bernheim, R. G., Childress, J. F., Bonnie, R. J., & Melnick, A. L. (2015). *Essentials of public health ethics.* Burlington, MA: Jones & Bartlett Learning.

Brotherhood, A., & Sumnall, H. (2011). European drug prevention quality standards: A manual for prevention professionals. Retrieved from Lisbon: www.emcdda. europa.eu/system/files/publications/646/TD3111250ENC_318193.pdf.

Childress, J. F., Faden, R. R., Gaare, R. D., Gostin, L. O., Kahn, J., Bonnie, R. J., … Nieburg, P. (2002). Public health ethics: Mapping the terrain. *Journal of Law, Medicine & Ethics, 30*(2), 170–178.

Christiansen, A. V., & Bojsen-Møller, J. (2012). "Will steroids kill me if I use them once?" A qualitative analysis of inquiries submitted to the Danish anti-doping authorities. *Performance Enhancement & Health, 1*(1), 39–47. doi: doi:10.1016/j. peh.2012.05.002.

European Monitoring Centre for Drugs and Drug Addiction. (2017). Cannabis legislation in Europe: An overview. Retrieved from Luxembourg: www.emcdda. europa.eu/system/files/publications/4135/TD0217210ENN.pdf.

Evans-Brown, M., & McVeigh, J. (2009). Anabolic steroid use in the general population of the United Kingdom. In V. Møller, M. McNamee, & P. Dimeo (Eds.), *Elite sport, doping and public health* (pp. 75–97). Odense, Denmark: University Press of Southern Denmark.

Havnes, I. A., Jorstad, M. L., & Wisloff, C. (2019). Anabolic-androgenic steroid users receiving health-related information: Health problems, motivations to quit and treatment desires. *Subst Abuse Treat Prev Policy, 14*(1), 20. doi: doi:10.1186/s13011-019-0206-5.

Kimergård, A., & McVeigh, J. (2014a). Environments, risk and health harms: a qualitative investigation into the illicit use of anabolic steroids among people using harm reduction services in the UK. *BMJ Open, 4*(6), e005275. doi: doi:10.1136/bmjopen-2014-005275.

Kimergård, A., & McVeigh, J. (2014b). Variability and dilemmas in harm reduction for anabolic steroid users in the UK: A multi-area interview study. *Harm Reduction Journal, 11*, 1–13. doi: doi:10.1186/1477-7517-11-19.

McVeigh, J., & Begley, E. (2017). Anabolic steroids in the UK: An increasing issue for public health. *Drugs: Education, Prevention and Policy, 24*(3), 278–285. doi: doi:10.1080/09687637.2016.1245713.

Oslo Universitetssykehus. (2019). Hormonlaboratoriet. Retrieved from: https:// oslo-universitetssykehus.no/avdelinger/klinikk-for-laboratoriemedisin/avdeling-for-medisinsk-biokjemi/hormonlaboratoriet.

Region Örebro Län. (2019). Dopningsmottagningen. Retrieved from: www.regionor ebrolan.se/dopningsmottagningen.

Retsinformation. (2013). Forslag til Lov om ændring af straffeloven (Forhøjet strafferamme for grov dopingkriminalitet) [Act on increased punishment for severe doping criminality]. Retrieved from: https://www.retsinformation.dk/eli/ft/201313L00008.

Rhodes, T., & Hedrich, D. (2010). Harm reduction and the mainstream. In T. Rhodes & D. Hedrich (Eds.), *Harm reduction: Evidence, impacts and challenges* (pp. 19–33). Luxembourg, Luxembourgh: European Monitoring Centre for Drugs and Drug Addiction.

Smit, D. L., & de Ronde, W. (2018). Outpatient clinic for users of anabolic androgenic steroids: An overview. *Neth J Med*, 76(4), 167.

Spaarne Gasthuis. (2019). Anabole steroïden. Retrieved from: https://spaarnegasthuis. nl/specialisme/interne-geneeskunde/anabole-steroiden.

Storm, R. K., Toft, D., & Bang, S. (2015). Motionsdoping i Danmark. Evaluering af indsatsen mod motionsdoping i kommercielle motions- og fitnesscentre (Use of IPEDs in Denmark. An evaluation of the intervention in commercial gyms in Denmark). Retrieved from København: www.idan.dk/vidensbank/downloads/m otionsdoping-i-danmark/382b209b-fd84-4c04-9a6a-a50f0113101b.

Vinther, A. S., & Christiansen, A. V. (2019). Different users, different interventions. On the ideal typology of anabolic-androgenic steroid use and its implications for prevention and harm reduction. In K. van de Ven, K. Mulrooney, & J. McVeigh (Eds.), *Human enhancement drugs* (pp. 249–263). London: Routledge.

Chapter 14

By way of conclusion

This book grew out of my aspiration to find out what makes young men in gym and workout communities use image- and performance-enhancing drugs (IPEDs) — given that few of them ever take part in bodybuilding or weightlifting competitions. I hope the analyses in the preceding chapters have offered answers that rise above the cliché that using such substances is merely a form of quick-fix cheating, perpetrated by self-engrossed muscle fanatics. What we have seen is that a person's decision to use anabolic steroids can be embedded in a wide variety of circumstances and be expressed in many different ways. These various motives and ambitions do, however, share general traits, and there are common denominators among steroid users that are psychological, social and cultural in nature.

That said, I seriously doubt the likelihood of ever formulating a single, comprehensive theory we can apply to this field. The following example illustrates one challenge. From the point of view of Western liberal societies, it may seem meaningful to understand the use of steroids as expressing "a crisis of masculinity," since some men in these fairly egalitarian countries, shaped by the impact of women's liberation and what is occasionally termed "the feminization of society," seek refuge in one of the most masculine activities around: cultivating the muscular body. However, this theory cannot explain the use of steroids in countries and areas that do not exhibit the same degree of gender equality as, say, Northwest Europe and Scandinavia do. Examples include Brazil and the Middle East, where some studies have found much higher prevalence rates for the use of anabolic steroids than those measured in Scandinavia, the UK and the US (Sagoe, Molde, Andreassen, Torsheim, & Pallesen, 2014). Steroid use in the former type of countries seems to be either based on more culture-specific explanations, which are rooted in a particular type of macho culture, or based on explanations that reflect a psychological, evolutionary component that is universally applicable.

Then again, the evolutionary-psychology angle suffers from precisely this universality, which means that it does not explain why "only" a small proportion of male inhabitants in Northwest Europe and the US have personal experience with steroid use. What helps us here, however, is the theory of precarious manhood (discussed in Chapter 10), which points out that men more often than women experience anxiety over their gender status. This, in turn, gives men who doubt their masculinity, or who feel it is threatened or weakened, a motivation to seek to regain, affirm and reinforce it through actions that can be confirmed by others. It is highly likely that in many cases these men overlap with the men Alan Klein describes as those driven by feelings of inferiority to build muscle mass. Further, the fact that some men are insecure about their masculinity may spring from the situation that although we live in an image-rich culture that offers loads of idealized male bodies — in whom men can mirror themselves — the male role itself has become unclear. The Norwegian researchers Bjørn Barland and Jan Ove Tangen have pointed out how Western culture has a paucity of clear-cut, positive male figures, as exemplified in the over-abundance of male film and computer-game roles that are culturally unambiguous, fantasy-based, devoid of content and lacking any reference whatsoever to real life (Barland & Tangen, 2009, p. 78).

Although it is hardly possible to formulate one comprehensive theory, the discussions in the preceding chapters contain two recurring elements. First, although we live in an intellectually enlightened and thoroughly rationalized society where we may imagine that legislative and regulatory equality has evened out the differences between us, sexually charged interactions among genders and individuals continue to have consequences for our psyche, our behavior and our norms — and in this context the body still plays a major role. Second, as Klein once put it, all men, whether consciously acknowledging it or not, have a sort of dialogue with muscle; a dialogue that is intimately linked with their perception of themselves as men (see Chapter 10).

To indicate the general direction of the studies I cover in this book, I initially set out three assumptions. The first was that the use of anabolic steroids must be understood in light of the identity-construction work that is a crucial element during every person's late teens to mid-twenties. The second was that the increased focus on competition in society also affects social relationships, and that as an extension of this the body has become an important indicator of personal success. The third assumption was that muscles play a particular role for men in this context, as muscles and masculine identity are connected. As I explained, these three assumptions are interlinked: The part of our identity associated with social recognition necessitates an effort on our part, producing situations where we also compete with others. And for some men, cultivating a well-muscled body becomes the central element in their life, at least for a time. While it is normal practice to test scientific hypotheses in various ways to either confirm or refute them, I have not subjected my three assumptions to this process. Rather, I have used them to guide the issues investigated and discussed in this book. Their applicability, their utility value if you will, ultimately depends on whether they have been able to contribute to new insights on the book's topic, and whether these can be integrated with findings in other relevant studies conducted in the wider research community.

The book's first four chapters laid the foundation for its analyses. Here, I introduced the topic and the problems raised; reviewed the dominant cultural and sociological theories in the field; outlined medical and biochemical research on anabolic steroids; and presented my understanding of the concept of identity. Working upwards and outwards from this foundation, we spent Chapter 5 looking at my informants' fascination with muscles and strength. The point of this was to study what had originally motivated them to begin strength training and, in some cases, to supplement their workouts and dietary regimes with IPEDs. It became clear that the bodily changes they underwent were not just some random aspect of their lives. Quite the opposite. These changes strongly influenced the way they interacted with their surroundings, by extension affecting their identity. One of my pivotal points concerning identity is that although each one of us must find, and continuously work on, our own identity, it is not fruitful to view identity merely as a social construct, or as something that is plastic, mutable and constantly up for renegotiation. As Anton (and other informants) explained, his relationship with the world around him changed immensely when he became larger, stronger and more muscular. This was not just because he began enacting his new-found identity as "a strong guy who worked out a lot," but because the people around him reacted to his appearance and physique, thereby accepting and confirming this new identity, which then began to take root in him. The analysis showed that the reactions in his environment were not arbitrary, but were based on a physical, bodily reality and a number of shared conditions for describing and interpreting peoples' experiences with that reality. Based on this, it is reasonable to say that our body image arises as we interact with our surroundings in a process that runs something like this: We are present in the world by virtue of our physical body. Our surroundings react to this body, and based on the reactions we get we develop our own personal learning strategies and interpretations of the social world, our place in it and our interactions with it. Consequently, our interpretations and learning strategies come to look different, depending on whether we have, for instance, a slight 60-kilo build or weigh in tall and muscular at 90 kilos. In that sense our body image and hence our identity are more than a social construction, as they are bound to the real, physical world and our interactions with it. This fact tempts some people to accelerate the pace of their body-altering efforts by supplementing their physical training with steroids.

We went on to look at specific examples of this in four very different personal accounts from the informants I call Jesper, Michael, Jonas and Adam. Their stories focused, respectively, on: (a) achieving a well-muscled body and minimizing the harmful effects of the drugs; (b) performance and competition; (c) partying to the max with sex, drugs and alcohol; and (d) promoting a particular lifestyle to increase physical well-being and social benefits. These descriptions served the dual purpose of demonstrating the diversity of steroid users' experiences, knowledge levels and deliberations, and paving the way for an ideal typology describing the use of anabolic steroids in workout communities. Bearing in mind these four accounts and other literature on the topic, we were able to set out a model in Chapter 7 that outlines four ideal-typical steroid users: the Expert type, the Well-being type, the YOLO type and the Athlete type. As noted several times, few people (if any) will fully align with one of these pure, idealized profiles. In the real world, people gradually change motives, goals and practices as they obtain new knowledge and pass through life. The typology is not meant as a device to fix individual users within a certain quadrant, or to peg them as a certain type. It is a theoretical framework and a tool we can use to investigate, describe and understand steroid use. My hope is that it will also serve as a practical analytical tool for researchers, health professionals, teachers, instructors, psychologists and others who work with IPED users.

The differences in risk profiles were also evident in Chapter 8, which dealt with how users felt and coped with side effects. One insight here was that the users' willingness to accept side effects did not stem from indifference to the actual side effects, or from a lack of concern about what could happen to them as a result. While some users believed they were personally capable of handling risks and side effects well, they were not convinced that others would also be able to do so. Rasmus, once a heavy steroid user, spoke of how he would not advise any future son of his to start using steroids, for fear that the young man might become addicted. Even so, for Rasmus personally, his body-sculpting project had carried more weight than the risk of the steroids causing harm.

Even when it came to the drugs affecting their sex lives, my informants were ambivalent. Several emphasized having a stronger sex drive while on steroids, which, combined with their experience of having an admirably toned body, greater self-confidence and reinforced masculinity, made for a positive situation. Meanwhile, this coincided with a real risk of their being unable to achieve or sustain an erection, or even becoming temporarily impotent after a cycle of steroids, as reported by several of my informants. The majority of users actually believe they can control their own steroid use, but paradoxically, although a more attractive, bulked-up body potentially gives them easier access to sex, they risk not feeling any desire, or not being able to perform sexually when an opportunity arises.

Diet, unlike side effects, can be controlled. Anyone wishing to increase their muscle volume and physical size must maintain a caloric surplus. People who work out hard will often have to eat quite a lot, and many prefer a specially planned diet, as described in Chapter 9. If, for some reason, a person cannot adhere to their workout schedule or strict dietary program, this can cause feelings of guilt. Such scenarios can be reminiscent of the obsessive preoccupation with food and exercise seen in people with eating disorders. Although there are no scientific grounds for classifying such conditions as actual eating disorders, patterns like this point to another paradoxical ambiguity in many of the informants who have contributed to this book. On the one hand, they are highly disciplined and steeled in their resolve when it comes to the training goals they set. On the other hand, they exhibit a certain psychological vulnerability or insecurity, which they seemingly have to veil behind grueling physical exercise and a rigidly ordered lifestyle. It was a similar observation that led Klein to identify bodybuilders as *Little Big Men* in his book of that name from 1993. My informants may well be extraordinary in their workout and diet regimes, but they still resemble most other people in the way they categorize others through "us-and-them" thinking: an ability to rationalize one's own unusual behavior while finding it hard to understand "strange" behavior in others.

We moved on to investigate, in Chapter 10, how strength training, bodybuilding and the athletic physique have a primal biological and psychological appeal as a part of our human nature. We did this to reach a better understanding of how the markets, the media and the organized fitness industry became so phenomenally successful in making us buy into the importance of having an athletic, well-toned body. This also helps us understand the allure of steroids. My main point here is, had the fitness marketeers had no biological and psychological scaffolding on which to brandish their message, their project to make us buy it would have been unsuccessful. Human beings are not simply cultural beings who can freely shift their focus of interest. We are also animals with an evolutionary history and various hard-wired preferences. For eons, males and females have played different roles in procreating and making sure their offspring survived so that they, in turn, could produce children and perpetuate our species. This has meant that certain general behaviors and norms prevail among men, and among women. Likewise, evolution has led to deep-seated aesthetic preferences in men and women when it comes to the appearance of the opposite sex. That is precisely why it is important to take evolutionary psychology on board if we want to understand why workout communities are so successful; why people prefer strong, muscular, symmetrical bodies; and, by extension, why steroids offer such a tantalizing proposition. This line of reasoning may seem obvious to some readers. All the more ironic, then, that these perspectives are largely absent from other literature on this phenomenon.

Because Denmark likely has the longest history of public authorities aiming to prevent IPED use in gyms, in Chapter 11 we looked at how the Danish strategies initially used to combat steroid use in gyms were largely based on rules and laws copied from the fight against sports doping. Furthermore, a brand of moral condemnation reminiscent of the general sentiment against sports doping was carried over into the country's public discourse about steroid use in non-athletic workout settings.

One example of how these two worlds became mingled, or mixed up, was a 2013 television documentary series from Danmarks Radio, the Danish broadcasting corporation, entitled *Doping Epidemien (The Doping Epidemic)*. The main character in the four-part series was the former professional cyclist Jesper Skibby, who, in a creative rendition into English of his colorful Danish wording, once conceded he had been "doped from his ass to his eyeballs." The series cast him, rather awkwardly, in the role of investigative, soul-searching journalist and show host, on a mission to expose the scourge of sports doping and its kingpins and middlemen. One particularly ill-conceived scene has a painfully earnest Skibby look straight into the camera after sneak-peeking into a gym where several brawny weightlifters are hard at work. Overly conscious of his own status as a role model, the host remorsefully confides in his viewers: "I really hope I'm not the one who made them start doping." Skibby, something of a European legend, has undoubtedly inspired many people to do many things. Still, it is hard to imagine a young man keen to bulk up, who suddenly gets the idea to use steroids after seeing Skibby and other wiry cycling pros in action.

As in cycling and other elite sports, a blend of checks, testing and control had been the main strategy to rid various sports of doping. In Denmark these elements also became an essential part of the strategy against steroid use among recreational and non-competitive exercise enthusiasts. One downside to this was a host of regulatory challenges, but the biggest problem was that the strategy severed all ties with the actual users of the prohibited substances. At the same time the gyms and the NADO, Anti Doping Danmark, were deeply frustrated at ending up in a stalemate. As a consequence of this, Anti Doping Danmark introduced a new strategy in 2012, which toned down doping control as the mainstay of its work to promote "cleaner" exercise environments. Changes were made to the Danish legislation, shifting the focus from testing and information campaigns towards dialogue and user involvement. These initiatives were welcomed by fitness centers and gyms and by their members. However, as discussed in Chapter 12, doping controls are still a part of the Danish strategy. Although many facilities and members approve of this, some users strongly object to testing, a practice that is difficult to justify as "necessary" from a health-promotion point of view.

Elsewhere, particularly in the United Kingdom, authorities have decided on a very different framework than the fair-play codex of sports in their attempts to handle steroid use in gyms. Chapter 13 explained how, in the UK, steroid use in gym settings is perceived much more as a health issue than as a moral issue reflecting poor sportsmanship. This has meant that authorities focus more on reducing harms than on exposing "cheaters." For a non-UK audience such a change of perspective can seem provocative, as this shift means saying goodbye to an ideal doping-free future where drug use in sports has been eradicated, and saying hello to pragmatically approaching users and the health repercussions of steroid use.

There is still no consensus on whether anabolic-steroid use is a personal-health issue for the few who use such drugs or a public-health problem that touches many lives. And how many lives are "enough lives" to make steroid (ab)use a public concern? In Chapter 2 we looked at the difficulties in accurately determining just how widespread steroid use is. One thing is certain: Steroid use does not necessarily become a public-health problem merely because researchers say it is. The hackneyed phrase that "further research is needed on this topic" — unabashedly used to round off countless scientific papers, almost as a matter of course — hints that some researchers may have motives besides promoting the greater good when seeking to classify an issue as a public-health problem.

Besides that, it is clear that other active substances are causing far greater problems in our societies than anabolic steroids are. In a high-profile article published in *The Lancet* in 2010, a group of experts ranked 20 of the most prevalent substances of potential abuse, based on two parameters: harm to the individual user, and harm to others. For individual users, the most harmful substance was heroin, followed by crack cocaine and methamphetamine, whereas alcohol, heroin and crack cocaine were the most harmful to others. An assessment combining both parameters put alcohol in first place as the most harmful substance of all, followed by heroin and crack cocaine. The combined assessment had tobacco in sixth place, cannabis in eighth place and anabolic steroids as far down as sixteenth place on the list (Nutt, King, & Phillips, 2010).[1] Obviously this does not mean steroids do *not* constitute a public-health problem. It simply means there are other substances that, all told, cause a good deal more damage than steroids do, to individuals and to society as a whole. What is more, it reminds us that in any effort to combat steroid use, we must consider the proportionality of the measures we put in place. Eager to do our best, and perhaps to make a political statement as well, we may find ourselves forfeiting our fundamental ethical principles and unintentionally doing more harm than good.

It is likewise important to regard the use of anabolic steroids in the proper context, which differs greatly from the context that applies to most other illicit or classified substances under scrutiny by the authorities. By and large, the activity of working with one's muscles is part of the male domain. It is an original, albeit atavistic, demonstration of a person's status as a man. Linking muscle-power ("brute force") to a person's masculine status may seem like a throwback to an earlier, premodern stage in human evolution, now apparent in an enlightened and thoroughly rationalized world. And yet, when such a seemingly anachronistic phenomenon has found its way into the mainstream of our world through the cracks in our rational thinking, we can only do it justice by taking it seriously.

I believe that asking the essential question of what "manhood" and "masculine status" means today, and studying how men handle their status, is the key to understanding the appeal of exercising and weightlifting to build a muscular body. It is also the backdrop for appreciating why Arnold Schwarzenegger, in his 1975 incarnation, still personifies the perfect body for many serious workout enthusiasts. This, in turn, can bring us closer to understanding the alluring but problematic aspects of using anabolic steroids in today's gym communities.

Note

1   This group assessed 20 substances in all, scoring their harmfulness based on 16 different criteria. While 9 criteria reflected the harm the substance caused in the individual, 7 reflected the harm caused to others (resulting from violence, traffic accidents, broken families and so forth). The fact that alcohol was ranked first naturally says more about the massive, pervasive use of alcohol than about the harmfulness of a single "dose" to a given individual. Clearly, heroin and crack cocaine are more harmful, in and of themselves, than alcohol is. However, they are much less prevalent, which affects their overall impact. Similar circumstances apply to anabolic steroids.

References

Barland, B., & Tangen, J. O. (2009). Kroppspresentasjon og andre prestasjoner – en omfangsundersøkelse om bruk av doping (2009:3). Retrieved from Oslo: https://a ntidoping.no/sitefiles/1/dokumenter/pdf/omfangsundersokelsen.pdf.

Nutt, D. J., King, L. A., & Phillips, L. D. (2010). Drug harms in the UK: A multicriteria decision analysis. *The Lancet*, 376, 1558–1565. doi:10.1016/S0140-6736(10)61462-6.

Sagoe, D., Molde, H., Andreassen, C. S., Torsheim, T., & Pallesen, S. (2014). The global epidemiology of anabolic-androgenic steroid use: A meta-analysis and meta-regression analysis. *Annals of Epidemiology*, 24(1873–2585 (Electronic)), 383–398.

Index

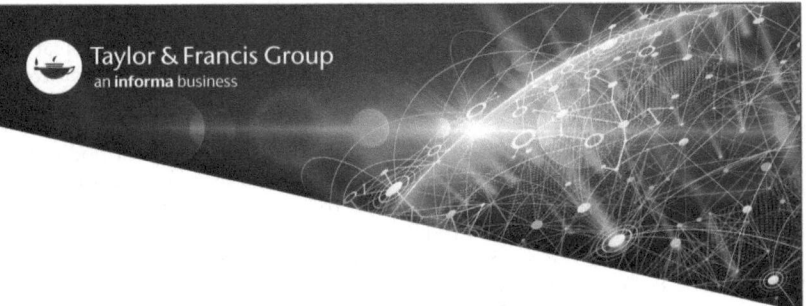
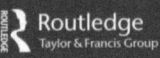 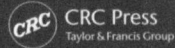